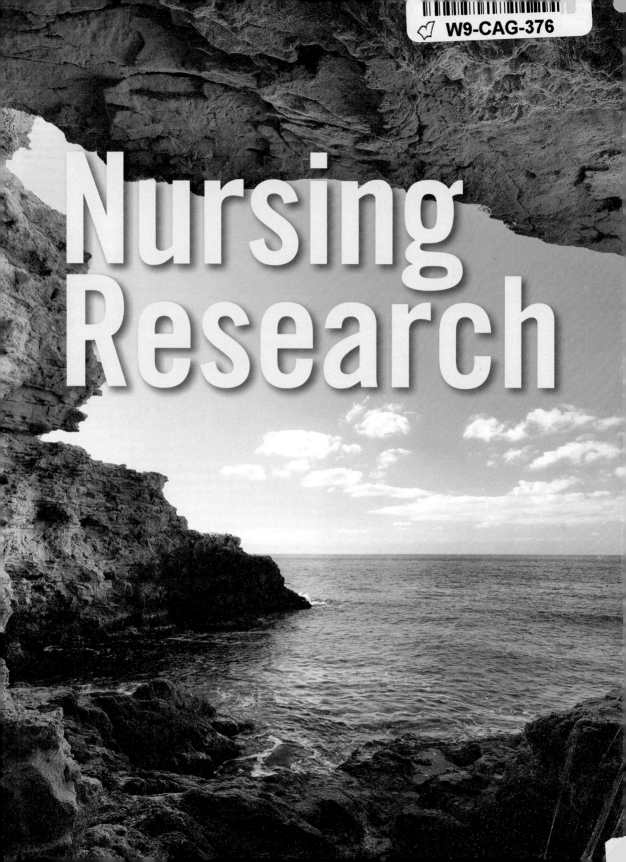

Nursing Research

the pedagogy

Nursing Research: Reading, Using, and Creating Evidence, Second Edition demonstrates how to use research as the basis for successful nursing practice. Fully updated and revised, this reader-friendly new edition provides students with the fundamentals of appraising and utilizing research. Organized around the different types of research in evidence-based practice, it addresses contemporary concerns, especially ethical and legal issues. Additionally, it explores both quantitative and qualitative traditions to encourage students to read, use, and participate in the research process. The pedagogical aids that appear in most chapters include the following:

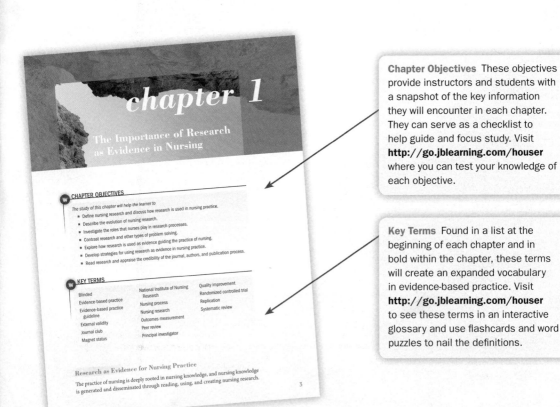

Chapter Objectives These objectives provide instructors and students with a snapshot of the key information they will encounter in each chapter. They can serve as a checklist to help guide and focus study. Visit **http://go.jblearning.com/houser** where you can test your knowledge of each objective.

Key Terms Found in a list at the beginning of each chapter and in bold within the chapter, these terms will create an expanded vocabulary in evidence-based practice. Visit **http://go.jblearning.com/houser** to see these terms in an interactive glossary and use flashcards and word puzzles to nail the definitions.

4

❝ *Voices from the Field* ❞

I was working as the clinical nurse specialist of a busy surgical intensive care unit (ICU) when we received a critically ill patient. He was fresh from cardiac surgery and quite unstable; he needed multiple drugs and an intra-aortic balloon pump just to maintain his perfusion status. He was so sick that we were not able to place him on a special bed for pressure relief. For the first 24 hours, we were so busy trying to keep him alive that we did not even get a chance to turn him.

About 36 hours into his ICU admission, he was stable enough to place on a low-air-loss mattress for pressure-ulcer prevention. When we were finally able to turn him, we noted he had a small stage II pressure ulcer on his coccyx. Despite the treatments that we used, the pressure ulcer evolved into a full thickness wound. He recovered from his cardiac surgical procedure but, unfortunately, required surgeries and skin grafts to close the pressure ulcer wound.

The experience I had with this patient prompted me to review the evidence-based practice guidelines we had in place to prevent pressure ulcers in critically ill patients. I wanted to make sure we could prevent this happening again, but I had a lot of questions. Could we preventively place high-risk patients on low-air-loss mattresses while they were still in the perioperative service? Did we even know the patients who were at risk for pressure ulcers? What assessment tools did nurses use to assess the patient's risk? When a high-risk patient was identified, what interventions did the nurses use to prevent pressure ulcers? How were the ulcers treated once they appeared?

I was fortunate that my chief nursing officer (CNO) was a strong advocate for evidence-based practice (EBP), and she encouraged me to initiate an EBP review of pressure ulcer prevention and treatment. Specifically, I wanted to find out what nursing interventions were supported by research evidence when we were trying to prevent pressure ulcers in the surgical ICU. So I contacted other inpatient units at the hospital to determine what they were doing.

I discovered that the surgical ICU was not different from the other inpatient units. There was no standard, evidence-based nursing practice for pressure ulcer prevention. Units were not consistently using the same skin assessment tools, so it was hard to objectively communicate risk from one unit to another. The tools we were using were not necessarily based on research. It was clear that we needed to identify the best available evidence and devise a protocol.

We started by establishing an evidence-based skin care council for the hospital. The team consisted of bedside nurses from all inpatient units and the perioperative service. Initially the council reviewed current nursing skin assessment forms, and we conducted a review of the literature on pressure ulcer prevention and interventions. We discovered the Association for Healthcare Research and Quality (AHRQ) guidelines on pressure ulcer prevention and treatment, a key source of evidence for healthcare practices.

Over the course of the next year, we revised our nursing policy and procedure, incorporating the AHRQ evidence into a treatment guideline. The guideline included a procedure for skin assessment and nursing documentation, and pressure ulcer assessment and treatment decision algorithms. We reviewed skin-care products and narrowed down the products to those that were supported by evidence. One algorithm helped staff make selections between products that

---

5

maximized prevention and treatment. Another algorithm guided nurses in the use of therapeutic surfaces (e.g., low-air-loss mattresses) to prevent pressure ulcers. To monitor our progress, we began quarterly pressure ulcer prevalence studies. As part of the implementation, we scheduled a skin-care seminar featuring a national expert on skin care.

At the beginning of our EBP skin-care journey, our pressure ulcer prevalence was 9 percent. Since implementing our EBP skin-care initiatives our pressure ulcer prevalence has dropped by two thirds. The EBP skin-care council continues to be active in our hospital. We meet monthly to seek out the best evidence to guide skin- and wound-care product decisions, practice guidelines, protocols, and policies. My initial search for a solution—based on my experience with one patient—led to improvements in practice that have benefited many patients since then.

Mary Beth Flynn Makic, PhD, RN

Professional nurses rely on research findings to inform their practice decisions; they use critical thinking to apply research directly to specific patient care situations. The research process allows nurses to ask and answer questions systematically that will ensure that decisions are based on sound science and rigorous inquiry. Nursing research helps nurses in a variety of settings answer questions about patient care, education, and administration. Research ensures that practices are based on evidence, rather than eloquence or tradition.

What Is Nursing Research?

Nursing research is a systematic process of inquiry that uses rigorous guidelines to produce unbiased, trustworthy answers to questions about nursing practice. Research is used as evidence in the evaluation and determination of best nursing practices. The aim of original nursing research is to generate new knowledge to inform the practice of nursing. However, nurses may use research to

Nursing research: A systematic process of inquiry that uses rigorous guidelines to produce unbiased, trustworthy answers to questions about nursing practice.

- Synthesize the findings of others into a coherent guide for practice
- Explore and describe phenomena that affect health
- Find solutions to existing and emerging problems
- Test traditional approaches to patient care for continued relevance and effectiveness

A variety of methods is used to generate new knowledge or summarize existing study results. Nurse researchers may measure observable characteristics, solicit perceptions directly from clients, assess words and phrases for underlying meaning, or analyze a group of study findings in aggregate. Nurse researchers have virtually limitless options for research design and may assume roles ranging from primary investigator for a large, multisite trial to staff nurse in a bedside science project. The goal, however, is always the same: to generate new knowledge that can be applied to improve nursing practice.

Regardless of the design, research is a rigorous endeavor that is subject to peer review and replication. These two characteristics are essential to ensure that research is unbiased

---

7

process and use evidence as a basis for practice. To maintain *Magnet* status, hospitals must show improved outcomes and clinical practice based on current evidence (Wise, 2009).

The Evolution of Research in Nursing

Nursing is a relatively young field when compared to fields such as philosophy or physics that have hundreds of years of historical study. Nursing has not always relied on profession-specific research as a basis for practice. However, if one reads contemporary nursing literature, it is clear that research is taking on fundamental importance as a source of evidence for practice.

Florence Nightingale introduced the concept of scientific inquiry as a basis for practice. Nightingale's work focused on collecting information about factors that affected soldier mortality and morbidity during the Crimean War. With scientific data, she was able to create change in nursing practice. Indeed, her work was so impressive that she was inducted into the Statistical Society of London.

The years following Nightingale's era offered relatively little scientific work in nursing, likely because nursing education was accomplished through apprenticeship rather than scholarly work. As more nursing education moved into university settings in the 1950s, research took on more prominence as a key nursing activity. Journals were initiated both in the United States and internationally that focused exclusively on publishing nursing research. More outlets for the publication of nursing research were established in the 1970s and 1980s, leading to the communication of research findings to a broader audience. The creation of the National Center for Research for Nursing within the National Institutes of Health (NIH) in 1986 was a seminal step in recognizing the importance of nursing research. In 1993, the center was given full institute status as the National Institute of Nursing Research (NINR). This move put nursing research on a par with medical research and the other health sciences, ensuring financial support and a national audience for disciplined inquiry in the field. The NINR and other national agencies guide the overarching research agenda that focuses nursing research on professional priorities. The mission of the NINR is to support clinical and basic research to establish a scientific basis for the care of individuals across the life span (NINR, 2010).

In the 1980s and 1990s, leaders in nursing research met periodically at a Conference on Research Priorities in Nursing Science (CORP) to identify research priorities for the nursing profession. These priorities were established as 5-year agendas. In the 1990s, advances in nursing research were coming so quickly that a more flexible approach was required. NINR research agenda planning now involves more frequent meetings of smaller groups that consist of nurse researchers, representa-

gray matter

Research is critical in nursing because
- The use of research is inherent to the definition of a profession.
- Nurses are accountable for outcomes.
- Consumers are demanding evidence-based care.

National Institute of Nursing Research (NNR): A federal agency responsible for the support of nursing research by establishing a national research agenda, funding grants and research awards, and providing training.

gray matter

Nurses may play a variety of roles in research, including the following:
- Informed consumer of research
- Participant in research-related activity, such as journal clubs
- Contributor to a systematic review process
- Data collector for a research project
- Principal investigator for a research study

Voices from the Field Often found at the beginning of a chapter, these features illustrate stories from practicing nurses and their real experiences with the research process.

New Term Found in the margins, these notes provide definitions of key terms when they first appear in the chapter.

Gray Matter Found in the margins, these notes cover information about key concepts for quick review.

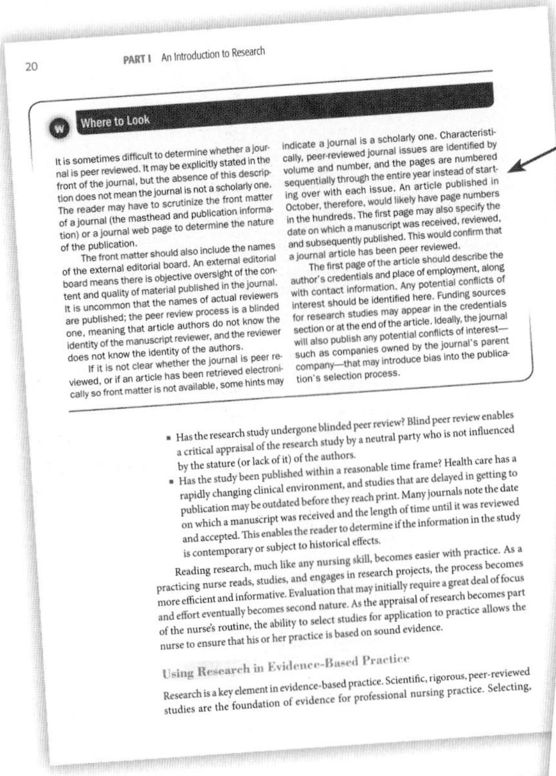

20 PART I An Introduction to Research

Where to Look

It is sometimes difficult to determine whether a journal is peer reviewed. It may be explicitly stated in the front of the journal, but the absence of this description does not mean the journal is not a scholarly one. The reader may have to scrutinize the front matter of a journal (the masthead and publication information) or a journal web page to determine the nature of the publication.

The front matter should also include the names of the external editorial board. An external editorial board means there is objective oversight of the content and quality of material published in the journal. It is uncommon that the names of actual reviewers are published; the peer review process is a blinded one, meaning that article authors do not know the identity of the manuscript reviewer, and the reviewer does not know the identity of the authors.

If it is not clear whether the journal is peer reviewed, or if an article has been retrieved electronically so front matter is not available, some hints may indicate a journal is a scholarly one. Characteristically, peer-reviewed journal issues are identified by volume and number, and the pages are numbered sequentially through the entire year instead of starting over with each issue. An article published in October, therefore, would likely have page numbers in the hundreds. The first page may also specify the date on which a manuscript was received, reviewed, and subsequently published. This would confirm that a journal article has been peer reviewed.

The first page of the article should describe the author's credentials and place of employment, along with contact information. Any potential conflicts of interest should be identified here. Funding sources for research studies may appear in the credentials section or at the end of the article. Ideally, the journal will also publish any potential conflicts of interest—such as companies owned by the journal's parent company—that may introduce bias into the publication's selection process.

- Has the research study undergone blinded peer review? Blind peer review enables a critical appraisal of the research study by a neutral party who is not influenced by the stature (or lack of it) of the authors.
- Has the study been published within a reasonable time frame? Health care has a rapidly changing clinical environment, and studies that are delayed in getting to publication may be outdated before they reach print. Many journals note the date on which a manuscript was received and the length of time until it was reviewed and accepted. This enables the reader to determine if the information in the study is contemporary or subject to historical effects.

Reading research, much like any nursing skill, becomes easier with practice. As a practicing nurse reads, studies, and engages in research projects, the process becomes more efficient and informative. Evaluation that may initially require a great deal of focus and effort eventually becomes second nature. As the appraisal of research becomes part of the nurse's routine, the ability to select studies for application to practice allows the nurse to ensure that his or her practice is based on sound evidence.

Using Research in Evidence-Based Practice

Research is a key element in evidence-based practice. Scientific, rigorous, peer-reviewed studies are the foundation of evidence for professional nursing practice. Selecting,

Where to Look These features provide guidance on where to look for the key elements of a research paper, the wording that might be used to describe them, and specific things to look for during the evaluation process. Visit **http://go.jblearning.com/houser** to find this guiding resource online.

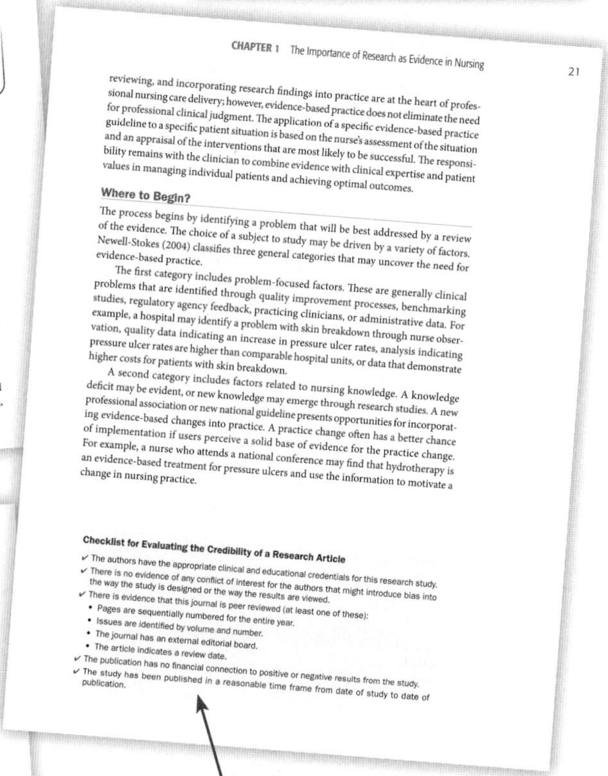

CHAPTER 1 The Importance of Research as Evidence in Nursing 21

reviewing, and incorporating research findings into practice are at the heart of professional nursing care delivery; however, evidence-based practice does not eliminate the need for professional clinical judgment. The application of a specific evidence-based practice guideline to a specific patient situation is based on the nurse's assessment of the situation and an appraisal of the interventions that are most likely to be successful. The responsibility remains with the clinician to combine evidence with clinical expertise and patient values in managing individual patients and achieving optimal outcomes.

Where to Begin?

The process begins by identifying a problem that will be best addressed by a review of the evidence. The choice of a subject to study may be driven by a variety of factors. Newell-Stokes (2004) classifies three general categories that may uncover the need for evidence-based practice.

The first category includes problem-focused factors. These are generally clinical problems that are identified through quality improvement processes, benchmarking studies, regulatory agency feedback, practicing clinicians, or administrative data. For example, a hospital may identify a problem with skin breakdown through nurse observation, quality data indicating an increase in pressure ulcer rates, analysis indicating pressure ulcer rates are higher than comparable hospital units, or data that demonstrate higher costs for patients with skin breakdown.

A second category includes factors related to nursing knowledge. A knowledge deficit may be evident, or new knowledge may emerge through research studies. A new professional association or new national guideline presents opportunities for incorporating evidence-based changes into practice. A practice change often has a better chance of implementation if users perceive a solid base of evidence for the practice change. For example, a nurse who attends a national conference may find that hydrotherapy is an evidence-based treatment for pressure ulcers and use the information to motivate a change in nursing practice.

Checklist for Evaluating the Credibility of a Research Article

- ✓ The authors have the appropriate clinical and educational credentials for this research study.
- ✓ There is no evidence of any conflict of interest for the authors that might introduce bias into the way the study is designed or the way the results are viewed.
- ✓ There is evidence that this journal is peer reviewed (at least one of these):
  - Pages are sequentially numbered for the entire year.
  - Issues are identified by volume and number.
  - The journal has an external editorial board.
  - The article indicates a review date.
- ✓ The publication has no financial connection to positive or negative results from the study.
- ✓ The study has been published in a reasonable time frame from date of study to date of publication.

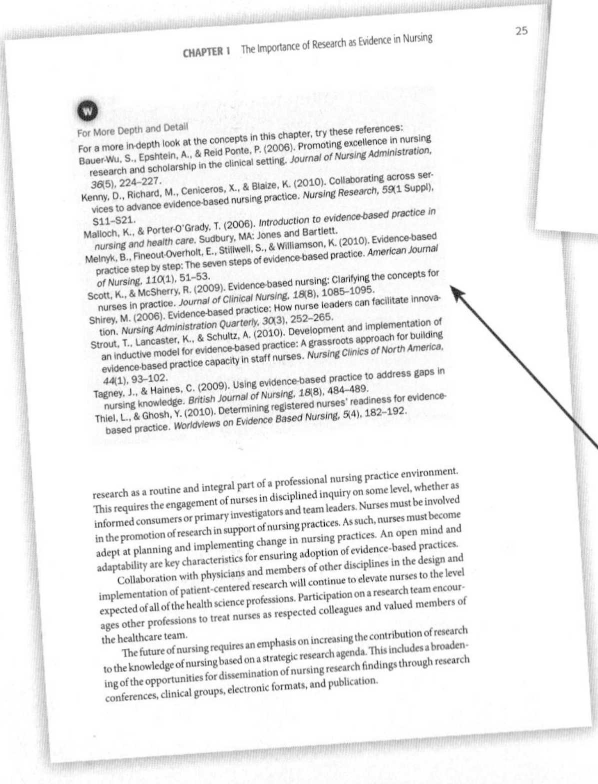

CHAPTER 1 The Importance of Research as Evidence in Nursing 25

For More Depth and Detail

For a more in-depth look at the concepts in this chapter, try these references:

Bauer-Wu, S., Epshtein, A., & Reid Ponte, P. (2006). Promoting excellence in nursing research and scholarship in the clinical setting. *Journal of Nursing Administration, 36*(5), 224–227.

Kenny, D., Richard, M., Ceniceros, X., & Blaize, K. (2010). Collaborating across services to advance evidence-based nursing practice. *Nursing Research, 59*(1 Suppl), S11–S21.

Malloch, K., & Porter-O'Grady, T. (2006). *Introduction to evidence-based practice in nursing and health care.* Sudbury, MA: Jones and Bartlett.

Melnyk, B., Fineout-Overholt, E., Stillwell, S., & Williamson, K. (2010). Evidence-based practice step by step: The seven steps of evidence-based practice. *American Journal of Nursing, 110*(1), 51–53.

Scott, K., & McSherry, R. (2009). Evidence-based nursing: Clarifying the concepts for nurses in practice. *Journal of Clinical Nursing, 18*(8), 1085–1095.

Shirey, M. (2006). Evidence-based practice: How nurse leaders can facilitate innovation. *Nursing Administration Quarterly, 30*(3), 252–265.

Strout, T., Lancaster, K., & Schultz, A. (2010). Development and implementation of an inductive model for evidence-based practice: A grassroots approach for building evidence-based practice capacity in staff nurses. *Nursing Clinics of North America, 44*(1), 93–102.

Tagney, J., & Haines, C. (2009). Using evidence-based practice to address gaps in nursing knowledge. *British Journal of Nursing, 18*(8), 484–489.

Thiel, L., & Ghosh, Y. (2010). Determining registered nurses' readiness for evidence-based practice. *Worldviews on Evidence Based Nursing, 5*(4), 182–192.

research as a routine and integral part of a professional nursing practice environment. This requires the engagement of nurses in disciplined inquiry on some level, whether as informed consumers or primary investigators and team leaders. Nurses must be involved in the promotion of research in support of nursing practices. As such, nurses must become adept at planning and implementing change in nursing practices. An open mind and adaptability are key characteristics for ensuring adoption of evidence-based practices.

Collaboration with physicians and members of other disciplines in the design and implementation of patient-centered research will continue to elevate nurses to the level expected of all of the health science professions. Participation on a research team encourages other professions to treat nurses as respected colleagues and valued members of the healthcare team.

The future of nursing requires an emphasis on increasing the contribution of research to the knowledge of nursing based on a strategic research agenda. This includes a broadening of the opportunities for dissemination of nursing research findings through research conferences, clinical groups, electronic formats, and publication.

Checklist These lists support the "Where to Look" features and provide students with an evaluation of specific research activities and issues.

For More Depth and Detail These reference lists are provided for a more in-depth look at the key concepts covered in each chapter. Visit **http://go.jblearning.com/houser** to find a list of these articles online.

26

Summary of Key Concepts

- The practice of nursing is founded on nursing knowledge, and nursing knowledge is generated and disseminated through reading, using, and creating nursing research.
- Nursing research is a systematic process of inquiry that uses rigorous, systematic approaches to produce answers to questions and solutions to problems in nursing practice. Research is designed so that it is free of bias and results are trustworthy. The hallmarks of research are peer review and replication.
- Nurses may use research to synthesize the findings of others, explore and describe phenomena, find solutions to problems, or test traditional approaches for efficacy.
- Research is fundamental to nursing practice because it is characteristic of a profession, and nurses are accountable for the care they deliver. Consumers and external agencies are demanding that healthcare professionals provide evidence for the effectiveness of interventions.
- Nursing is a relatively young profession, but there is still a history of disciplined inquiry by its practitioners. The National Institute of Nursing Research gives nursing research national stature and financial support, and also establishes a national agenda of priorities for nursing research.

CRITICAL APPRAISAL EXERCISE

Retrieve the following full text article from the Cumulative Index to Nursing and Allied Health Literature, or a similar search database:

Ortiz, J., McGilligan, K., & Kelly, P. (2004). Duration of breast milk expression among working mothers enrolled in an employer-sponsored lactation program. *Pediatric Nursing*, 30(2), 111–118.

Review the article, including information about the authors and sponsors of the study. Consider the following appraisal questions in your critical review of this research article:

1. Do the authors have the appropriate clinical and educational credentials for this research study? What are the strengths and weaknesses of this research team?
2. Is there evidence of any conflict of interest that might introduce bias into the way the study is designed or the way the results are viewed? Do the authors have any potential financial gain from the results of this study?
3. What is the evidence that this journal is peer-reviewed? Find the home page of this journal on the web. Does the journal have an editorial board?
4. Does the journal have anything to gain by publishing positive or negative results from this study?
5. Has the study been published in a reasonable time frame? Were the data that were used for the study based on a relatively recent sampling time frame?
6. Is there evidence of bias in the way the study was designed or implemented? If so, how does it affect the nurses' use of these data in the practice setting?

Summary of Key Concepts Found at the end of each chapter, these lists compile the most pertinent concepts and information for quick review and later reference.

Critical Appraisal Exercises Found at the end of each chapter, these exercises direct readers to apply the chapter concepts to a full-length research report. Visit **http://go.jblearning.com/houser** where you can complete your answers to each question.

Where to Look

Where to look for information about the research question or hypothesis:

- The research question may be explicitly stated in the research abstract but is commonly only implied by the title of the article, purpose statement, or objectives for the study.
- Ideally, the question is discussed at the beginning of the article, often at the end of the introduction. When it is stated early, it is followed by evidence from the literature review to support why this question is important to investigate further. It may be written as a statement instead of a question. If not at the beginning, look for the question at the end of the literature review.
- The null and alternate hypotheses are often found in the methods section where statistical methods are discussed, along with the rationale for the statistical tests used to test the hypotheses. Hypotheses are typically easy to find and are explicitly identified as such.
- Sometimes a separate section is created for a formal statement of the problem, the purpose of the study, and the research question. It may be labeled "Purpose," "Aims," or "Objectives." The research question may similarly have its own heading.
- If the researcher used any inferential statistical tests, which most quantitative studies do, then there were hypotheses, whether they are stated or not. Sometimes the reader is left to infer what the hypotheses were based on the tests that were reported.

SKILL Builder | Write Stronger Research Questions

The most important part of the research process is getting the question right. How the problem is stated determines what measures will be used, what data will be collected, the kind of analysis that will be used, and the conclusions that can be drawn. It is worth the time, then, to carefully consider how this element of the research study is developed. A thoughtful process does not necessarily mean a complicated process, however. Here are some simple suggestions for creating strong research questions:

- Answer the "why" question first. With a solid understanding of the reason for the study, the specifics of the research question are easier to identify.
- Review the literature before finalizing the question. Do not hesitate to replicate the question of a research study that accomplishes similar goals. It is flattering to a researcher—even established, well-known ones—to have their work replicated. Be sure to give credit where credit is due.
- Focus, focus, focus. Refine the research question, mull it over for a bit, and then refine it again. The effort spent to get the question just right will be worth it, because there will be less confusion later as to how to answer the question.
- That said, do not wait until the question is perfect to begin the design of the study. The question is, to some extent, a work in progress as the specifics of the research unfold. The question can, and likely will, be revised as new information, resources, and constraints come to light.
- Keep the research questions focused; do not include more than one major concept per question. Compound questions are hard to study and make it harder to isolate the effects of a single independent variable. Multiple research questions should be used instead of multiple parts of a single question.

Skill Builder Found in select chapters, these features provide practical advice for finding research, reading it critically, and strengthening research skills.

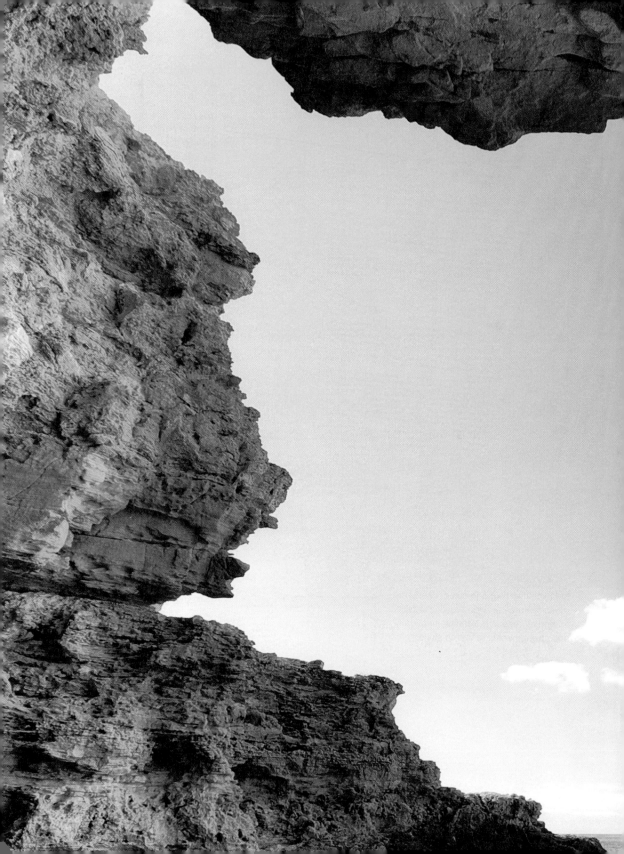

Nursing Research

Reading, Using, and Creating Evidence

SECOND EDITION

Janet Houser, PhD, RN

Academic Dean
Rueckert-Hartman College for Health Professions
Regis University
Denver, Colorado

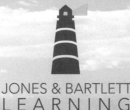

JONES & BARTLETT
LEARNING

World Headquarters

Jones & Bartlett Learning
40 Tall Pine Drive
Sudbury, MA 01776
978-443-5000
info@jblearning.com
www.jblearning.com

Jones & Bartlett Learning Canada
6339 Ormindale Way
Mississauga, Ontario L5V 1J2
Canada

Jones & Bartlett Learning International
Barb House, Barb Mews
London W6 7PA
United Kingdom

Jones & Bartlett Learning books and products are available through most bookstores and online booksellers. To contact Jones & Bartlett Learning directly, call 800-832-0034, fax 978-443-8000, or visit our website, www.jblearning.com.

The author, editor, and publisher have made every effort to provide accurate information. However, they are not responsible for errors, omissions, or for any outcomes related to the use of the contents of this book and take no responsibility for the use of the products and procedures described. Treatments and side effects described in this book may not be applicable to all people; likewise, some people may require a dose or experience a side effect that is not described herein. Drugs and medical devices are discussed that may have limited availability controlled by the Food and Drug Administration (FDA) for use only in a research study or clinical trial. Research, clinical practice, and government regulations often change the accepted standard in this field. When consideration is being given to use of any drug in the clinical setting, the health care provider or reader is responsible for determining FDA status of the drug, reading the package insert, and reviewing prescribing information for the most up-to-date recommendations on dose, precautions, and contraindications, and determining the appropriate usage for the product. This is especially important in the case of drugs that are new or seldom used.

Production Credits

Publisher: Kevin Sullivan
Acquisitions Editor: Amanda Harvey
Editorial Assistant: Sara Bempkins
Production Editor: Amanda Clerkin
Associate Marketing Manager: Katie Hennessy
V.P., Manufacturing and Inventory Control: Therese Connell

Composition: Publishers' Design and Production Services, Inc.
Cover Design: Scott Moden
Cover Image: © djgis/ShutterStock, Inc.
Printing and Binding: Courier Kendallville
Cover Printing: Courier Kendallville

To order this product, use ISBN: 978-1-4496-3173-4

Library of Congress Cataloging-in-Publication Data
Houser, Janet, 1954–
    Nursing research : reading, using, and creating evidence / Janet Houser. — 2nd ed.
        p. ; cm.
    Includes bibliographical references and index.
    ISBN 978-0-7637-8014-2 (pbk.)
    1. Nursing—Research—Methodology.   2. Evidence-based nursing.   I. Title.
    [DNLM: 1. Clinical Nursing Research—methods.   2. Evidence-Based Nursing.   3. Research Design. WY 20.5]
    RT81.5.H72 2012
    610.73072—dc22
                                2011000986
6048

Printed in the United States of America
15   14   13   12   11   10 9 8 7 6 5 4 3

dedication

Dedicated to my husband, Floyd, my partner in the pursuit of dreams.

contents

acknowledgments

It is a bit misleading to conclude that a book is produced solely by the person whose name appears on the cover. Help and support are needed from many people on both professional and personal fronts to complete a project of this size. The help of editorial staff is always welcome; advice from Kevin Sullivan was invaluable in merging the interests of writing with those of producing a book that others will want to read. My family—my husband, Floyd; my sisters, Anne and Ande; my niece, Stef; and mini-me, Amanda—provided me with enough encouragement to keep going even as they reminded me there is life beyond the pages of a book.

I must thank Regis profusely for providing me with inspirational colleagues and a place that supports my work. Thank you in particular to Phyllis Graham-Dickerson, Maureen McGuire, Mike Cahill, and Sheila Carlon, for kicking in their own contributions, often above and beyond what I expected. Pat Ladewig, as always, provided pragmatic advice and guidance from her impressive experience publishing her own texts. My contributors and reviewers each provided a unique viewpoint and help in discovering the best way to help students "get it." Most of all, I have to thank my dad, Glen. As always, his quiet pride inspires me, and he reminds me that life really happens around the dinner table.

contributors

J. Susan Andersen, PhD, FNP, BC
Texas Tech University Health Science Center
Lubbock, Texas
Chapter 19: Translating Research into Practice

Barbara W. Berg, DNP, CNS, PNP, CNE
Regis University
Denver, Colorado
Feature Contributor

Michael Cahill, MS
Centura Health
Parker, Colorado
Chapter 14: Summarizing and Reporting Descriptive Data

Sheila Carlon, PhD, RHIA, FAHIMA
Regis University
Denver, Colorado
Chapter 3: Ethical and Legal Considerations in Research

Karen Harris Frith, PhD, RN, NEA-VC
University of Alabama in Huntsville
Huntsville, Alabama
Chapter 13: Summarizing and Reporting Descriptive Data

Phyllis Graham-Dickerson, PhD, RN, CNS
Regis University
Denver, Colorado
Chapter 16: Qualitative Research Questions and Procedures
Chapter 17: Analyzing and Reporting Qualitative Results

LeeAnn Hanna, PhD, RN, CPHQ, FNAHQ
Centennial Medical Center
Nashville, Tennessee
Chapter 4: Finding Problems and Writing Questions

Deborah A. Jasovsky, PhD, MSN, NEA-BC
Loyola University Medical Center
Maywood, Illinois
Chapter 11: Enhancing the Validity of Research

Mary Kamienski, PhD, APRN-C, FAEN, CEN
University of Medicine and Dentistry of New Jersey School of Nursing
Newark, New Jersey
Chapter 11: Enhancing the Validity of Research

Cheryl Kruschke, EdD, MS, RN
Regis University
Denver, Colorado
Online Resources

Jan Loechell-Turner, MS, MA
Regis University, Dayton Memorial Library
Denver, Colorado
Chapter 5: The Successful Literature Review

Maureen McGuire, PhD, RN
Regis University
Denver, Colorado
Chapter 10: Data Collection Methods

Yvonne C. Shell, MS, RN
Kaiser-Permanente
Littleton, Colorado
Chapter 12: Descriptive Research Questions and Procedures

Cheryl Wagner, PhD, RN, MSN/MBA
Kaplan University
Chapter 6: Theoretical Frameworks

preface

This nursing research textbook is based on the idea that research is essential for nurses as evidence for practice. The contents are intended to be relevant for undergraduate nursing students, RNs that are returning to school, and practicing nurses that must apply evidence to practice. All nurses should be able to read research, determine how to use it in their practice, and participate in the research process in some way during their career as a professional. This text is intended to support all these efforts.

Evidence-based practice is one of the most exciting trends in nursing practice in decades. However, its integration into daily practice requires a solid understanding of the foundations of research design, validity, and application. This book is intended as a reader-friendly approach to a complex topic so that beginners can grasp the fundamentals of appraising research, experienced nurses can use research in practice, and practicing nurses can gain skills to create bedside science projects or participate effectively on research teams.

This text is presented in an uncluttered, straightforward manner. Although this text uses many bulleted lists to make the material visually interesting, sidebars, figures, and tables are limited to those that truly illustrate important concepts. This format allows the reader to grasp the information quickly and to read efficiently. Margin Notes provide definitions of new terms when they first appear, and the Gray Matter features cover information about key concepts that are of particular importance.

This book differs in its approach from traditional textbooks in that it does not focus primarily on interpreting inferential research; rather, it focuses on imparting a fundamental understanding of all types of research that may be used as evidence. This textbook also addresses contemporary concerns for today's nurses, including ethical and legal issues. Although both ethics and legal issues are mentioned in many research texts, a full chapter is devoted to these topics in this textbook so the intricacies of these issues can be thoroughly considered. In an era of HIPAA and numerous ethical quandaries, a thorough discussion of ethics and legal issues is essential.

This book covers the research process with an integrated discussion of both quantitative and qualitative traditions. Most nurse researchers have learned to appreciate the need to consider all paradigms when approaching a research question; separating the two approaches when discussing the fundamental interests of researchers results in a polarized view. Intuitively, nurses know that the lines between quantitative and qualitative designs are not so clear in practice and that they should consider multiple ways of knowing when evaluating research questions. The planning process covered in this book helps the novice researcher consider the requirements of both approaches in the context of sampling, measurement, validity, and other crucial issues they share. Detailed descriptions of the procedures for each type of design are given attention in separate chapters.

The chapters are organized around the types of research processes that make up the evidence base for practice. The first section of the book provides information that is applicable to all research traditions, whether descriptive, quantitative, or qualitative. Part I provides an overview of issues relevant to all researchers: understanding the way research and practice are related, the ways that knowledge is generated, and legal and ethical considerations. Part II describes the processes that go into planning research. The chapters in Part III present decisions that must be made in each phase of the research process.

The evidence generated by descriptive, survey, and qualitative designs is placed in the context of both the definition of evidence-based practice and application in practice guidelines. In Parts IV, V, and VI, each major classification of research is explored in depth through review of available designs, guidelines for methods and procedures, and discussion of appropriate analytic processes. Brief examples of each type of research are provided, along with notes explaining the features demonstrated in each case in point. Finally, Part VII details the processes used to communicate research through symposia and publication, and translate research into clinical practice.

Many chapters begin with a feature called "Voices from the Field" that relates a real-life story of a nurse's experience with the research process, illustrating the way that the material covered in that chapter might come to life. The main content for each chapter is broken into five parts:

- A thorough review of the topic under consideration is presented. This lays out the fundamental knowledge that is the basis for the topic.
- The text helps the nurse consider the aspects of a study that should be appraised when reading research. All nurses—regardless of their experience—should be able to read research critically and apply it appropriately to practice. Added features include guidance on where to look for the key elements of a research paper, the wording that might be used to describe them, and specific things to look for during the evaluation process. Evaluation checklists support this process in each chapter.
- The third section is using research in practice. This section supports the nurse in determining if and how research findings might be used in his or her practice.
- The fourth section is for nurses who may be involved on teams that are charged with creating research or who may plan bedside science projects to improve practice. This section gives practical advice and direction in the design and conduct of a realistic, focused nursing research project.
- The final section of each chapter contains summary points and a critical appraisal exercise so that the nurse can immediately apply the chapter concepts to a real research report.

Online materials provide support for both students and faculty. An online workbook is available to support students or nurses as they study the material or to use directly as a learning exercise in an electronic environment. These materials also provide novel support through discussion threads or topics available for posting on electronic discussion boards or in course chat rooms for online courses. Teachers can find slide presentations, suggested in-class exercises, and web resources to support the instructional process.

All these features are intended to help the reader gain a comprehensive view of the research process as it is used as the evidence for professional nursing practice. The use of this text as a supportive resource for learning and for ongoing reference in clinical practice is planned into the design of each element of the text. The goal is to stimulate nurses to read, use, and participate in the process of improving nursing practice through the systematic use of evidence. Accomplishing this goal improves the profession for all of us.

part I

An Introduction to Research

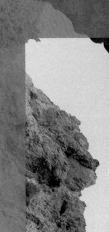

chapter 1

The Importance of Research as Evidence in Nursing

 ## CHAPTER OBJECTIVES

The study of this chapter will help the learner to

- Define nursing research and discuss how research is used in nursing practice.
- Describe the evolution of nursing research.
- Investigate the roles that nurses play in research processes.
- Contrast research and other types of problem solving.
- Explore how research is used as evidence guiding the practice of nursing.
- Develop strategies for using research as evidence in nursing practice.
- Read research and appraise the credibility of the journal, authors, and publication process.

KEY TERMS

Blinded	National Institute of Nursing Research	Quality improvement
Evidence-based practice		Randomized controlled trial
Evidence-based practice guideline	Nursing process	Replication
	Nursing research	Systematic review
External validity	Outcomes measurement	
Journal club	Peer review	
Magnet status	Principal investigator	

Research as Evidence for Nursing Practice

The practice of nursing is deeply rooted in nursing knowledge, and nursing knowledge is generated and disseminated through reading, using, and creating nursing research.

❝❝ Voices from the Field ❞❞

I was working as the clinical nurse specialist of a busy surgical intensive care unit (ICU) when we received a critically ill patient. He was fresh from cardiac surgery and quite unstable; he needed multiple drugs and an intra-aortic balloon pump just to maintain his perfusion status. He was so sick that we were not able to place him on a special bed for pressure relief. For the first 24 hours, we were so busy trying to keep him alive that we did not even get a chance to turn him.

About 36 hours into his ICU admission, he was stable enough to place on a low-air-loss mattress for pressure-ulcer prevention. When we were finally able to turn him, we noted he had a small stage II pressure ulcer on his coccyx. Despite the treatments that we used, the pressure ulcer evolved into a full thickness wound. He recovered from his cardiac surgical procedure but, unfortunately, required surgeries and skin grafts to close the pressure ulcer wound.

The experience I had with this patient prompted me to review the evidence-based practice guidelines we had in place to prevent pressure ulcers in critically ill patients. I wanted to make sure we could prevent this happening again, but I had a lot of questions. Could we preventively place high-risk patients on low-air-loss mattresses while they were still in the perioperative service? Did we even know the patients who were at risk for pressure ulcers? What assessment tools did nurses use to assess the patient's risk? When a high-risk patient was identified, what interventions did the nurses use to prevent pressure ulcers? How were the ulcers treated once they appeared?

I was fortunate that my chief nursing officer (CNO) was a strong advocate for evidence-based practice (EBP), and she encouraged me to initiate an EBP review of pressure ulcer prevention and treatment. Specifically, I wanted to find out what nursing interventions were supported by research evidence when we were trying to prevent pressure ulcers in the surgical ICU. So I contacted other inpatient units at the hospital to determine what they were doing.

I discovered that the surgical ICU was not different from the other inpatient units. There was no standard, evidence-based nursing practice for pressure ulcer prevention. Units were not consistently using the same skin assessment tools, so it was hard to objectively communicate risk from one unit to another. The tools we were using were not necessarily based on research. It was clear that we needed to identify the best available evidence and devise a protocol.

We started by establishing an evidence-based skin care council for the hospital. The team consisted of bedside nurses from all inpatient units and the perioperative service. Initially the council reviewed current nursing skin assessment forms, and we conducted a review of the literature on pressure ulcer prevention and interventions. We discovered the Association for Healthcare Research and Quality (AHRQ) guidelines on pressure ulcer prevention and treatment, a key source of evidence for healthcare practices.

Over the course of the next year, we revised our nursing policy and procedure, incorporating the AHRQ evidence into a treatment guideline. The guideline included a procedure for skin assessment and nursing documentation, and pressure ulcer assessment and treatment decision algorithms. We reviewed skin-care products and narrowed down the products to those that were supported by evidence. One algorithm helped staff make selections between products that maximized prevention and treatment. Another algorithm guided nurses in the use of therapeutic surfaces (e.g., low-air-loss mattresses) to prevent pressure ulcers. To monitor our progress, we began quarterly pressure ulcer prevalence studies. As part of the implementation, we scheduled a skin-care seminar featuring a national expert on skin care.

At the beginning of our EBP skin-care journey, our pressure ulcer prevalence was 9 percent. Since implementing our EBP skin-care initiatives our pressure ulcer prevalence has dropped by two thirds. The EBP skin-care council continues to be active in our hospital. We meet monthly to seek out the best evidence to guide skin- and wound-care product decisions, practice guidelines, protocols, and policies. My initial search for a solution—based on my experience with one patient—led to improvements in practice that have benefited many patients since then.

Mary Beth Flynn Makic, PhD, RN

Professional nurses rely on research findings to inform their practice decisions; they use critical thinking to apply research directly to specific patient care situations. The research process allows nurses to ask and answer questions systematically that will ensure that decisions are based on sound science and rigorous inquiry. Nursing research helps nurses in a variety of settings answer questions about patient care, education, and administration. Research ensures that practices are based on evidence, rather than eloquence or tradition.

What Is Nursing Research?

Nursing research is a systematic process of inquiry that uses rigorous guidelines to produce unbiased, trustworthy answers to questions about nursing practice. Research is used as evidence in the evaluation and determination of best nursing practices. The aim of original nursing research is to generate new knowledge to inform the practice of nursing. However, nurses may use research to

> **Nursing research:** A systematic process of inquiry that uses rigorous guidelines to produce unbiased, trustworthy answers to questions about nursing practice.

- Synthesize the findings of others into a coherent guide for practice
- Explore and describe phenomena that affect health
- Find solutions to existing and emerging problems
- Test traditional approaches to patient care for continued relevance and effectiveness

A variety of methods is used to generate new knowledge or summarize existing study results. Nurse researchers may measure observable characteristics, solicit perceptions directly from clients, assess words and phrases for underlying meaning, or analyze a group of study findings in aggregate. Nurse researchers have virtually limitless options for research design and may assume roles ranging from primary investigator for a large, multisite trial to staff nurse in a bedside science project. The goal, however, is always the same: to generate new knowledge that can be applied to improve nursing practice.

Regardless of the design, research is a rigorous endeavor that is subject to peer review and replication. These two characteristics are essential to ensure that research is unbiased and applicable to the real world. A study is subjected to peer review when experts in the field evaluate the quality of the research and determine whether it warrants presentation at a conference or publication in a professional journal. These reviews are generally blinded, meaning the reviewer is unaware of the researcher's identity. In blind peer review, a research report is subjected to appraisal by a neutral party who is unassociated with the research and unaware of the authorship. Reviewers determine whether the study process and outcome are of acceptable quality for communication to the broader professional community. Replication ensures that findings can be duplicated in different populations and at different times. This characteristic provides the nurse with confidence that the findings are not limited to a single sample, but that study outcomes will likely be similar in other patient populations.

Research: A Fundamental Nursing Skill

Although many students and practitioners of nursing consider research to be the purview of academics and graduate students, in reality, research is fundamental to professional nursing practice. There are many reasons why research is critical for the nurse in any role. Nursing is a profession, and along with advanced education and self-regulation, research is one of the central tenets that defines a profession. For nurses to function on the healthcare team as colleagues with therapists, physicians, and other caregivers, they must speak the language of science and use the best available research evidence as a basis for collaborating in planning patient care.

As professionals, nurses are accountable for the outcomes they achieve and the effectiveness of interventions that are applied and recommended to patients. Accountability is based on a solid understanding and evaluation of the best available evidence as a basis for decision making and patient counseling. In current healthcare practice, access, cost, and patient safety are all areas that clearly benefit from nursing research.

Consumer demands require that nurses are accountable for their practice as well. Consumers and their families are often well informed about the evidence that reveals the effectiveness of care. The baby boom generation is entering the years that typically yield higher healthcare use, and this generation is better educated, is healthier, and has better access to information than any generation in history. The Internet has given consumers unprecedented access to health information—some of it questionable, but much of it of high quality—that enables them to evaluate the basis for their own healthcare decisions.

In recent years, external agencies and purchasers of healthcare services are requiring that organizations collect and report information about the quality of care that is delivered and the outcomes that are achieved. These external regulators frequently require that organizations report the evidence they use to make nursing practice decisions. Many nursing organizations are in the process of pursuing or maintaining Magnet status, which requires that staff nurses understand the research

Peer review: The process of subjecting research to the appraisal of a neutral third party. Common processes of peer review include selecting research for conferences and evaluating research manuscripts for publication.
Blinded: The peer reviewer is unaware of the author's identity, so personal influence is avoided.
Replication: Repeating a specific study in detail on a different sample. When a study has been replicated several times and similar results are found, the evidence can be used with more confidence.
Magnet status: A designation for organizations that have characteristics that make them attractive to nurses as workplaces.

process and use evidence as a basis for practice. To maintain *Magnet* status, hospitals must show improved outcomes and clinical practice based on current evidence (Wise, 2009).

The Evolution of Research in Nursing

Nursing is a relatively young field when compared to fields such as philosophy or physics that have hundreds of years of historical study. Nursing has not always relied on profession-specific research as a basis for practice. However, if one reads contemporary nursing literature, it is clear that research is taking on fundamental importance as a source of evidence for practice.

Florence Nightingale introduced the concept of scientific inquiry as a basis for practice. Nightingale's work focused on collecting information about factors that affected soldier mortality and morbidity during the Crimean War. With scientific data, she was able to create change in nursing practice. Indeed, her work was so impressive that she was inducted into the Statistical Society of London.

The years following Nightingale's era offered relatively little scientific work in nursing, likely because nursing education was accomplished through apprenticeship rather than scholarly work. As more nursing education moved into university settings in the 1950s, research took on more prominence as a key nursing activity. Journals were initiated both in the United States and internationally that focused exclusively on publishing nursing research. More outlets for the publication of nursing research were established in the 1970s and 1980s, leading to the communication of research findings to a broader audience. The creation of the National Center for Research for Nursing within the National Institutes of Health (NIH) in 1986 was a seminal step in recognizing the importance of nursing research. In 1993, the center was given full institute status as the **National Institute of Nursing Research (NINR)**. This move put nursing research on a par with medical research and the other health sciences, ensuring financial support and a national audience for disciplined inquiry in the field. The NINR and other national agencies guide the overarching research agenda that focuses nursing research on professional priorities. The mission of the NINR is to support clinical and basic research to establish a scientific basis for the care of individuals across the life span (NINR, 2010).

In the 1980s and 1990s, leaders in nursing research met periodically at a Conference on Research Priorities in Nursing Science (CORP) to identify research priorities for the nursing profession. These priorities were established as 5-year agendas. In the 1990s, advances in nursing research were coming so quickly that a more flexible approach was required. NINR research agenda planning now involves more frequent meetings of smaller groups that consist of nurse researchers, representa-

gray matter

Research is critical in nursing because
- The use of research is inherent to the definition of a profession.
- Nurses are accountable for outcomes.
- Consumers are demanding evidence-based care.

National Institute of Nursing Research (NNR): A federal agency responsible for the support of nursing research by establishing a national research agenda, funding grants and research awards, and providing training.

gray matter

Nurses may play a variety of roles in research, including the following:
- Informed consumer of research
- Participant in research-related activity, such as journal clubs
- Contributor to a systematic review process
- Data collector for a research project
- Principal investigator for a research study

tives of other NIH groups, and experts from the larger multidisciplinary community to identify pressing issues, research opportunities, and gaps in knowledge. This approach allows the NINR to set both long- and short-term goals for the national nursing research agenda. Some examples of recent NINR nursing research priorities appear in **Table 1.1**.

The 1990s and early twenty-first century saw a shift in emphasis on research as an academic activity to one that is a basis for nursing practice. The impetus for this shift was partially due to external influences that created demands for accountability, effectiveness, and efficiency. Internal influences in the profession also played a key role in this shift, as nursing professionals strive to create a norm of professional practice that is firmly grounded in best demonstrated practice.

Table 1.1

National Institute of Nursing Research Proposed Strategic Objectives for Nursing Research, 2011–2020

Objective	Examples
Advance health promotion and disease prevention	■ Study the behavior of systems that promote health, e.g., family units, populations, and organizations ■ Improve the understanding of health behavior patterns and incentives for behavior change ■ Determine the effects of models of preventive care ■ Create communication strategies that promote health and improve health literacy ■ Translate scientific research that will positively affect health behaviors ■ Incorporate interprofessional partnerships in the conduct of health behavior research
Improve quality of life by managing the symptoms of chronic illness	■ Improve knowledge of the biological basis for symptoms ■ Test interventions that reduce the development and/or impact of symptoms of chronic illness ■ Develop strategies that improve symptom management in chronic illness ■ Design strategies that help patients manage symptoms over the course of a disease
Improve end of life and palliative care	■ Enhance the scientific knowledge of issues and choices underlying end of life and palliative care ■ Develop and test interventions that provide palliative care across the lifespan ■ Develop strategies to minimize the burden of caregivers ■ Determine the impact of provider training on outcomes ■ Create communication strategies to promote end of life care
Enhance innovation in nursing research	■ Develop technologies and informatics-based solutions for health problems ■ Expand knowledge and application of telehealth interventions ■ Extend preventive interventions to underserved groups ■ Mobilize technology to form global partnerships to facilitate research and exchange of information

Source: National Institute of Nursing Research. Retrieved January 30, 2011, at http://www.ninr .nih.gov/NewsAndInformation/StrategicPlan2011.htm

Contemporary Nursing Research Roles

The nurse may be an effective team member on any number of research projects and may assume roles ranging from data collection to research design. The broad number of potential roles provides nurses with the chance to participate at an individual comfort level while learning increasingly complex research skills. The professional clinician has both opportunities and responsibilities to use research in a variety of ways to improve practice. Table 1.2 contains the statement from the American Nurses Association that describes the expected roles of nurses in research processes.

Most nurses are first exposed to clinical research as informed consumers. The informed consumer of research is able to find appropriate research studies, read them critically, evaluate their findings for validity, and use the findings in practice. Nurses may also participate in research-related activities, including journal clubs or groups that meet periodically to critique one another's research studies. Attending research presentations and discussing posters at conferences also expose the nurse to a variety of research studies.

> **Journal club:** A formally organized group that meets periodically to share and critique contemporary research in nursing, with a goal of both learning about the research process and finding evidence for practice.

Table 1.2	

Research Roles for Nurses

Educational Level	Research Role
Baccalaureate	Have a basic understanding of the processes of research.
	Apply research findings from nursing and other disciplines to practice.
	Work with others to identify research problems.
	Collaborate on research teams.
Masters	Evaluate research findings to develop EBP guidelines.
	Form and lead teams focused on evidence-based practice.
	Identify practices and systems that require study.
	Collaborate with nurse scientists to initiate research.
Practice-based doctorates	Translate scientific knowledge into complex clinical interventions tailored to meet individual, family, and community health needs.
	Use advanced leadership knowledge and skills to translate research into practice.
	Collaborate with scientists on new health research opportunities.
Research-focused doctorates	Pursue intellectual inquiry and conduct independent research for the purpose of extending knowledge.
	Plan and carry out an independent program of research.
	Seek support for initial phases of a research program.
	Involve others in research projects and programs.

Adapted from: American Association of Colleges of Nursing. (2006). *AACN position statement on nursing research.*

As the nurse becomes more proficient in the research process, involvement in a systematic review is a logical next step. Conducting a systematic review resulting in an evidence-based practice guideline requires the ability to develop research questions methodically, write inclusion criteria, conduct in-depth literature searches, and review the results of many studies critically. This participation also leads to facilitating changes in clinical practice on a larger scale and requires the nurse to use leadership and communication skills.

Involvement in actual research studies does not require complete control or in-depth design abilities. Assisting with data collection can take the form of helping measure outcomes on subjects or personally participating as a subject. Clinicians are frequently recruited to participate in studies or collect data directly from patients or their records. Collecting data for the studies of other researchers can give the nurse valuable insight into the methods used to maximize reliability and validity, which helps later if the nurse chooses to design an experiment.

Most nurses do not immediately start with an individual research study, but serve on a research team. As part of a team, the nurse can learn the skills needed to conduct research while relying on the time and expertise of a group of individuals. Serving on a team gives the nurse the opportunity to participate in research in a collegial way, collaborating with others to achieve a mutual goal.

The most advanced nurses are principal investigators, or producers of research, designing and conducting their own research projects. It is rare that individuals are able to accomplish research projects on their own, so it is more likely that the nurse will lead a research team. This requires not only research and analytical skill, but also skill in leading groups, managing projects, and soliciting organizational commitment.

Research Versus Problem Solving

Research is distinct from other problem-solving processes. Many processes involve inquiry. In an organizational setting, quality improvement, performance improvement, and outcomes measurement all involve systematic processes and an emphasis on data as a basis for decisions. For an individual nurse, the nursing process requires that the nurse gather evidence before planning an intervention and subsequently guides the nurse to evaluate the effectiveness of care objectively. Although both organizational and individual problem-solving processes may be systematic and objective, these are not synonymous with research in intent, risks, or outcome (Newhouse et al., 2006).

The intent of quality improvement is to improve processes for the benefit of patients or customers within an organizational context. It is basically a management tool that is used to ensure continuous improvement and a focus on quality. Research, on the other hand, has a broader intent. The goal of research is to benefit the profession of nursing and to make a contribution to the knowledge base for practice. Research is more beneficial because it becomes more broadly applied; quality improvement is beneficial specifically because of its specificity to a single organization.

The risk for a subject in a quality improvement study is not much more than the risk associated with clinical care. These studies are frequently descriptive or measure relationships that are evidenced by existing data. Often, patients who are the subjects of study for a quality improvement project are unaware they are even in a study. In a research project, however, subjects are clearly informed at the beginning of the project of the risks and benefits associated with participating in the study, and they are allowed to withdraw their information at any time. Upfront and informed consent is central to the research process.

> **Nursing process:** A systematic process used by nurses to identify and address patient problems. Includes the stages of assessment, planning, intervention, and evaluation.

Finally, the outcomes of a quality improvement study are intended to benefit a specific clinical group and so are reviewed by formal committees and communicated internally to organizational audiences. Research findings are subjected to rigorous peer review by neutral, external reviewers, and findings are expected to stand up to replication. When quality improvement projects are planned with an expectation of publication, the distinction becomes less clear. Is the goal of publication to share perspective on a process or to generalize the results to a broader group of patients? If the latter is the goal, then quality improvement projects should be subjected to the same rigorous review and control as a research project.

The intent when an individual nurse applies the nursing process for problem solving is even more specific. The nursing process requires an individual nurse to gather data about a patient, draw conclusions about patient needs, and implement measures to address those needs. Data collected from the patient are used to evaluate the effectiveness of care and make modifications to the plan. These steps mirror the research process, but at an individual level. Research is useful within the nursing process as a source of knowledge about assessment procedures, problem identification, and effective therapeutics, but simply using the nursing process does not constitute research.

Research as Evidence in Nursing Practice

It would seem a foregone conclusion that effective nursing practice is based on the best possible, rigorously tested evidence. Yet it is only in the past two decades that an emphasis on evidence as a basis for practice has reached the forefront of professional nursing. Although it may be surprising that the scientific basis for nursing practice has been this long in coming, there are many reasons why evidence-based nursing practice is a relatively recent effort. The past decade has seen unprecedented advances in information technology, making research and other types of evidence widely available to healthcare practitioners. Whereas a nurse practicing in the 1980s may have read one or two professional journals a month and attended perhaps one clinical conference in a year, contemporary nursing professionals have access to a virtually unlimited bank of professional journal articles and other sources of research evidence via the Internet. Technology has supported the communication of best practices and afforded consumers open access to healthcare information

> **gray matter**
>
> The research process is distinct from other problem-solving processes in that
> - Research contributes to the profession of nursing, not just a single organization or patient.
> - Research involves an explicit process of informed consent for subjects.
> - Research is subjected to external peer review and replication.

as well. As a result, evidence-based practice is quickly becoming the norm for effective nursing practice.

Evidence-Based Practice

What Evidence-Based Practice IS

Evidence-based practice: The use of the best scientific evidence, integrated with clinical experience and incorporating patient values and preferences in the practice of professional nursing care.

Evidence-based practice is the use of the best scientific evidence, integrated with clinical experience and incorporating patient values and preferences in the practice of professional nursing care. All three elements are important. As illustrated in **FIGURE 1.1**, the triad of rigorous evidence, clinical experience, and patient preferences must be balanced to achieve clinical practices that are both scientifically sound and acceptable to the individuals applying and benefiting from them.

Although healthcare practitioners have long used research as a basis for practice, a systematic approach to the translation of research into practice has been introduced in relatively recent times. The impetus for evidence-based practice was a 1990 comment by a Canadian physician on the need to "bring critical appraisal to the bedside." The first documented use of the term *evidence-based practice* appeared less than two decades ago when a clinical epidemiology text (Sackett et al., 1991) used the term to describe the way students in medical school were taught to develop an attitude of "enlightened skepticism" toward the routine application of diagnostic technologies and clinical interventions in their daily practice. The authors described how effective practitioners rigorously review published studies to inform clinical decisions. The goal stated in this publication was an

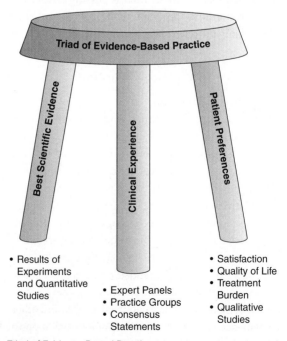

FIGURE 1.1 The Triad of Evidence-Based Practice

awareness of the evidence on which professional practice is based and a critical assessment of the soundness of that evidence.

The term entered the U.S. literature in 1993 when an article in the *Journal of the American Medical Association* described the need for an established scientific basis for healthcare decisions (Oxman, Sackett, & Guyatt, 1993). The authors of the article noted that the goal of evidence-based practice is to help practitioners translate the results of research into clinical practice, and they recognized that the scientific practice of health care required sifting through and appraising evidence to make appropriate decisions.

Even with the relatively recent birth of the term, evidence-based practice has rapidly become an international standard for all healthcare practitioners. Using the best scientific evidence as a basis for practice makes intuitive sense and places nursing in the company of the other science-based health professions in using evidence as a foundation for clinical decision making.

What Evidence-Based Practice Is NOT

A wide range of activities contribute to evidence-based practice. Many of these activities—reviewing research, consulting expert colleagues, considering patient preferences—are common in nursing practice. However, many such activities are not considered evidence-based practice, but rather other forms of decision making used to solve problems.

Evidence-Based Practice Is Not Clinical Problem Solving

Although evidence-based practice is a mechanism for solving clinical problems and making decisions about interventions, it is distinct from traditional problem-solving approaches in health care. Conventional decision making about clinical practices relied on expert opinion—sometimes achieved by consensus, but rarely through experimentation—combined with standard practice. Evidence-based practice is a systematic process of critically reviewing the best available research evidence and then incorporating clinical experience and patient preferences into the mix.

Evidence-Based Practice Is Not Solely Randomized Controlled Trials

Evidence-based practice does not mean choosing only those interventions supported by **randomized controlled trials**—although these studies are clearly important in providing guidance for effective practices. A somewhat tongue-in-cheek article by Smith and Pell (2006) suggested that we did not need a randomized trial to inform practitioners of the importance of a parachute as a measure of preventing death when jumping from an airplane (and, in fact, noted the difficulty in recruiting a control group for such a trial!). Evidence-based practice does not rely solely on one type of evidence, but rather is founded on a hierarchy of evidence, with individual studies rated from "strongest" to "weakest" based on the type of design and quality of execution. Evidence can come from many different types of studies in addition to randomized trials.

> **Randomized controlled trial:** A typical experiment in which subjects are randomly assigned to groups, one of which gets an experimental treatment while another is a control group. The experiment has high internal validity so the researcher can draw conclusions regarding the effects of treatments.

Evidence-Based Practice Is Not "Cookbook Medicine"

Guidelines based on the best available evidence do not mean the practitioner has an edict to practice in a single way. In fact, evidence alone is never sufficient to make a specific clinical decision about a specific patient. The nurse needs evidence plus good judgment, clinical skill, and knowledge of the patient's unique needs to apply evidence to a specific patient care situation. The definition of evidence-based practice, in fact, holds evidence as only one element of the triad of decision making. Clinical judgment and patient values must be considered when applying the evidence to a particular situation.

Evidence Is Not the Same as Theory

Theoretical effects must be tested and retested to be determined effective. As late as the early twentieth century, physicians still believed that bloodletting was an effective treatment for a host of disorders. This belief was based on the empirical observation that a patient's pulse rate slowed when he or she was bled and the theory that a slower pulse reduced irritation and inflammation. Although the empirical observations were accurate—the patient's pulse would slow, indeed, but due to ensuing hypovolemic shock—the theoretical relationship to a therapeutic response was ill founded. Many contemporary healthcare interventions are, unfortunately, based on similar theoretical relationships that have been untested for years. Recent research has refuted many of these theoretical assumptions, including the protective value of hormone-replacement therapy, the use of rubbing alcohol to prevent infection in a neonate's umbilical cord, and the relative harmlessness of margarine, among many others.

Evidence-Based Nursing Is Not Evidence-Based Medicine

The nature and processes of research are likely to be unique for any given profession. Medicine and nursing have different philosophical roots and approaches to patient care. Medicine relies on an extensive scientific basis that is primarily concerned with the cause of disease and effects of treatment. The evidence for medical care, by necessity, focuses on scientific studies that quantify these effects. Medical evidence has been criticized, however, for its sometimes artificial nature. It is a research paradox that the more an experiment is controlled, the less applicability the results will have in the real world. Randomized controlled trials, then, may provide the most rigorous scientific evidence, but that evidence may not apply well to individual patients with a broad range of physical, psychological, and behavioral conditions.

Nursing, on the other hand, requires a holistic approach to the care of individuals with physical, psychosocial, and/or spiritual needs. This care is founded on the nurse–patient relationship and the nurse's appreciation for the patient's unique needs. The evidence for nursing care, then, will require a broad range of methodologies as a basis for care. This is not to imply that these sources of evidence are not subjected to healthy skepticism and systematic inquiry, but rather that a broader range of evidence is considered as a basis for practice.

The Importance of Evidence-Based Practice in Nursing

Evidence-based practice is important to the nurse for many reasons. At the top of this list is the contribution of evidence to the effective care of patients. Studies have supported that patient outcomes are substantially improved when health care is based on evidence from well-designed studies versus tradition or clinical expertise alone. Leufer and Cleary-Holdforth (2009) aggregated outcomes studies related to evidence-based practice changes. A wide range of effects were found in multiple specialties including orthopedic, cardiovascular, respiratory, and obstetrical outcomes. Evidence-based practices in obstetrics and neonatal care reduced morbidity and mortality, sometimes dramatically. The use of corticosteroids in premature labor, for example, reduced the risk of premature infant death by 20 percent. A seminal meta-analysis by Heater, Becker, and Olson (1988) demonstrated the impact of evidence-based practices on a range of behavioral, physiological, and psychosocial aspects of patient well-being. The linkage between evidence-based interventions and outcomes is an important one, and determining the scientific support for a practice prior to its implementation makes intuitive sense.

Although quantitative studies of cause and effect are limited, there are indications that evidence as a basis for process improvement and leadership practices may benefit the organization as well as its patients (Stetler & Caramanica, 2007). Changes in attitudes, knowledge, and skills related to evidence-based practices have been demonstrated through testing educational interventions (Varnell et al., 2008). Evidence-based practice may soon become the norm for both the way care is delivered and the way organizations operate.

Healthcare providers operate in an era of accountability, in which quality issues, patient safety, and cost concerns are primary drivers of patient care processes. Using evidence to guide practice streamlines patient care (Newhouse, 2007). Practices that are unnecessary are eliminated; ineffective practices are replaced with practices that result in desired outcomes.

Existing practices may even be unintentionally harming patients (as was found in the hormone-replacement studies), so it is ethically unjustified to continue using untested interventions. Evidence can help healthcare professionals avoid making errors in decision making relative to patient care. Using research decreases the need for trial and error, which is time-consuming and may be counterproductive. In any case, time is not wasted on practices that may be ineffective or unnecessarily time-intensive.

> **gray matter**
>
> Evidence-based practice is important in nursing practice because research has shown that
> - Patient outcomes are better when evidence is used as a basis for practice.
> - Nursing care is more efficient as ineffective processes are replaced.
> - Errors in decision making become less frequent.
> - Consumers want evidence-based information to make decisions.

Consumers are well-informed about their options for personal health care and often resist the traditional, paternalistic approach to health interventions. The public expects that care is based on scientific evidence and believes that care processes should routinely lead to high quality outcomes that are physically and mentally desirable (Aarons et al., 2009). Healthcare professionals must be able to respond to their patients' questions about the scientific merit of interventions and about the relative benefit of treatment options.

Evidence might come in the form of journal articles, policies, guidelines, professional consensus statements, and standards of practice as well as formalized research. Although evidence-based practice implies scientific evidence, the words *relevant* and *rigorous* might be better adjectives to describe the kind of evidence needed by healthcare professionals. Critical skills include the ability to judge both the *type of evidence* that is needed and the *value of that evidence.*

Healthcare practitioners do not practice in professional isolation, but rather explore what works and does not work using empirical methods. An increased emphasis on evidence-based practice can be viewed as a response to these broader forces in the context of healthcare delivery and a logical progression toward the utilization of research as a basis for patient care decisions.

How Can Evidence Be Used in Health Care?

At its best, evidence provides the basis for effective, efficient patient care practices. At a minimum, an evidence-based approach can enhance practice by encouraging reflection on what we know about virtually every aspect of daily patient care. The evidence-based practice (EBP) process need not be onerous, and basically entails five elements: (1) formulating an appropriate question, (2) performing an efficient literature search, (3) critically appraising the best available evidence, (4) applying the best evidence to clinical practice, and (5) assessing outcomes of care (Noteboom et al., 2008). The original question can come from a variety of sources in a healthcare setting and, likewise, there is a wide range of organizational processes for which evidence can improve outcomes.

Evidence as a Basis for Healthcare Processes

Evidence can be incorporated into virtually every phase of the healthcare process. Evidence exists for best practices in

- Assessment of patient conditions
- Diagnosis of patient problems
- Planning of patient care
- Interventions to improve the patient's function or condition, or to prevent complications
- Evaluation of patient responses to intervention

Evidence as a Basis for Policies and Procedures

Although healthcare professionals from different educational programs, backgrounds, and experience may have different ways of delivering patient care, few can argue with the need for best practices. Evidence-based practice provides the foundation for policies and procedures that are tested and found effective, as opposed to "the way we've always done it."

Evidence as a Basis for Patient Care Management Tools

The evidence that is revealed through systematic review of research and other sources provides an excellent basis for patient care management tools such as care maps, critical paths, protocols, and standard order sets. One of the benefits of patient care management tools is the reduction of variability in practices, and evidence serves as a rational basis for standardized practices.

Evidence as a Basis for Care of the Individual

The complexity of patients that need care in the healthcare system can make the clinician wonder if evidence can ever be applied to an individual patient. It is easy to consider the question, "Is my patient so different from those in the research that results will not help me make a treatment decision?" This question, more than any other, may stand in the way of applying evidence to individual patient care situations. In fact, one study found that the more familiar a patient was to a practitioner, the *less likely* the clinician was to use evidence as a basis for that person's care (Summerskill & Pope, 2002).

As practitioners, though, we must ask whether these assumptions about the uniqueness of patients are in their best interests when it comes to clinical care. Uncertainty is inherent in the healthcare process; evidence helps to quantify that uncertainty. Concern for the uniqueness of the individual patient is not a reason to ignore the evidence, but rather to learn to critically apply it appropriately. Evidence is not intended to be rigid, but rather—as our definition makes explicit—to be *integrated* with clinical experience and a patient's unique values to arrive at optimal outcomes.

Evidence in clinical practice is not solely limited to patient care, however. Healthcare professionals might be interested in evidence as it relates to team functioning, the best way to communicate change, organizational models for research utilization, or even the effects of insurance on healthcare usage. Evidence in health care abounds on a variety of topics, and research utilization can improve patient care in a multitude of ways.

> **gray matter**
>
> Evidence can be used in nursing practice as a basis for
> - Nursing care processes such as assessment, diagnosis, treatment, and evaluation
> - Policies and procedures that guide nursing practice within an organization
> - Patient care management tools such as care maps, standard order sets, and critical paths
> - Care decisions regarding individual patient needs

Strategies for Implementing Evidence-Based Practice

Considering the benefits of basing clinical nursing practice on evidence, it would make sense for evidence-based nursing practice to be the norm. Unfortunately, this is not the case. There are many reasons why evidence-based practices are the exception rather than the rule, including limitations created by evidence-based practice systems themselves. Some barriers are related to human factors, and still others are related to the organizations within which nursing care is delivered. Table 1.3 lists some of the common barriers to using evidence as a basis for practice.

Organizations do not commonly have systems in place to support clinicians in the development of evidence-based practice tools. Although there has been a surge in the resources available for practitioners who want to participate in the development of practice guidelines, there has been little in the way of operational models to guide healthcare organizations that want to implement pervasive evidence-based practice (Salbach et al., 2007).

Table 1.3	

Barriers to Using Evidence in Clinical Practice

Limitations in evidence-based practice systems	▪ Overwhelming amount of information in the literature ▪ Sometimes contradictory findings in the research
Human factors that create barriers	▪ Lack of knowledge about evidence-based practice ▪ Lack of skill in finding and/or appraising research studies ▪ Negative attitudes about research and evidence-based care ▪ Perception that research is "cookbook medicine" ▪ Perception that research is for medicine, not nursing ▪ Patient expectations (e.g., demanding antibiotics)
Organizational factors that create barriers	▪ Lack of authority for clinicians to make changes in practice ▪ Peers emphasize status quo practice because "we've always done it this way" ▪ Demanding workloads with no time for research activities ▪ Conflict in priorities between unit work and research ▪ Lack of administrative support or incentives

The complexities of changing practice based on evidence are daunting indeed. Pagoto et al. (2007) studied the barriers and facilitators of evidence-based practice as perceived by healthcare professionals. Seven themes were used to describe both barriers and facilitators:

- Training and educational support
- Attitudes toward EBP and research
- Consumer demand for evidence-based care
- Logistical and organizational considerations
- Institutional and leadership support
- Policies and procedures
- Access to appropriate evidence

Strategies for Overcoming Barriers

Although little can be done to reduce the complexity of contemporary clinical care, there are some strategies that can help improve the rate at which healthcare professionals utilize research as a basis for their practice.

Begin the process by specifically *identifying the facilitators of and barriers to EBP practices.* Use of a self-assessment such as that tested by Gale and Schaffer (2009) can help identify organizational strengths and limitations in preparation for an EBP effort.

Education and training can improve knowledge and strengthen practitioners' beliefs about the benefits of EBP (Varnell et al., 2008). Clinicians may fear they will appear to lack competence, and knowledge will give them confidence in determining an evidence base for their practice.

One of the most helpful—and difficult—strategies is to *create an environment that encourages an inquisitive approach* about clinical care. The first step in identifying opportunities for best practices is questioning current practice. This can be accomplished by creating a culture in which EBP is valued, supported, and expected.

Despite the barriers inherent in implementing evidence-based practice in clinical practice, it is imperative to create structures and processes that reduce these obstacles. Regardless of the system within which the clinician practices, there is a systematic approach to finding and documenting the best possible evidence for practice. The process involves defining a clinical question, identifying and appraising the best possible evidence, and drawing conclusions about best practice.

Reading Research for Evidence-Based Practice

Reading research as evidence requires that the professional nurse have a basic understanding of research processes and can apply that understanding to the critical appraisal of individual studies. This is a systematic process of assessing the reliability, validity, and trustworthiness of studies, which will be explored in detail throughout this text. The appraisal process begins by determining if the journal, authors, and publication process are credible.

Consider the following key issues when assessing credibility:

- Does the author have the appropriate clinical and educational credentials for the research study? If not, have team members been recruited who have the requisite knowledge and skill? Teams give strength to a research project by providing diversity of perspectives and enlarging the expertise that is accessible to the team members.
- Is there evidence of a conflict of interest that may introduce bias into the study? For example, does the financial sponsor of the study have something to gain by positive or negative results? Sponsors may unintentionally impose expectations on a study and a researcher that may introduce bias into the study. Do the authors have an association with any of the entities in the study? If the authors are employed by an agency being tested in the study, then researcher bias may be a potential influence on the interpretation of data or the selective reporting of findings.
- Is the journal unbiased? In other words, does the publication have anything to gain by publishing positive or negative results? The publication should be one that has an external editorial board and a cadre of reviewers who are not associated financially with the publication. The names and credentials of the editorial board should be accessible in the publication.

Where to Look

It is sometimes difficult to determine whether a journal is peer reviewed. It may be explicitly stated in the front of the journal, but the absence of this description does not mean the journal is not a scholarly one. The reader may have to scrutinize the front matter of a journal (the masthead and publication information) or a journal web page to determine the nature of the publication.

The front matter should also include the names of the external editorial board. An external editorial board means there is objective oversight of the content and quality of material published in the journal. It is uncommon that the names of actual reviewers are published; the peer review process is a blinded one, meaning that article authors do not know the identity of the manuscript reviewer, and the reviewer does not know the identity of the authors.

If it is not clear whether the journal is peer reviewed, or if an article has been retrieved electronically so front matter is not available, some hints may indicate a journal is a scholarly one. Characteristically, peer-reviewed journal issues are identified by volume and number, and the pages are numbered sequentially through the entire year instead of starting over with each issue. An article published in October, therefore, would likely have page numbers in the hundreds. The first page may also specify the date on which a manuscript was received, reviewed, and subsequently published. This would confirm that a journal article has been peer reviewed.

The first page of the article should describe the author's credentials and place of employment, along with contact information. Any potential conflicts of interest should be identified here. Funding sources for research studies may appear in the credentials section or at the end of the article. Ideally, the journal will also publish any potential conflicts of interest—such as companies owned by the journal's parent company—that may introduce bias into the publication's selection process.

- Has the research study undergone blinded peer review? Blind peer review enables a critical appraisal of the research study by a neutral party who is not influenced by the stature (or lack of it) of the authors.
- Has the study been published within a reasonable time frame? Health care has a rapidly changing clinical environment, and studies that are delayed in getting to publication may be outdated before they reach print. Many journals note the date on which a manuscript was received and the length of time until it was reviewed and accepted. This enables the reader to determine if the information in the study is contemporary or subject to historical effects.

Reading research, much like any nursing skill, becomes easier with practice. As a practicing nurse reads, studies, and engages in research projects, the process becomes more efficient and informative. Evaluation that may initially require a great deal of focus and effort eventually becomes second nature. As the appraisal of research becomes part of the nurse's routine, the ability to select studies for application to practice allows the nurse to ensure that his or her practice is based on sound evidence.

Using Research in Evidence-Based Practice

Research is a key element in evidence-based practice. Scientific, rigorous, peer-reviewed studies are the foundation of evidence for professional nursing practice. Selecting, reviewing, and incorporating research findings into practice are at the heart of professional nursing care delivery; however, evidence-based practice does not eliminate the need for professional clinical judgment. The application of a specific evidence-based practice guideline to a specific patient situation is based on the nurse's assessment of the situation and an appraisal of the interventions that are most likely to be successful. The responsibility remains with the clinician to combine evidence with clinical expertise and patient values in managing individual patients and achieving optimal outcomes.

Where to Begin?

The process begins by identifying a problem that will be best addressed by a review of the evidence. The choice of a subject to study may be driven by a variety of factors. Newell-Stokes (2004) classifies three general categories that may uncover the need for evidence-based practice.

The first category includes problem-focused factors. These are generally clinical problems that are identified through quality improvement processes, benchmarking studies, regulatory agency feedback, practicing clinicians, or administrative data. For example, a hospital may identify a problem with skin breakdown through nurse observation, quality data indicating an increase in pressure ulcer rates, analysis indicating pressure ulcer rates are higher than comparable hospital units, or data that demonstrate higher costs for patients with skin breakdown.

A second category includes factors related to nursing knowledge. A knowledge deficit may be evident, or new knowledge may emerge through research studies. A new professional association or new national guideline presents opportunities for incorporating evidence-based changes into practice. A practice change often has a better chance of implementation if users perceive a solid base of evidence for the practice change. For example, a nurse who attends a national conference may find that hydrotherapy is an evidence-based treatment for pressure ulcers and use the information to motivate a change in nursing practice.

Checklist for Evaluating the Credibility of a Research Article

✔ The authors have the appropriate clinical and educational credentials for this research study.
✔ There is no evidence of any conflict of interest for the authors that might introduce bias into the way the study is designed or the way the results are viewed.
✔ There is evidence that this journal is peer reviewed (at least one of these):
   • Pages are sequentially numbered for the entire year.
   • Issues are identified by volume and number.
   • The journal has an external editorial board.
   • The article indicates a review date.
✔ The publication has no financial connection to positive or negative results from the study.
✔ The study has been published in a reasonable time frame from date of study to date of publication.

The third category includes factors such as new equipment, technology, or products that become available to the nurse. All of these present opportunities to use evidence in practice to improve outcomes.

Once the need is identified for a change in practice, the way the research is gathered and used may take a variety of forms.

Processes for Linking Evidence to Practice

Evidence can be used as a basis for practice through several processes. An individual nurse may appraise research studies and share findings with colleagues. A specific question may be answered by reviewing the literature or attending research presentations at conferences.

Although reviewing research studies is a good beginning for establishing evidence for nursing practice, it is possible to introduce bias into the selection of the articles to review. Nurses may consciously or unconsciously select only those articles that support their point of view while ignoring studies that do not. A systematic review process controls the potential for this bias. A systematic review process is a structured approach to a comprehensive research review. A systematic review begins by establishing objective criteria for finding and selecting research articles, combined with documentation of the rationale for eliminating any study from the review.

Research studies that are selected for inclusion in the review are subjected to careful and thorough appraisal of study quality and validity. Studies are graded based on the strength of evidence they provide as well as design and quality criteria. There is some variability in the rating scales that are commonly used to evaluate a research study's strength as evidence. It is important to understand that one rating system is not necessarily better than another. Individual values, the nature of the practice question, and the kind of knowledge needed drive the choice of a rating system. Most grading systems have between four and six levels. Table 1.4 depicts a rating system for levels of evidence that is a composite of the works of Armola et al. (2009), Ahrens (2005), and Rice (2008).

Using this scale, for example, a randomized trial of the use of aromatherapy in a postanesthesia care unit to reduce nausea would be the strongest level of evidence if it were from a large study with definitive results or if it were successfully replicated several times at several sites. The same study conducted in a single setting with a small sample of convenience would provide evidence that was less authoritative. Weaker still would be the evidence that was generated through observation or expert opinions.

It must be noted that these rating scales apply primarily to the evaluation of treatments, interventions, or the effectiveness of therapies. Recall the definition of evidence-based practice: practice based on the best demonstrated evidence combined with clinical experience and patient preferences. The hierarchy of evidence may look quite different depending on the nature of the practice under study.

Review and rating of the evidence should result in recommendations for practice. The strength of these recommendations is commensurate with the level of evidence and the quality of the study. The link between the strength of the evidence and the strength of the

Table 1.4	

Rating Systems for Grading Levels of Evidence

Level of Rating	Type of Study
Level I	▪ Multiple randomized controlled trials (RCTs) reported as meta-analysis, systematic review, or meta-synthesis, with results that consistently support a specific intervention or treatment
	▪ Randomized trials with large sample sizes and large effect sizes
Level II	▪ Evidence from well-designed controlled studies, either randomized or nonrandomized, with results that consistently support a specific intervention or treatment
Level III	▪ Evidence from studies of intact groups
	▪ Ex-post-facto and causal-comparative studies
	▪ Case–control or cohort studies
	▪ Evidence obtained from time series with and without an intervention
	▪ Single experimental or quasi-experimental studies with dramatic effect sizes
Level IV	▪ Evidence from integrative reviews
	▪ Systematic reviews of qualitative or descriptive studies
	▪ Theory-based evidence and expert opinion
	▪ Peer-reviewed professional organization standards with supporting clinical studies

resulting recommendation is the way in which varying levels of evidence are incorporated into a single practice guideline. **Table 1.5** depicts the way that the American Academy of Pediatrics (2004) recommends that evidence be linked to a subsequent system of recommendations. Based on the strength of the evidence and the preponderance of benefit or harm, recommendations are generated that are classified as strongly recommended, optional, or recommended. Some evidence results in no recommendation because a conclusion cannot be definitively drawn. Some evidence that shows harm to the patient may result in not recommended status.

The systematic review process is an involved and time-consuming one and should be undertaken only when no existing evidence-based practice guidelines exist. The effort is warranted, though, when no clear guidance exists for specific practices, or when the development of a guideline is likely to be affected by practitioner bias.

Creating Evidence for Practice

Nurses are commonly the primary investigators for studies that focus on the needs of patients and the effectiveness of nursing interventions. When a nurse conceives of, designs, and implements a research project, he or she is designated as a primary

Table 1.5

The Link Between Evidence and Recommendations for Practice

Type of Evidence	Clear Evidence of Benefit or Harm	Benefit and Harm Are Balanced
Well-designed, randomized controlled trials (RCTs) or reports of multiple RCTs	Strong recommendation for or against the intervention.	Action is optional.
RCTs with limitations of quasi-experimental studies	Recommendation for or against the intervention.	Action is optional.
Observational and descriptive studies, case controls, and cohort designs	Recommendation for or against the intervention.	Action is optional.
Expert opinion, case studies	Action is optional.	No recommendation for or against the intervention.

Source: Levin, R. F., & Feldman, H. R. (2006). *Teaching evidence-based nursing.* New York: Springer.

investigator. The primary investigator is responsible for all aspects of a research study's conduct and outcome, even if a team is involved. The primary investigator also has the right to be the first author noted on a research publication.

The design of a research study is an advanced and complex skill that requires experience in the clinical processes under study as well as an understanding of the complexity of research design and analysis. That is not to say that the professional nurse cannot gain the skill and experience needed to be a primary investigator, only that becoming a nurse researcher is an evolutionary process that occurs over time. It is the rare nurse who is able to design and conduct a study on the first attempt. More commonly, a nurse learns the process by being involved in the research of others in some way—either in data collection, team participation, or even as a subject. Only gradually does he or she gain the ability to conceive of and lead a research project.

Creating nursing research is a systematic, rigorous process. The remainder of this text will guide the nurse as he or she gains the foundation needed to read, use, and create evidence.

Future Directions for Nursing Research

It is clear that nursing research will continue to assume a prominent role in supporting the professional practice of nursing. The future of nursing research is exciting and requires that all nurses accept responsibility for seeking and using evidence as a basis for practice. It can be expected that research as part of nursing's future includes focusing on

For More Depth and Detail

For a more in-depth look at the concepts in this chapter, try these references:

Bauer-Wu, S., Epshtein, A., & Reid Ponte, P. (2006). Promoting excellence in nursing research and scholarship in the clinical setting. *Journal of Nursing Administration, 36*(5), 224–227.

Kenny, D., Richard, M., Ceniceros, X., & Blaize, K. (2010). Collaborating across services to advance evidence-based nursing practice. *Nursing Research, 59*(1 Suppl), S11–S21.

Malloch, K., & Porter-O'Grady, T. (2006). *Introduction to evidence-based practice in nursing and health care.* Sudbury, MA: Jones and Bartlett.

Melnyk, B., Fineout-Overholt, E., Stillwell, S., & Williamson, K. (2010). Evidence-based practice step by step: The seven steps of evidence-based practice. *American Journal of Nursing, 110*(1), 51–53.

Scott, K., & McSherry, R. (2009). Evidence-based nursing: Clarifying the concepts for nurses in practice. *Journal of Clinical Nursing, 18*(8), 1085–1095.

Shirey, M. (2006). Evidence-based practice: How nurse leaders can facilitate innovation. *Nursing Administration Quarterly, 30*(3), 252–265.

Strout, T., Lancaster, K., & Schultz, A. (2010). Development and implementation of an inductive model for evidence-based practice: A grassroots approach for building evidence-based practice capacity in staff nurses. *Nursing Clinics of North America, 44*(1), 93–102.

Tagney, J., & Haines, C. (2009). Using evidence-based practice to address gaps in nursing knowledge. *British Journal of Nursing, 18*(8), 484–489.

Thiel, L., & Ghosh, Y. (2010). Determining registered nurses' readiness for evidence-based practice. *Worldviews on Evidence Based Nursing, 5*(4), 182–192.

research as a routine and integral part of a professional nursing practice environment. This requires the engagement of nurses in disciplined inquiry on some level, whether as informed consumers or primary investigators and team leaders. Nurses must be involved in the promotion of research in support of nursing practices. As such, nurses must become adept at planning and implementing change in nursing practices. An open mind and adaptability are key characteristics for ensuring adoption of evidence-based practices.

Collaboration with physicians and members of other disciplines in the design and implementation of patient-centered research will continue to elevate nurses to the level expected of all of the health science professions. Participation on a research team encourages other professions to treat nurses as respected colleagues and valued members of the healthcare team.

The future of nursing requires an emphasis on increasing the contribution of research to the knowledge of nursing based on a strategic research agenda. This includes a broadening of the opportunities for dissemination of nursing research findings through research conferences, clinical groups, electronic formats, and publication.

Summary of Key Concepts

- The practice of nursing is founded on nursing knowledge, and nursing knowledge is generated and disseminated through reading, using, and creating nursing research.
- Nursing research is a systematic process of inquiry that uses rigorous, systematic approaches to produce answers to questions and solutions to problems in nursing practice. Research is designed so that it is free of bias and results are trustworthy. The hallmarks of research are peer review and replication.
- Nurses may use research to synthesize the findings of others, explore and describe phenomena, find solutions to problems, or test traditional approaches for efficacy.
- Research is fundamental to nursing practice because it is characteristic of a profession, and nurses are accountable for the care they deliver. Consumers and external agencies are demanding that healthcare professionals provide evidence for the effectiveness of interventions.
- Nursing is a relatively young profession, but there is still a history of disciplined inquiry by its practitioners. The National Institute of Nursing Research gives nursing research national stature and financial support, and also establishes a national agenda of priorities for nursing research.

 CRITICAL APPRAISAL EXERCISE

Retrieve the following full text article from the Cumulative Index to Nursing and Allied Health Literature, or a similar search database:

Ortiz, J., McGilligan, K., & Kelly, P. (2004). Duration of breast milk expression among working mothers enrolled in an employer-sponsored lactation program. *Pediatric Nursing, 30*(2), 111–118.

Review the article, including information about the authors and sponsors of the study. Consider the following appraisal questions in your critical review of this research article:

1. Do the authors have the appropriate clinical and educational credentials for this research study? What are the strengths and weaknesses of this research team?
2. Is there evidence of any conflict of interest that might introduce bias into the way the study is designed or the way the results are viewed? Do the authors have any potential financial gain from the results of this study?
3. What is the evidence that this journal is peer-reviewed? Find the home page of this journal on the web. Does the journal have an editorial board?
4. Does the journal have anything to gain by publishing positive or negative results from this study?
5. Has the study been published in a reasonable time frame? Were the data that were used for the study based on a relatively recent sampling time frame?
6. Is there evidence of bias in the way the study was designed or implemented? If so, how does it affect the nurses' use of these data in the practice setting?

- Nurses may fulfill a variety of roles in contemporary nursing research practice, ranging from informed consumers to data collectors to primary investigators. As nurses become more proficient in nursing research, their roles may broaden and involve projects of increasing complexity.

- Research is not synonymous with problem solving; it is intended to benefit the profession as a whole. A systematic approach and upfront, informed consent of subjects are hallmarks of a research process.

- The benefit of research to nurses is its use as evidence for practice. Evidence-based practice is the use of the best scientific evidence integrated with clinical experience, and incorporating patient values and preferences in the practice of professional nursing care. A variety of types of research is required to accomplish this goal.

- Evidence-based practice is important in nursing because outcomes are improved, care is more efficient and effective, and errors are reduced when practitioners use evidence as a standard of care. Consumers are asking for evidence to help them make decisions about their treatment options, and nurses are in a unique position to provide them with appropriate evidence.

- Evidence can be used as a basis for nursing practice in assessment of the patient's condition, diagnosis of patient problems, planning patient care, evaluating interventions, and evaluating patient responses.

- Barriers to using evidence as a basis for nursing practice may be related to the nature of evidence in practice, individual issues, or organizational constraints. Nurses must identify barriers to the use of evidence in practice and implement strategies to overcome them.

- Translation of research into practice is based on a careful evaluation of the characteristics of a patient population, matched with an assessment of the credibility and external validity of studies relative to patient needs.

> **External validity:** A study that can be confidently generalized to people, places, or situations other than those in the experiment.

- Future directions in nursing research include focusing on research as an integral part of nursing practice in a collaborative environment. Collaboration with other healthcare team members in research enhances the value of the profession and garners respect for its practitioners.

For a full suite of assignments and additional learning activities, use the access code located in the front of your book to visit this exclusive website: http://go.jblearning .com/houser. If you do not have an access code, you can obtain one at the site.

References

Aarons, G., Wells, R., Zagursky, K., Fettes, D., & Palinkas, L. (2009). Implementing evidence-based practice in community mental health agencies: A multiple stakeholder analysis. *American Journal of Public Health, 99*(11), 2087–2095.

Ahrens, T. (2005). Evidence-based practice: Priorities and implementation strategies. *AACN Clinical Issues, 16*(1), 36–42.

American Academy of Pediatrics. (2004). Policy statement: Classifying recommendations for clinical practice guidelines. *Pediatrics, 114*(3), 874–877.

American Association of Colleges of Nursing. (2006). AACN Position Statement on Nursing Research. Retrieved January 31, 2001, from www.aacn.nche.edu

Armola, R., Bourgault, A., Halm, M., Board, R., Bucher, L., et al. (2008). AACN's levels of evidence: What's new? *Critical Care Nurse, 29*(4), 70–73.

Gale, B., & Schaffer, M. (2009). Organizational readiness for evidence-based practice. *Journal of Nursing Administration, 39*(2), 91–97.

Heater, B., Becker, A., & Olson, R. (1988). Nursing interventions and patient outcomes: A meta-analysis of studies. *Nursing Research, 37*(5), 303–307.

Leufer, T., & Cleary-Holdforth, J. (2009). Evidence-based practice: Improving patient outcomes. *Nursing Standard, 23*(32), 35–39.

National Institute of Nursing Research. (2010, January). About NINR: Mission statement. Retrieved January 31, 2010, from http://www.ninr.nih.gov/AboutNINR/NINRMissionandStrategicPlan/

Newell-Stokes, G. (2004). Applying evidence-based practice: A place to start. *Journal of Infusion Nursing, 27*(6), 381–385.

Newhouse, R. (2007). Creating infrastructure supportive of evidence-based nursing practice: Leadership strategies. *Worldviews on Evidence-Based Nursing, 4*(1), 21–29.

Newhouse, R., Pettit, J., Poe, S., & Rocco, L. (2006). The slippery slope: Differentiating between quality improvement and research. *Journal of Nursing Administration, 36*(4), 211–219.

Noteboom, J., Allison, S., Cleland, J., & Whitman. J. (2008). A primer on selected aspects of evidence-based practice to questions of treatment. Part 2: Interpreting results, application to clinical practice, and self-evaluation. *Journal of Orthopaedic and Sports Physical Therapy, 28*(8), 485–501.

Oxman, A., Sackett, D., & Guyatt, G. (1993). Users' guides to the medical literature: I. How to get started. *Journal of the American Medical Association, 270,* 2093–2095.

Pagoto, S., Spring, B., Coups, E., Mulvaney, S., Coutu, M., et al. (2007). Barriers and facilitators of evidence-based practice perceived by behavioral science health professionals. *Journal of Clinical Psychology, 63*(7), 695–705.

Rice, M. (2008) Evidence-based practice in psychiatric care: Defining levels of evidence. *Journal of the American Psychiatric Nurses Association, 14*(3), 181–187.

Sackett, D., Haynes, R., Guyatt, G., & Tugwell, P. (1991). *Clinical epidemiology: A basic science for clinical medicine* (2nd ed.). Boston: Little, Brown.

Salbach, N., Jaglal, S., Korner-Bitensky, N., Rappolt, S., & Davis, D. (2007). Practitioner and organizational barriers to evidence-based practice of physical therapists for people with stroke. *Physical Therapy, 87*(10), 1284–1305.

Smith, G., & Pell, J. (2006). Parachute use to prevent death and major trauma related to gravitational challenge: Systematic review of randomized controlled trials. *International Journal of Prosthodontics, 19*(2), 126–128.

Stetler, C., & Caramanica, L. (2007). Evaluation of an evidence-based practice initiative: Outcomes, strengths, and limitations of a retrospective, conceptually-based approach. *Worldviews on Evidence-Based Nursing, 4*(4), 187–199.

Summerskill, W., & Pope, C. (2002). An exploratory qualitative study of the barriers to secondary prevention in the management of coronary heart disease. *Family Practitioner, 19*, 605–610.

Varnell, G., Haas, B., Duke, G., & Hudson, K. (2008). Effect of an educational intervention on attitudes toward an implementation of evidence-based practice. *Worldviews on Evidence-Based Nursing, 5*(4), 172–181.

Wise, N. (2009). Maintaining Magnet status: Establishing an EBP committee. *AORN Journal, 90*(2), 205–213.

chapter 2

The Research Process and Ways of Knowing

CHAPTER OBJECTIVES

The study of this chapter will help the learner to

- Discuss the philosophical orientations that influence the choice of a research design.
- Contrast the characteristics of quantitative and qualitative research.
- Review the steps involved in the research process.
- Determine the way that a design is linked to the research question.
- Classify research based on characteristics related to intent, type, and time.

KEY TERMS

Applied research	Mixed methods	Quasi-experimental studies
Basic research	Paradigm	Retrospective studies
Cross-sectional methods	Prospective studies	
Experimental research	Qualitative research	
Longitudinal studies	Quantitative research	

Introduction

What is the nature of truth? It is hard to think of a more difficult question to answer. This fundamental question must be considered, however, to ensure that the research process is successful in answering the research question. Research is about the search for truth. There are, however, multiple approaches for determining and describing truth. Critical to a successful research process is understanding which approach is effective for the particular research problem to be solved. The key is to consider assumptions about the nature of the world, the question to be answered, and the intent of the researcher.

❝❝ *Voices from the Field* ❞❞

I was at yet another meeting to talk about emergency department (ED) waiting room issues. We were part of a hospital-wide strategic initiative to address patient flow. During the meeting I realized we had addressed multiple ED patient flow issues with many time studies, but not one had examined some of the more "touchy feely" thoughts that patients and families might have with the waiting room itself. As one of the ED leaders, I wanted to know more about what patients and families thought about the "front door" to our hospital.

I pulled a multidisciplinary team together, and we began meeting on a monthly basis. Our first task was to search the literature about how others had evaluated the waiting room environment. We found several good waiting room satisfaction studies, but other than using general satisfaction surveys, we did not find any reliable or valid questionnaires. Many of the studies also looked at "time-to" issues or looked at satisfaction with the entire waiting room experience, but did not address the environment of the waiting room itself. My goal was to find a way to adequately look at all aspects of the waiting room environment that we could improve. I also knew that these might be some unique opportunities for our evaluation because we had plans to build a new waiting room in the near future.

Our research question started out very general and became more focused as we discussed our project. It was refined to ask the following question: What ED waiting room factors are associated with low satisfaction in ED patients and their families? We realized we also had a second question we hoped to answer: Were there other factors that we had not yet identified about the ED waiting room that ED patients and their families felt we should address?

Our hospital ethnographer had helped a team in the ICU evaluate its waiting room and had created a brief questionnaire we thought would be appropriate for our study as well. It had some basic demographic information about the person filling out the questionnaire (patient, family, or friend) and then about 10 five-point Likert scale questions about how satisfied they were with certain aspects of the waiting room environment, such as noise, temperature, and the comfort of the chairs. After talking with our leadership team and several staff members, we also added several open-ended questions about location, parking, and the waiting room in general. As a team, we realized that our research questions would drive our study design and that we weren't just looking for "quantitative data," we also wanted "qualitative information." We expanded our study to include random 30- to 60-minute observations of the waiting room during the same time period that we gave out our questionnaires.

The resulting study design was a mixed method, pre- and postobservation study that provided valuable information to the study team and to our ED leadership. We were able to identify what changes to make and then track the impact of those changes because of our mixed method study design.

Anne Panik, RN, MSN, CNAA

The most fundamental questions to be answered in the beginning of a research process are philosophical, but necessary ones: What constitutes knowledge? What is the nature of the world, and how can this research reflect that nature? The researcher should carefully consider these issues before proceeding with the design of the inquiry. It is a mistake to jump from research question to design without considering the philosophical foundation on which the study will be built.

These philosophical considerations, however, must represent more than the researcher's view of the world. They must be carefully matched to a design that will address the specific nature of the research question. The goal is to produce knowledge that is relevant and applicable to the body of nursing knowledge that becomes evidence for practice.

The Research Process

Regardless of the philosophical assumptions, some characteristics are universal to a research study. Research by its nature is systematic and rigorous; it is about a disciplined search for truth. Systematic is not synonymous with preplanned, but rather implies that decisions are carefully considered, options weighed, and a rational basis can be documented to support the choices that are made. Those decisions and choices help form the foundation and build a research study. These choices make up phases of study that are more or less completed in sequence. These phases are depicted in **FIGURE 2.1**:

- *Define a research problem:* Identify a gap in the knowledge of nursing practice that can be effectively addressed with evidence.
- *Scan the literature:* Complete a systematic review of the literature to determine basic knowledge about the problem and to identify relevant previous research problems.
- *Select a theoretical framework:* Determine an appropriate theoretical basis for the way the researcher thinks about the study of the problem.
- *Determine an appropriate design:* Select a design that is appropriate for the philosophical assumption, the nature of the question, the intent of the researcher, and the time dimension.
- *Define a sampling strategy:* Design a sampling plan that details both how subjects will be recruited and assigned to groups, if appropriate, and how many subjects will be needed.
- *Collect data:* Gather the data using appropriate data collection protocols and reliable, valid methods.
- *Analyze data:* Apply analytic techniques that are appropriate for the type of data collected and that will answer the question.
- *Communicate the findings:* Disseminate the findings to the appropriate audiences through conferences and publication.
- *Use the findings to support practice:* Promote the uptake of the research by linking it to specific guidelines for nursing practice.

These phases may look as if they make up steps, with the end of one phase leading to the beginning of another. It is, however, misleading to call the research process a series of

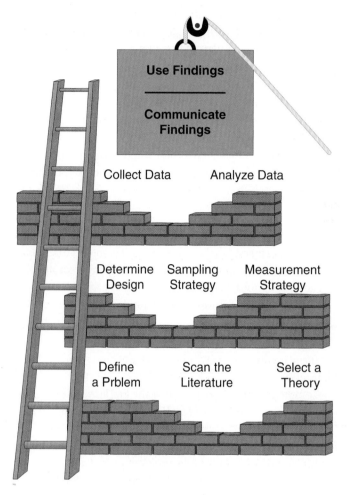

FIGURE 2.1 The Research Process: Building a Study

steps. This description implies that the steps are done in a particular sequence and that the components are distinct and mutually exclusive. In reality, the design of a research study is a fluid process, one that may be considered a work in progress until the final plan is complete. The process may resemble an elaborate game of Chutes and Ladders more than anything else. In this game, progress is made until one reaches a chute, which will take one back to a lower level. In research, several things may happen more or less at the same time, for example, the search for a theoretical framework, the literature review, and construction of the research question. Although the researcher may complete most of these tasks and move on to design, occasionally a situation will arise that makes the researcher reconsider the phrasing of the question, or new literature may be published. The phases may be conducted out of sequence, or the researcher may go back and forth between phases. The phases may overlap, or some phases may not be used at all. So many varieties of research are possible that any depiction of the research process must come with the caveat that it is a general guide that is adapted to the particular situation at hand.

In quantitative research, decisions are usually finalized before data collection begins, although emergent issues may, even then, require adaptation of the research plan. In the type of research called qualitative, the research plan adapts to both the data generated by the respondents and the nature of that data. Qualitative decisions may not be completed until the final report is written.

The research process, then, should not be considered a series of steps, but a series of thoughtful decisions about alternative approaches on a continuum of choices. Decisions are based on careful consideration of options, issues, and consequences. The decisions are then followed by a systematic series of actions to solve the original research problem.

In general, the way the research process emerges and the particular phases that are in a research study are based on many characteristics of both the research problem and the researcher. These characteristics and assumptions lend themselves to several general classifications of research. The choice of an overall research classification is the first step in determining the specifics of a research design.

Classification of Research by Philosophical Assumptions About the Nature of the World

The philosophical assumptions that drive the design of a study are rooted in the paradigms of those who are doing the studying. A paradigm is an overall belief system, a view of the world that strives to make sense of the nature of reality and the basis of knowledge. The disciplined study of nursing phenomena is rooted in two broad paradigms, both of which are relevant for nursing research. These two broad paradigms reflect methods that are primarily quantitative (based on the measurement of observable phenomena) or qualitative (based on the analysis of the meaning of events as depicted in the words and actions of others).

> **Paradigm:** An overall belief system or way of viewing the nature of reality and the basis of knowledge.

Quantitative Research

Quantitative research is the traditional approach to scientific research. It is rooted in the philosophical assumptions of positivism and determinism. Positivism assumes that features of the environment have an objective reality; the world is viewed as something available for study in a more or less unchanging form. A related assumption for the scientific method is that of determinism, a belief that events are not random, but have antecedent causes. Because of these beliefs—the existence of an objective reality, in which events can be linked to an associated cause—the researcher's task is to understand the reasons for human phenomena. The task of positivist scientific inquiry, then, is to make unbiased observations of the natural and social world.

> **Quantitative research:** A traditional approach to research in which variables are identified and measured in a reliable and valid way.

Quantitative research involves identifying the variables that represent characteristics of interest and then measuring them in a reliable, valid way. Quantitative research is characterized by a tightly controlled context that enables the researcher to rule out extraneous effects. The way subjects are selected and the protocols for the study are designed to eliminate bias. Statistical analysis is used to establish the amount of confidence in the results and to rule out the effects of random error. These conclusions, then, constitute the contribution to scientific knowledge.

There is no doubt that the scientific study of cause and effect in nursing practice is necessary and important; quantitative approaches are particularly suited for answering questions about the nursing actions that can influence outcomes. These studies produce some of the strongest evidence for the benefits of an intervention. But nurses pose many questions that are not adequately addressed by a strict adherence to measurement of an objective reality. The single adherence to a positivist view has come under considerable criticism from nurse researchers, and many of these criticisms are legitimate. The nature of nursing care involves helping others attain their health goals, many of which are defined by the individual, not the nurse. Perceptions of quality of life, the meaning of a life event, and the willingness to endure side effects for a therapeutic result are all based on the patient's construction of reality, not the nurse's. Many related questions are better addressed with a process of naturalistic inquiry.

Qualitative Research

Qualitative research: A naturalistic approach to research in which the focus is on understanding the meaning of an experience from the individual's perspective.

Qualitative research is based on a naturalistic paradigm. This belief system is represented by a view of reality that is constructed by the individual, not the researcher. In the naturalistic view, reality is not a fixed entity, but rather in the context of what the research participant believes it to be. Qualitative researchers believe that many different views of reality are possible, and all of them are right. An associated belief for the naturalistic researcher is relativism, or the belief that there are always multiple interpretations of reality, and that these interpretations can only exist within an individual. The qualitative researcher, then, believes there is no process in which the ultimate basis for a singular truth can be identified.

Qualitative methods focus on an understanding of the meaning of an experience from the individual's perspective. Extended observation of participants, in-depth interviews or focus groups, case studies, and studies of social interaction are characteristic of qualitative methods. The inquiry process focuses on verbal descriptions and observable behaviors as a basis for analysis and conclusions.

Qualitative methods are appropriate for questions in which the meaning of the patient's experience is central to understanding the best therapeutic approach. Issues of behavior change, motivation, compliance with a regimen, and tolerance of a treatment are all examples of topics in which the patient's perception is central to assisting the patient to a healthy state. The analysis of themes that describe the meaning of the experience for the patient is based on words and observations, rather than measurable phenomena. The researcher establishes a relationship with the subject, and bias is considered an inherent part of the research process. The findings from qualitative studies are used to enhance evidence-based practice by incorporating the patient's preferences and values into guides for nursing practice.

The differences in philosophy, roles, and methods between quantitative and qualitative research are depicted in Table 2.1. These contrasts are made to help the student understand the variations between these two overall approaches. In reality, both types of research have many characteristics in common, including:

- A disciplined, rigorous approach based on external evidence
- Methods that require samples and the cooperation of individuals
- A focus on the rights of human subjects and ethical guidelines
- An ultimate aim of discovering new knowledge that can be used to improve nursing practice

Many nurse researchers assume they have to select only one approach and carry out the study in a pure and inflexible way. In fact, it is the rare study that is purely one approach or the other. The choices made in research design are probably less about qualitative or quantitative and more along a continuum of choices that may overlap from one approach to the other. Many quantitative studies involve asking the subjects to respond to questions or give opinions in which the words are later analyzed to enhance

Table 2.1

A Contrast of Quantitative and Qualitative Characteristics

Element	Quantitative	Qualitative
View of reality	Reality is objective and can be seen and measured.	Reality is constructed by the individual.
View of time	Reality is relatively constant.	Reality is continuously constructed.
Context	Reality can be separated from context.	Reality is embedded in its context.
Researcher approach	Objective, detached.	Personally involved.
Populations studied	Samples that represent overall populations as subjects.	Individual cases, represented as informants.
Measures	Human behavior or other observable phenomena.	Study the meanings that individuals create.
Observations	Analyze reality as definable variables.	Make holistic observations of the total context.
Design	Preconceived and highly controlled.	Emergent and fluid, adaptable to informants' views.
Analysis	Descriptive and inferential statistics.	Analytic induction to determine meaning.
Generalization	Use inference to generalize from a sample to a defined population.	Transfer knowledge from case analysis to similar cases.
Reports	Objective, impersonal reports in which the researcher's opinions are undetectable.	Interpretive reports that reflect the researcher's reconstruction of the meaning of the data.

the statistical findings. Experimental researchers may rate subject behaviors using scales that have subjective elements, or they may record their own observations of behaviors. Conversely, many qualitative studies use measurement to determine the reliability of multiple raters in determining themes and to verify the trustworthiness of conclusions. A basic qualitative validation method is triangulation, or the search for multiple sources to confirm the same finding, in which numbers are often retrieved to confirm verbal data. There are many situations in which a blend of methods is appropriate, and these mixed method designs are becoming more common.

Mixed Methods

Mixed methods: A research approach that combines quantitative and qualitative elements; it involves the description of the measurable state of a phenomenon and the individual's subjective response to it.

Mixed methods are becoming an important tool in nursing research, particularly in evaluation research. Evaluation research is the application of research methods to the study of programs, projects, or phenomena. Increasingly, the question is not whether mixed methods are appropriate, but rather how they should be used.

Mixed methods are often applied in an ad hoc way, meaning the study begins by using a primarily quantitative or qualitative method, and elements of the alternative approach are integrated as an afterthought. The most effective use of mixed methods, however, is when they are employed in a systematic way (Miller & Fredericks, 2006). As a precursor to design, a thoughtful consideration of the elements of a study can establish sound reasons for employing mixed methods and is a helpful tactic for ensuring that the final study is a strong one meeting both quantitative and qualitative standards.

Mixed methods are commonly used in descriptive studies. Mixed methods may be used to describe both the measurable state of a phenomenon and the individual responses to it. For example, a mixed method might be used to

- Describe the rate of hand washing on a nursing unit (quantitative) as well as the nurses' perceptions about the importance of hand washing (qualitative)
- Measure the presence of bacteria on a nurse's hands after washing (quantitative) and observe the hand-washing steps the nurse used (qualitative)
- Count the number of times a nurse washed his or her hands between patients (quantitative) and record the nurse's report on the convenience of hand-washing facilities (qualitative)

Consider the following elements prior to choosing a research design:
- Philosophical orientation of the researcher
- Nature of the research question or problem
- Skills, abilities, and preferences of the researcher
- Resources and sample access

Reasons for Choosing a Design

There are many considerations that go into the choice of a general approach to research design. The philosophical orientation of the researcher is only one element. The nature of the research question, the skills and abilities of the researcher, and access to resources and samples all are important elements to consider prior to choosing the research methodology.

Of primary importance to the selection of an approach is the nature of the research question. Research questions that focus on the effectiveness of an intervention require a scientific approach (assuming effectiveness is defined as an objectively measured outcome). For example, determination of the effectiveness of a skin-care regimen in preventing pressure ulcers is best studied by applying the proposed regimen to one group of patients, applying a standard regimen to another group of patients, and then measuring the rate of pressure ulcer development in both groups. If the regimen is effective, then the subjects getting the new regimen will have a lower pressure ulcer rate than those with the standard regimen. This is the traditional experiment, and it is still one of the most common research designs in health care.

On the other hand, research questions that focus on the acceptability of an intervention may require a qualitative approach. The new regimen may be effective, but it may be painful, have an unpleasant smell, or involve a cream that sticks to the clothing. These attributes, which will almost certainly affect whether a patient complies with the regimen, require asking the patients about their preferences for the treatment, and whether the outcome outweighs the unpleasant side effects.

Some of the considerations when choosing an approach are researcher driven. Many researchers have a personal preference for one approach over another. When the research question may be answered in several different ways, or when various aspects of a phenomenon require study before evidence can be deduced, then the researcher's personal preference may drive the selection of an approach. The skills that are required for quantitative research include the capacity to define variables, recruit subjects, use random assignment methods, create reliable and valid measurements, and analyze results with statistical techniques. The skills that are required for qualitative researchers are quite different. These include the ability to find and select subjects who can best inform the question, observe and record actions and interactions in detail, skillfully interview subjects or focus groups, and distill meaning from large amounts of word-based data. Both skill sets can require years of development. It is natural, then, that most researchers find themselves specializing in one approach or the other.

There is a host of practical considerations when selecting an approach. Quantitative methods require measurement tools, subjects who are willing to be subjected to experimental treatments (or the risk of no treatment), statistical software, and access to individuals knowledgeable in statistical analysis and interpretation. Qualitative methods require less in the way of tools and software, but require informants who are willing to be observed or interviewed, often for extended periods of time. The particular individuals who are accessible as well as the material resources required may drive the selection of a feasible research approach.

A host of thoughtful decisions must be made in choosing the right approach for a particular research problem. The key word is *thoughtful*. These decisions should be based on a sound rationale, and the researcher should be able to articulate the basis for these decisions.

gray matter

The following skills are required for quantitative research:
- Defining variables
- Recruiting subjects
- Using random assignment methods
- Creating reliable and valid measurements
- Analyzing results with statistical techniques

gray matter

The following skills are required for qualitative research:
- Finding and selecting subjects appropriate for the question
- Observing and recording actions and interactions in detail
- Interviewing subjects skillfully
- Distilling meaning from large amounts of word-based data

Classifications of Research by the Intent of the Researcher

Research is classified by the basic belief system that drives its design features, but it must also reflect the intent of the researcher. There are two kinds of goals for research: one is to provide new knowledge for the foundation of nursing, and the other is to provide knowledge that can be immediately applied to the practice of nursing. The first of these is referred to as *basic research* and the latter as *applied research*.

Basic research is commonly referred to as theoretical, pure, fundamental, or bench research. One might think of the work done by scientists in laboratories as basic research. It is used to test theories and to build the body of knowledge that forms the foundation for practice, but does not directly apply to the practice setting. Examples of basic research are measuring neuromuscular responses to stimuli or studying the effects of circulatory volume on neonatal cardiac function.

Applied research is undertaken with the single goal of improving nursing practice. The findings are intended to contribute in some way to a modification of nursing practice. Examples of applied research are investigating the effects of topical drugs on phlebitis or determining the efficacy of specific counseling techniques after the death of a spouse.

> **Basic research:** Theoretical, pure, fundamental, or bench research done to advance knowledge in a given subject area.
> **Applied research:** Research conducted to gain knowledge that has a practical application and contributes in some way to a modification of practice.

Both basic and applied research may use quantitative, qualitative, or mixed methods. Most clinical nursing research is considered applied research, and the research that is generated as evidence for practice is exclusively of an applied nature. This is not to imply that basic research is not valuable. Indeed, one must have a clear understanding of the underlying theoretical and physiological basis for a given nursing practice to understand its mechanisms of effect.

Classifications of Research by the Nature of the Design

Another classification of research is associated with the nature of the design. Experimental research refers to studies of cause and effect, usually applied to determine the effectiveness of an intervention. In an experimental design, using some type of randomization method, subjects are selected or assigned to groups according to how well they represent the population of interest. The researcher manipulates some aspect of the patient's treatment in a highly controlled setting and compares the outcomes to a group that has had no treatment or a standard treatment. If the outcomes are different, the researcher assumes the difference is a result of the treatment because all other variables have been controlled. Experimental designs are characterized by highly structured protocols for sample selection and assignment, intervention, measurement, and analysis. Design is aimed at eliminating bias and controlling rival explanations for the outcome.

> **Experimental research:** Highly structured studies of cause and effect, usually applied to determine the effectiveness of an intervention. Subjects are selected and randomly assigned to groups to represent the population of interest.
> **Quasi-experimental studies:** Studies of cause and effect similar to experimental design but using convenience samples or existing groups to test interventions.

Nonexperimental designs cover a broad range of studies that do not share these characteristics and, therefore, cannot test cause and effect. Quasi-experimental studies mimic experimental designs in most ways except the selection and assignment of subjects. Quasi-experimental studies often use convenience samples or existing groups to test interventions. For example, a quasi-experimental study might involve testing an intervention between the population in one nursing home and another, where one group gets the treatment and the other does not. However, subjects are not assigned to the nursing homes randomly.

Other nonexperimental designs include descriptive research, correlation research, and predictive research. Descriptive research involves the study of a particular situation or event that already exists. The researcher does not manipulate any variables, although the study itself is systematic and thorough. Correlation research focuses on the existing relationships between variables. A correlation study may be applied to the search for a relationship between a single variable in two populations. (For example, do teens with mothers who had teen pregnancies have a higher teen pregnancy rate themselves?) Correlation studies may also search for relationships between two variables in the same sample. (For example, do overweight teens have higher pregnancy rates?) Predictive research takes correlation one step further, searching for relationships in which the values of one variable can be used to predict the values of another. (For example, do certain family characteristics predict the risk of a teen pregnancy?) Predictive research is particularly helpful in public health studies and research involving the determination of whether a risk factor will lead to a particular health condition.

Classifications of Research by the Time Dimension

A final classification of research studies is by the time dimension chosen for the studies. These may fall into categories that are in the past or future, referred to as retrospective or prospective. Retrospective studies are those that are conducted using data that have already been collected about events that have already happened. For nursing research, these data often come from chart review. The researcher is unable to control most aspects of variable definition and data collection because the data have already been collected. The researcher conducting a retrospective study relies on the accuracy and completeness of this secondary data, or data that were originally collected for a purpose other than the research study. For example, a nurse might conduct a retrospective study to determine differences in the ventilator-associated pneumonia rate between patients who received oral care every 4 hours and those who did not. The diagnosis of ventilator-associated pneumonia and the timing of oral care could both be retrieved from patient charts, a convenient source of reliable data. However, in this case, the nurse researcher is dependent upon the staff nurses' documentation of the timing and extent of oral care. If the chart does not have a record of oral care in a 4-hour period, is it because it was not done or because it was not recorded? If oral care is recorded, was the care rendered according to current standards? The nurse researcher must balance the convenience of secondary data with the risks of inaccuracy and incompleteness.

Prospective studies are those conducted by the researcher. This enables the researcher to control most aspects of research design and implementation, and primary data are collected (that is, data are collected by the researcher for the specific study at hand). As a result, prospective studies are generally more reliable than retrospective studies due to the greater control afforded the researcher. For

Retrospective studies: Studies conducted using data that have already been collected about events that have already happened. Secondary data were originally collected for a purpose other than the current research.

Prospective studies: Studies planned by the researcher for collection of primary data for the specific research and implemented in the future.

example, a nurse might conduct a prospective study of oral care and ventilator-associated pneumonia by experimenting with different time periods, methods, or durations of oral care and measuring the rate of ventilator-associated pneumonia in the study patients. In this case, the procedures could be highly controlled and the outcomes reliably measured and recorded accurately. The study would be difficult to design and carry out, though, involving ethical questions, sampling challenges, and substantial time demands. The accuracy and completeness of data would be at the expense of considerable complexity and effort.

Studies may also be characterized by whether they are conducted over time or at a single point in time. Such studies are referred to as longitudinal or cross-sectional studies.

Longitudinal studies are conducted over time—often very long time periods—to study the emergence of disease or the long-term effects of treatments. Subjects are followed over a period of time with data collection occurring at prescribed intervals over the period. An advantage of longitudinal studies is the capacity to determine the effects of risk factors or interventions over time. A disadvantage is the potential for attrition as subjects are lost to the study over the duration of the study. There may also be effects from the act of repeatedly measuring the same individuals over time. An example of a longitudinal study would be monitoring the children of smokers over time to measure the emergence of pulmonary disease.

Cross-sectional methods focus on collecting data at a single point in time. No follow-up is intended or built into the design. The result is a comprehensive picture of the existence of a phenomenon in the present, without concern for how it will look in the future. Cross-sectional methods often look at a single phenomenon across multiple populations at a single point in time. These methods have the advantage that they are completed in a limited amount of time and may yield valuable information about how different populations respond to the same disease or treatment. The primary disadvantage is that the effects of time are not evaluated and cannot be analyzed. An example of a cross-sectional study would be determining the prevalence and distribution of pulmonary diseases in a sample of children who have a parent smoker in the home at a given point in time.

Longitudinal and cross-sectional studies are frequently used in public health and epidemiology to study the distribution and determinants of disease over time or across populations. These methods can also be used in nursing research to study the effects of risk factors, interventions, or nursing practice changes as they unfold at different times and for different people.

Longitudinal studies: Studies conducted by following subjects over a period of time with data collection occurring at prescribed intervals.
Cross-sectional methods: Studies conducted by looking at a single phenomenon across multiple populations at a single point in time with no intent for follow-up in the design.

Reading Research for Evidence-Based Practice

Although it is relatively easy to categorize research by its approach, type, time dimension, and other distinctions in a research textbook, in reality, these distinctions are not quite so tidy. Reading a research study while trying to classify its characteristics often results in frustration. Just as a research process must be viewed as a fluid process that articulates decisions on a continuum, reading a research study challenges the nurse not to determine whether the right design has been selected, but whether the researcher has made the right choices.

Often, qualitative researchers will make explicit in the introduction of a study their reasoning for a particular design choice. In general, a qualitative study will state that it is a qualitative approach somewhere in the abstract, introduction, or initial methods sections. This is not usually the case with quantitative research. It is often up to the reader to determine the specific decisions the researcher made and to try to deduce the reasoning behind those decisions.

The reader can pick up some hints early in the abstract and the methods section that will provide clues to the time dimension of the study. Comments about the use of "secondary data" or "using data collected for another study" will indicate the study is retrospective. In this case, the critical reader should be looking for evidence that the researchers accounted for the lack of accuracy and specificity that accompanies retrospective studies, or at least acknowledged its existence. Researchers will rarely identify primary data explicitly as such, but the inclusion of an intervention protocol or a measurement procedure indicates that the data were prospectively gathered.

It is usually relatively easy to determine if a study is longitudinal or cross-sectional. The reader can look for measures that were collected repeatedly on the same individuals as a clue that a study is longitudinal. The researcher might use words such as *paired sample*, *dependent data*, or *repeated measures* to indicate that data were collected over time from the same subjects. When it is clear that data were collected once from individuals at a single point in time, then the study is a cross-sectional one.

It is important to categorize the type of study before using it as evidence. The hierarchy of evidence (see Chapter 1) encompasses a variety of research designs, but the connection to the strength of a practice recommendation is based, to a great extent, on the type of study. Listed below are some of the points to appraise when reading a research study to determine whether the authors used the appropriate approach:

- Does the research question match the specific approach that was chosen?
- If an intervention was being tested, was a quantitative approach used?
- If patient preferences and values were being assessed, was a qualitative or mixed method used?
- Does the researcher articulate a rationale for decisions about the research approach?
- Does the author provide logical reasoning for the specific design selected? If not, can it be deduced from the characteristics of the study?

The initial review of a research study for its approach, type, and time dimension is useful in determining the level of evidence that can be attributed to its findings. This ensures that the nurse will use the research results appropriately in supporting evidence-based nursing practice.

Using Research in Evidence-Based Practice

Although it would seem obvious that applied research is the most helpful for evidence-based practice, basic research may also be used. The hierarchy of evidence considers basic research about physiology and pathophysiology to be legitimate considerations, on a par with professional expert opinion and descriptive research. When developing a research-based practice guideline, a good starting place is a basic foundation of the existing knowledge about the physiological and psychological forces that may be in play in a given nurse practice situation.

Both quantitative and qualitative research are useful in evidence-based practice. Although it is clear that randomized controlled trials (experimental designs)—both singularly and in aggregate—provide the strongest evidence for practice, they do not provide the only evidence for practice. Well-designed quasi-experimental, descriptive, correlation, and predictive designs can provide evidence that can be used to determine whether an action can be recommended, optional, or not recommended.

Qualitative and mixed methods are primarily useful in determining the preferences and values of the patient. They may, however, be used to theorize what interventions might be effective, particularly when little research is found or when the subject is one that is behavioral, psychological, or spiritual. Exploratory studies often give rise to theories that subsequently can be tested with quantitative methods, improving on the evidence for practice. The best practice guidelines are those that incorporate a variety of research studies and methods into a single guideline so the needs of patients can be addressed in a comprehensive, evidence-based manner.

For More Depth and Detail

For a more in-depth look at the concepts in this chapter, try these references:

Blegen, M. (2009). Qualitative or quantitative is beside the point. *Nursing Research, 58*(6), 381.

Happ, M. (2009). Mixed methods in gerontological research: Do the qualitative and quantitative data "touch"? *Research in Gerontological Nursing, 2*(2), 122–127.

Hopper, K. (2008). Qualitative and quantitative research: Two cultures. *Psychiatric Services, 59*(7), 71.

Kroll, T., & Morris, J. (2009). Challenges and opportunities in using mixed method designs in rehabilitation research. *Archives of Physical Medicine and Rehabilitation, 90*(11 Suppl 1), S11–S16.

Lipscomb, J. (2008). Mixed method nursing studies: A critical realist critique. *Nursing Philosophy, 9*(1), 32–45.

Nicholls, D. (2009). Qualitative research: Part one—philosophies. *International Journal of Therapy and Rehabilitation, 16*(10), 526–533.

Pluye, P., Gagnon, M., Griffiths, F., & Johnson-Lafleur, J. (2009). A scoring system for appraising mixed methods research. *International Journal of Nursing Studies, 46*(4), 529–546.

Rolfe, G. (2006). Validity, trustworthiness and rigour: Quality and the idea of qualitative research. *Journal of Advanced Nursing, 53*(3), 304–310.

Weaver, K., & Olson, J. (2006). Understanding paradigms for nursing research. *Journal of Advanced Nursing, 53*(4), 459–469.

Creating Evidence for Practice

Given all these approaches, types, and dimensions of research, outlining a specific research study may seem daunting. A systematic approach to making the decisions that are required, however, helps narrow the choices relatively quickly and makes the process a manageable one. Using criteria for each step in the decision-making and design process can help ensure that the right choices are made for the right reasons.

Criteria for Selecting an Approach

The primary consideration for selecting an approach is a match between the problem and the approach chosen to provide a solution. If the question is one that relates to the effectiveness of an intervention, identifies factors that influence a patient's outcome, or finds the best predictors for a patient condition, then clearly a quantitative approach is needed. If the problem is one that requires an in-depth understanding of the patient's experience and the meaning of a phenomenon, then qualitative research is required. Either type of research may be used for exploratory research or for subjects on which there is little existing research. However, a qualitative or descriptive study is often a good way to start an exploration of a phenomenon in which little or no existing literature is available.

A mixed method is best to capture the outcomes of both approaches. Mixed methods are complex, however, and require that the researcher have a command of both quantitative and qualitative skills. It is rare that a mixed method would be used by a novice researcher for a single problem. Mixed methods are often reserved for evaluation of complex issues or for developing and testing models of action and interaction.

A careful self-assessment of personal experiences and abilities will also help the researcher arrive at a feasible study method. Reflection about one's propensity toward quantitative or qualitative methods is time well spent in preparing for a research study. Using a method that is not supported by the researcher's nature can be frustrating and result in poorly executed research. If a researcher knows that a particular approach is difficult for him or her, then he or she may want to join a research team to learn more about the process and to gain the mentorship and support that comes from individuals who are competent and passionate about the approach. A pragmatic self-assessment of available time, software, resources, and competency is also useful before arriving at a conclusion about a study design.

Finally, the nurse researcher should consider the expectations of the audience he or she is trying to reach. That audience may include fellow nurses, healthcare team members, or administrators. The nurse researcher will do well to consider other audiences that must be addressed to communicate the results effectively, such as journal editors, conference attendees, graduate committees, or professors. The needs and interests of these audiences may be as important as those of fellow practitioners to ensure that the research results are communicated broadly enough to be used in practice.

Summary of Key Concepts

- Research is about the search for truth, but there are multiple ways to determine and describe truth. The key to a successful research process is to understand which approach is appropriate for the particular problem to be solved.
- The research process is a fluid, dynamic one that includes multiple processes. These processes may be in sequence or may overlap; some phases even may be skipped. These phases include defining the research problem, scanning the literature, selecting a theoretical framework, determining an appropriate design, defining a sampling strategy, collecting and analyzing data, communicating the findings, and using the findings to support practice.
- Philosophical assumptions drive the fundamental design of a study and are rooted in the paradigms of quantitative or qualitative methods. Quantitative studies employ measurement to produce an objective representation of relationships and effects. Qualitative studies use verbal reports and observations to arrive at an interpretation of the meaning of a phenomenon.
- Mixed methods may involve elements of both quantitative and qualitative research, but the standards for both approaches must be met. Mixed methods are most effective for evaluation research and for developing and testing models of action and interaction.
- A design is chosen based on the nature of the research question and the preferences and skills of the researcher, as well as practical considerations such as access to subjects, software, and other resources.

 CRITICAL APPRAISAL **EXERCISE**

Retrieve the following full text article from the Cumulative Index to Nursing and Allied Health Literature or similar search database:

Thomas, L. (2009). Effective dyspnea management strategies identified by elders with end-stage chronic obstructive pulmonary disease. *Applied Nursing Research, 22*(2), 79–85.

Review the article, focusing on the design of the study. Consider the following appraisal questions in your critical review of this research article:

1. What is the author's rationale for using a mixed method for the study of this subject?
2. Discuss the link between the purpose of the study and this design.
3. Classify this study with respect to each of the following dimensions:
   a. The intent of the researcher
   b. The type of study
   c. The time dimension of the study
4. What characteristics did this study possess that were quantitative in nature?
5. What characteristics did this study possess that were qualitative in nature?
6. Describe the reasons you think a mixed method approach was the most appropriate for this population and research goals.

- Research can be classified by the intent of the researcher. Basic research reflects intent to contribute to the fundamental body of knowledge that is nursing. Applied research reflects the sole intention of providing evidence that can be directly applied to the practice of nursing.
- The nature of research design can be categorized as experimental or nonexperimental. Experimental designs are highly controlled, with a goal of testing cause and effect. Nonexperimental designs can be descriptive, correlation, or predictive. Both types of designs provide evidence for nursing practice, but the recommendations from experimental designs are considered stronger.
- Research can be categorized by its time dimension as retrospective or prospective. Retrospective studies use secondary data that have already been collected. Prospective studies use real-time processes to collect primary data explicitly for the study.
- Studies can also be classified as longitudinal or cross-sectional. Longitudinal studies involve measures on the same subjects over time, whereas cross-sectional studies measure a characteristic from multiple populations at a single point in time.

For a full suite of assignments and additional learning activities, use the access code located in the front of your book to visit this exclusive website: http://go.jblearning .com/houser. If you do not have an access code, you can obtain one at the site.

References

Creswell, J. (2003). *Research design: Qualitative, quantitative, and mixed methods* (2nd ed.). Thousand Oaks, CA: Sage.

Fain, J. (2004). *Reading, understanding, and applying nursing research* (2nd ed.). Philadelphia: F.A. Davis.

Gall, M., Gall, J., & Borg, W. (2007). *Educational research: An introduction* (8th ed.). Boston: Pearson.

Locke, L., Silverman, S., & Spirduso, W. (2004). *Reading and understanding research* (2nd ed.). Thousand Oaks, CA: Sage.

Miller, S., & Fredericks, M. (2006). Mixed-methods and evaluation research: Trends and issues. *Qualitative Health Research, 16*(4), 567–569.

chapter 3

Ethical and Legal Considerations in Research

CHAPTER OBJECTIVES

The study of this chapter will help the learner to

- Describe fundamental ethical concepts applicable to human subjects research.
- Discuss the historical development of ethical issues in research.
- Describe the components of valid informed consent.
- Identify the populations that are considered vulnerable from a research context.
- Discuss statutes and regulations related to conducting clinical research.
- Describe the history, functions, and processes related to the institutional review board.
- Identify the three levels of review conducted by institutional review boards.
- Discuss the major provisions of the privacy rule (HIPAA) that affect data collection for research.

KEY TERMS

A priori	Full review	Nontherapeutic research
Beneficence	HIPAA	Respect for persons
Ethics	Informed consent	Right of privacy
Exempt review	Institutional review board (IRB)	Therapeutic research
Expedited review		Vulnerable populations
Full disclosure	Justice	

Introduction

Ethics: A type of philosophy that studies right and wrong.

Ethics is the study of right and wrong. It explores what one might do when confronted with a situation where values, rights, personal beliefs, or societal norms may be in conflict. In everyday life, we are often faced with ethical situations when we must decide a course of action and ask the question: What is the right thing to do in this particular situation?

Ethical considerations tell us how we should conduct research. There are directives for the ethical conduct of nursing research, and these are applied through personal decision making and guided by the researcher's integrity. Legal guidelines, on the other hand, tell us how we are *required* to conduct research. These guidelines are found in laws and regulations that are provided by agencies external to the nurse researcher. The two are often inextricably intertwined. In the end, it does not matter if an ethical guideline or a legal regulation provides guidance to the nurse researcher: They are equally important for quality research.

Researchers face ethical and legal situations in almost every step of the research process, from selecting participants to data collection to reporting findings at the conclusion of the study. This chapter explores the history of ethical issues in research practice, the development of ethical guidelines for researchers, the elements of an ethical study, and the laws and regulations to consider when conducting research.

Learning from the Past, Protecting the Future

When humans participate as subjects in research studies, care must be taken to preserve their rights: their right to be informed of the study process and potential risks, their right to be treated in a fair and transparent manner, and their right to withdraw from a study at any time for any reason without question or negative consequences (Layman, 2009).

Unfortunately, breaches of ethical conduct have a long history. In the aftermath of World War II, disclosure of Nazi experimentation on prison camp detainees revealed the need for consideration of basic human rights in research involving human subjects. In this country, the revelation of the deception and nontreatment of men of color with syphilis during the Tuskegee syphilis study (1932–1972) and, more recently, the Gelsinger case at the University of Pennsylvania and the Roche case at Johns Hopkins (discussed later in this chapter) demonstrate that ethical breaches are not solely of historical interest. Research that involves human subjects requires careful consideration of the rights of those subjects.

Although the primary investigators for these research activities were physicians, evidence suggests that nurses were aware of deceit in participant recruitment and delivery of nontherapeutic treatment, at least within the Tuskegee syphilis study. Why are these events historically important to nurses? Reflection and careful thought about the roles of nurses in research—from data collector to principal investigator—and the responsibility nurses have to humankind mandate that we learn from the past and, in doing so, protect the future.

❝ *Voices from the Field* ❯❯

As soon as I identify an idea for a research project, I start thinking about the legal implications of this study or how this study will look in the eyes of our institutional review board (IRB). When I was a novice researcher, the IRB seemed like a big hurdle to overcome. Now that I am an experienced researcher, I view it as a significant asset to the research process.

The IRB is made up of a wide variety of professionals who evaluate a study from their area of expertise. There is a lot of research experience on the IRB. They pay particular attention to the risks and benefits of each study, and it is clear their focus is on protecting the rights of subjects. But they can also give you excellent advice and suggestions to make your study stronger and ensure it is ethical. They also give good feedback about the soundness of the overall study design and ability of the study team to perform this particular research.

This became very clear to me when I had to consider the legal implications of a recent study that I helped design. The study itself seemed quite benign. The research question was, "Do two 15-minute foot massages done on two consecutive days decrease anxiety in inpatient cancer patients?" We chose to answer this question using a randomized controlled trial (RCT) study design. The two co-primary investigators (PIs) were bedside nurses on our inpatient cancer unit who cared deeply about their patients and wanted to do a study that would help lessen the stress of being hospitalized. The study team included an oncologist who was also the chief of Oncology Services, several clinical nurse specialists, the unit director, an experienced massage therapist, and me in my role as medical epidemiologist and nurse researcher. As a team we designed a study that we felt adequately addressed our study question.

The IRB saw it differently. They were concerned that we had not adequately addressed the risks of a foot massage; although rare, they still needed to be expressed in both the protocol and consent. We needed to inform potential subjects that there was a risk of dislodging a clot, causing severe pain or discomfort, or irritating or damaging the skin. Further, the board suggested that our control group (no massage) would be a better comparison group if we offered some type of therapeutic nurse interaction for the same amount of time as our foot massage. This would help overcome any placebo effect from the treatment. They had concerns about our measurement tools and our enrollment methods as well. Our simple little study suddenly wasn't so simple—and we had to admit their suggested changes would improve the study in a lot of ways.

So, instead of becoming discouraged, we took the IRB's recommendations and began to redesign our study. We realized we needed to better communicate how we had identified and addressed risks in our IRB documents, so we rewrote our consent form. We asked for advice from a variety of sources and wrote a better protocol that included a comparison therapy. We identified a stronger instrument and cleaned up our sampling procedure. In retrospect, I'm relieved we were stopped when we were—we honestly hadn't considered the risks carefully enough, and the IRB made us do that.

In retrospect, we should have asked for feedback from clinical and scientific colleagues outside of our team before submitting our project for IRB review. Lessons learned. Even though it was small and seemingly benign, we needed to be more aware of the risks involved.

Joanna Bokovoy, RN, DrPH

Medical Epidemiologist

Ethical Issues: A Historical Overview

The ethics of human subjects research and federal control have evolved since the mid-twentieth century. Professional organizations and international associations alike have developed codes of ethics that apply to research involving human subjects. In this chapter, the ethical foundation of research is examined, considering both recent and remote examples of scientific transgressions that helped form current research practices. What society has legislatively imposed in the context of research regulation also is discussed.

Nazi Medical Experimentation

From 1933 until 1945 and the liberation of the death camps in Europe, atrocities were inflicted on concentration camp detainees in the name of science. Adhering to a goal of the Third Reich in Europe, the Nazis conducted medical experiments to produce a race of pure Aryans who would rule the world.

Under the guise of benefiting soldiers of the Third Reich, Nazi physicians carried out experiments to test the limits of human endurance. For example, prisoners were submerged for days at a time in a tank of cold water. The goal was to test how long German pilots, who had to parachute into the cold North Sea, would survive. Different types of clothing were tested, as well as different methods for resuscitating the experimental subjects who survived. Other prisoners were burned with phosphorus to track wound healing. Surgery was performed without anesthesia to gauge pain levels; in-utero surgery was carried out to determine fetal growth and development during stages of pregnancy, and surgical gender changes were accomplished. Many of the subjects in these experiments did not survive.

These experiments were not randomly carried out by only a few scientists; they were regarded as fulfillment of governmental policy in support of the war effort. These atrocities in the name of scientific experimentation made clear that international oversight of the rights of human subjects in research was necessary.

The Tuskegee Study

It is tempting to consider the Nazi studies to be examples of outrageous acts that could not occur in our society. Unfortunately, the U.S. Public Health Service has its own record of egregious treatment of experimental subjects. A study undertaken in 1932 by the Public Health Service set out to determine the natural history of syphilis. Called the

"Tuskegee Study of Untreated Syphilis in the Negro Male," the study initially involved 600 black men—399 with syphilis and 201 without. The study was conducted without informed consent. While the subjects were led to believe they were being treated for a blood disorder, in reality the progress of their syphilis was allowed to unfold without treatment. Although originally projected to last 6 months, the study went on for 40 years. In 1972, a news story about the study caused a public outcry that led the government to appoint an ad hoc advisory panel to investigate the study. The panel concluded that the Tuskegee Study was "ethically unjustified" and ordered reparations for the men and their families (CDC, 2011).

As a result of these violations of basic human rights both international and national guidelines for the ethical treatment of research subjects were developed.

International Guides for the Researcher

Two major international codes and reports guide researchers in carrying out ethical research. They are the Nuremberg Code and the Declaration of Helsinki.

The Nuremberg war crimes trials, which were held from 1945 to 1947, were focused on crimes against humanity. They were presided over by judges from the four Allied powers—the United States, Great Britain, France, and the Soviet Union. The city of Nuremberg was purposely chosen for the trials because, after 11 Allied air strikes during the war, the city was declared 90 percent dead. During the trials, a large-scale prosecution of Nazi officials took place, many of whom pleaded a defense that they were following their superiors' orders. Their crimes included inhumane acts on civilians, initiating and waging aggressive acts of war, murder, near extermination of a race, slavery, ill treatment of prisoners, plunder, and destruction.

As a result, the Nuremberg Code was developed in 1949. This code contained guidelines requiring voluntary, informed consent to participate in medical experimentation. It further specified that the research must serve a worthy purpose, that the desired knowledge was unobtainable by other means, and that the anticipated result justified the performance of the experiment. All unnecessary physical and mental suffering was to be avoided. A little-known fact is that the Nuremberg Code led to the notion of substituting animal experimentation in advance of or in lieu of human experimentation.

The Nuremberg Code further guaranteed that no experiments are to be permitted when death or disability is an expected outcome, "except, perhaps, in those experiments where the experimental physicians also serve as subjects." Risks were to be commensurate with the importance of the problem, and human subjects were to be protected from even a remote possibility of harm. Experiments were to be conducted only by properly qualified scientists, and the subject had the right to stop the experiment at any time. Further, the scientist in charge was obligated to stop the experiment if injury, disability, or death was

gray matter

The Nuremberg Code, developed in 1949, contains research guidelines stipulating that

- Consent is voluntary and informed for subjects who participate in medical experimentation.
- The research serves a worthy purpose.
- Knowledge gained is unobtainable by any other means.
- Anticipated results justify performance of the experiment.
- Unnecessary physical and mental suffering or harm is avoided.
- Death or disability is not an expected outcome.
- Properly qualified scientists conduct the experiments.

Therapeutic research: Studies in which the subject can be expected to receive a potentially beneficial treatment. **Nontherapeutic research:** Studies that are carried out for the purpose of generating knowledge. They are not expected to benefit the research subject, but may lead to improved treatment in the future.

likely to result. The code may be viewed online at http://ohsr.od.nih.gov/guidelines/nuremberg.html.

From an extension of the Nuremberg Code came the Declaration of Helsinki, adopted in 1964 by the World Medical Association and amended and updated most recently in 2008. The Declaration of Helsinki expanded the principles of the Nuremberg Code to differentiate therapeutic research from nontherapeutic research. Therapeutic research is expected to confer on the study subject an opportunity to receive a treatment that might be beneficial. Nontherapeutic research is carried out for the purpose of generating knowledge and is not expected to benefit the study subject, but it might lead to improved treatment in the future.

Similar to the Nuremberg Code, the Declaration of Helsinki requires informed consent for ethical research, while allowing for surrogate consent when the prospective research subject is incompetent, physically or mentally incapable of providing consent, or a minor. Furthermore, the Declaration of Helsinki states that research within these groups should be conducted only when this research is necessary to promote the health of the representative group and when this research cannot otherwise be performed on competent persons. For more information on the declaration, visit http://ohsr.od.nih.gov/guidelines/helsinki.html.

National Guidelines for the Nurse Researcher

In 1974, Congress passed the National Research Act, which resulted in the formation of the National Commission for the Protection of Human Subjects of Biomedical and Behavioral Research. Members of the national commission wrote the Ethical Principles and Guidelines for the Protection of Human Subjects of Research (commonly known as the Belmont Report). The Belmont Report was published in 1978 and has become the cornerstone statement of ethical principles on which regulations for protection of human subjects are based (U.S. Department of Health, Education, and Welfare [HEW], 1979).

The Belmont Report (which can be viewed online at http://ohsr.od.nih.gov/guidelines/belmont.html) begins by stating, "Scientific research has produced substantial social benefits. It has also posed some troubling ethical questions. Public attention was drawn to these questions by reported abuses of human subjects in biomedical experiments . . ." (HEW, 1979, p. 1). As a result, state and national regulations, as well as international and professional codes, have been developed to guide researchers. These rules are based on broader ethical principles that provide a framework to evaluate investigators' judgment when designing and carrying out their research. Three foundational ethical principles relevant to the ethics of human subjects are described in the Belmont Report. These basic principles are respect for persons, beneficence, and justice.

Respect for persons: A basic principle of ethics stating that individuals should be treated autonomously, as capable of making their own decisions. Persons with limited autonomy or who are not capable of making their own decisions should be protected.

Respect for Persons

Respect for persons, the first principle, incorporates two ethical convictions: that individuals should be treated autonomously, capable of making their own decisions, and that persons with diminished autonomy or those not capable of making their own decisions should be protected. The extent of protection to those incapable of self-determination will depend on the risks, harms, and benefits of the study. The principle of respect for persons thus divides into two separate moral requirements: the requirement to acknowledge a person's autonomy and the requirement to protect those with diminished autonomy.

Persons with diminished autonomy sometimes are regarded as vulnerable or as a member of a vulnerable population. These are groups that may contain some individuals who possess limited autonomy (that is, they cannot fully participate in the consent process). Such groups may include children, individuals with dementia and other cognitive disorders, prisoners, and pregnant women. Some ethicists regard older persons, terminally ill persons, and other hospitalized persons, as well as those who are homeless, students, or transgender, as deserving of special consideration by researchers.

> **Vulnerable populations:** Groups of people with diminished autonomy who cannot participate fully in the consent process. Such groups may include children, individuals with cognitive disorders, prisoners, and pregnant women.

Special consideration for research studies that may include vulnerable populations involve ensuring the following:

- The risks of participating would be acceptable to volunteers in the general public.
- Selection of subjects is fair and unbiased.
- The written consent form is understandable given the subject's expected level of function and comprehension.
- Adequate follow-up is provided (Mehlman and Berg, 2008).

Beneficence

One of the most fundamental ethical principles in research is beneficence or "do no harm." According to the Belmont Report, "Persons are treated in an ethical manner not only by respecting their decisions and protecting them from harm, but also by making efforts to secure their well-being. Two general rules have been formulated as complementary expressions of beneficent actions (1) do no harm and (2) maximize possible benefits and minimize possible harms" (HEW, 1979, §B.2).

> **Beneficence:** A basic principle of ethics that states that persons should have their decisions respected, be protected from harm, and have steps taken to ensure their well-being.

Human subjects can be harmed in a variety of ways, including physical harm (e.g., injury), psychological harm (e.g., worry, stress, and fear), social harm (e.g., loss of friends or one's place in society), and economic harm (e.g., loss of employment). Researchers must strive to minimize harm and to achieve the best possible balance between the benefits to be gained from participation and the risks of being a participant.

The Belmont Report tells us that the assessment of the risks and benefits of a study presents an opportunity to gather comprehensive information about the proposed research. The investigator strives to design a study that will answer a meaningful question. A review committee will determine whether risks inherent in participation are justified. Prospective subjects will make an assessment, based on their understanding of risks and benefits, as to whether to participate in the study.

> **gray matter**
>
> During research, human subjects can suffer harm in the following ways:
> - Physically (injury)
> - Psychologically (worry, stress, or fear)
> - Socially (loss of friends or place in society)
> - Economically (loss of employment)

Table 3.1

Ethical Principles and Research Design

This Ethical Principle	Is Managed with This Design Principle
Respect for persons	Informed consent process
	Subject selection process
	Adequacy of follow-up systems
Beneficence	Assessment of risk and benefit
Justice	Subject selection process

Justice

Justice: A basic principle of ethics that incorporates a participant's right to fair treatment and fairness in distribution of benefit and burden.

The third broad principle found in the Belmont Report is justice. The principle of justice incorporates participants' right to fair treatment and fairness in distribution of benefit and burden. According to the report, an injustice would occur when a benefit to which a person is entitled is denied or when some burden is unduly imposed. For example, the selection of research subjects needs to be closely scrutinized to determine whether some subjects (for example, welfare patients, racial and ethnic minorities, or persons confined to institutions) are being systematically selected because of their easy accessibility or because of their compromised position. The application of justice also requires that research should not unduly involve persons from groups unlikely to be beneficiaries of the results of the research. However, members of diverse groups also should be included, and not excluded, without a prior knowledge of their suitability to participate.

Certain diverse groups, such as minorities, the economically disadvantaged, the homeless, the very sick, and those persons who have a compromised ability to provide consent, should be protected against the danger of being recruited for a study solely for the researcher's convenience. In short, this means that researchers may not use underprivileged persons to benefit those who are privileged. Table 3.1 links the ethical principles to the elements of research design.

The ethical nurse researcher considers all these principles as a research study is designed and carried out. The failure to identify and resolve ethical issues can place both the conduct and the results of a research study in jeopardy (Oberle, 2006).

The Ethical Researcher

Bad behavior in the name of science has given rise to the need for laws, regulations, and safeguards. The public's perception of research, its benefits, and its risks is shaped by the way research is conducted and by the way results are reported. Researchers, then, should abide by the ethical guidelines cited in the Nuremberg Code, the Belmont Report, and the Helsinki Declaration. Additionally, there are other guidelines specific to research funded by the federal government or foundations. These groups use guidelines to uphold the public's confidence in research and its contribution to knowledge for the greater good. These guidelines state that the ethical researcher should

- Adhere to principles of beneficence by doing no harm, maximizing benefits, and minimizing possible harms
- Respect the autonomy of the participants in the consent process
- Employ the principle of justice in subject selection
- Explain the research procedures to the participants
- Obtain proper and informed consent
- Ensure the confidentiality of participants
- Maintain appropriate documentation of the research process
- Adhere to research protocols
- Report results in a fair and factual manner (National Academy of Sciences, 1995)

One way to ensure that the study meets these criteria is to select the most appropriate participants for the study. They must also understand their role in the research. Most important in this process is for the researcher to secure the participants' informed consent.

Informed Consent

Informed consent is more than a form or a signature; it is a process of information exchange that includes recruitment materials, verbal dialogue, presentation of written materials, questions and answers, and an agreement that is documented by a signature. According to the Belmont Report, the consent process contains three components: information, comprehension, and voluntariness. Participants should be able to ask questions, understand the risks and benefits, and be assured that if they choose to participate they may withdraw at any time without consequences.

To judge how much information should be disclosed to a prospective subject, the "reasonable subject" standard should be used. This standard requires that the extent and nature of the information provided be sufficient for a reasonable person to decide whether or not to participate (Mayo & Wallhagen, 2009).

> **Informed consent:** A process of information exchange in which participants are provided understandable information needed to make a participation decision, full disclosure of the risks and benefits, and the assurance that withdrawal is possible at any time without consequences. This process begins with recruitment and ends with a signed agreement document.

Organization of the Informed Consent

Prospective subjects who are fully informed about the nature of the research and its associated risks and benefits are positioned to make an educated decision on whether to participate. Essential content for informed consent in research can be found in the U.S. Department of Health and Human Services Code of Federal Regulations (CFR 45, Part 46.106). Accordingly, it is useful to remember that these guidelines emanated from the Nuremberg Code. Information that is essential for informed consent can be found in Table 3.2.

Deception or Incomplete Disclosure

When explaining the research procedures to the prospective subject, the researcher must explain all the information that is known about risks and benefits. The subject needs

---

Table 3.2

Elements of the Informed Consent Form

- Title of study and name(s) of investigator(s)
- Introduction and invitation to participate
- Basis for selection
- Explanation of study purpose and procedures
- Duration of participation
- Reasonably foreseeable risks/unforeseen risks
- Benefits of participation/cost of participation
- Appropriate alternatives to participation
- Voluntary withdrawal from study
- Payments/compensation
- Confidentiality of records
- Contact person
- Funding statement/conflict of interest statement
- Statement of voluntary participation
- Signature lines

Full disclosure: Reporting as much information about the research as is known at the time without threatening the validity of the study. This allows the subject to make an informed decision as to whether to participate.

to know if the treatment, drug, or procedure used in the study is not necessary for his or her care and that it may have outcomes that are questionable or not completely understood. Full disclosure, or reporting as much information as is known at the time, is crucial so the participant can make an informed decision as to whether to participate.

Some participants may not be informed of some aspects of the research because it likely impairs the validity of the research. This threat to validity—called the Hawthorne effect, treatment effects, or placebo effects—may lead subjects to behave differently simply because they are being treated. This might happen in a study involving experimental drugs or complementary therapies. Balancing the expectations of participants for the care they will receive with the purpose of the research may be challenging (Kapp, 2007). This is most often addressed by using vague, rather than deceptive, language. However, incomplete disclosure is generally allowable under three circumstances:

1. The incomplete disclosure is necessary for the goals of the research.
2. The undisclosed risks are minimal.
3. There is a plan to debrief the subjects and discuss the results with the participants as soon as results are apparent.

Incomplete disclosure should never be used to enroll participants in a study or to elicit cooperation and participation from reluctant subjects by masking or minimizing potential risks.

Table 3.3

Ethical Responsibilities of a Nurse Researcher

- To respect individuals' autonomy in consenting to participate in research
- To protect those prospective subjects for whom decisional capacity is limited
- To minimize potential harm and to maximize possible benefits for all subjects enrolled
- To ensure that benefits and burdens associated with the research protocol are distributed equally when identifying prospective subjects
- To protect privacy, to ensure confidentiality, and to guarantee anonymity when promised
- To notify institutional officials of breaches of research protocols and incidents of scientific misconduct
- To maintain competence in one's identified area of research
- To maintain proficiency in research methods

Comprehension

Because a person's informed consent to participate is based on his or her understanding of benefits and risks, in addition to the overall importance of the area under study, the researcher acts as a communicator and evaluator when ensuring that the prospective subject understands the intent of the study. When developing the informed consent form, the investigator may use institutional boilerplate templates to communicate all necessary information in an organized fashion. It is important to avoid the use of healthcare jargon and technical terms and to use simple language. For participants from a general population (for example, hospitalized patients), the wording of the consent form should be at the seventh- or eighth-grade level. Readability formulas, based on length of sentences and number of syllables per word, can be found in Microsoft Word. These formulas are based on the Flesch Reading Ease Score developed in the 1940s and the Flesch-Kincaid Grade Level score developed for educational purposes in the 1970s (Flesch, 1948; Kincaid et al., 1975).

Ethical Practices in Human Subject Research

Relatively recent events have renewed societal concerns about ethical practice in research and the responsibilities of researchers for subject welfare. The following three cases demonstrate tragedies experienced by subjects in research.

Case #1: Jesse Gelsinger

Gene therapy is viewed as having the potential to produce highly impressive advances in medical treatment. In 1992, an investigator with an excellent reputation as a genetic researcher founded a company with the intent to commercialize successful gene therapies. Corporate investors contributed millions of dollars to the company. Following the establishment of the business venture, the investigator designed a clinical trial in which a genetically engineered cold virus was used to deliver genes to correct a genetic liver disorder. This virus had been tested in animals, but not yet in humans, prior to the beginning of this trial. The investigator's original proposal involved testing this gene therapy on terminally ill newborns, but this plan was rejected by the institutional bioethicist. Following this setback, the investigator modified the proposed research protocol and decided to test the gene therapy on stable patients with the previously identified genetic liver disorder. Institutional approval was provided in 1995, and the trial commenced at multiple study sites. In 1999, Jesse Gelsinger, an 18-year-old subject who had the genetic liver disorder, but was asymptomatic and living a normal life, was enrolled in this gene therapy clinical trial at the University of Pennsylvania.

At the same time, researchers from other study sites began to contact the investigator expressing concern about the safety of the use of the cold virus. The trial continued, and Jesse Gelsinger, the next to last patient enrolled in the clinical trial, received a dose that was 300 times the dose received by the first patient. Gelsinger died from a massive immune system response to the gene therapy. The Food and Drug Administration (FDA) immediately shut down all gene therapy research at the University of Pennsylvania. After Gelsinger's death, 921 adverse events in this and other gene therapy trials were reported to the FDA and to the National Institutes of Health (NIH) (Stolberg, 1999).

Questions Raised by the Death of Jesse Gelsinger
- Should high-risk research be conducted on "healthy, stable" persons?
- Was this particular research protocol ready for human trials?
- Were adverse events ignored? Misinterpreted? Apparent only in retrospect?
- Did a financial conflict of interest (the investigator owned the gene therapy company) bias the researcher's judgment?

Case #2: Ellen Roche

In April 2001, Ellen Roche, a healthy 24-year-old laboratory employee at Johns Hopkins Asthma and Allergy Center, was recruited as a normal volunteer to participate in an NIH-funded research study at her workplace. The aim of this study was to determine factors leading to airway irritation in asthma patients. The protocol required the use of inhaled hexamethonium to induce asthma-like effects. The pulmonary toxicity associated with oral, intramuscular, and/or subcutaneous hexamethonium administration for hypertension was first reported in 1953. Between that time and 1960, 11 articles that included individual case reports and a small series of autopsied cases were published. In 1970, a review article on the use of hexamethonium listed six references from the 1950s.

Johns Hopkins used a stronger concentration of hexamethonium than that used in the case reports from the 1950s and 1960s. The first volunteer developed a cough; the second volunteer experienced no ill effects. Roche, the third volunteer, developed irreversible lung damage after receiving 1 gram of hexamethonium by inhalation, and died approximately 1 month later. While Ellen Roche lay in the ICU, the trial continued, with six additional volunteers enrolled. However, none of these six volunteers reached the point in the protocol when hexamethonium would be inhaled. The study was stopped when Roche died. Later, it was found that this specific study had not been part of the original grant application to NIH, but it was mentioned as a planned study in continuation applications (requests for additional funding and extension of time for carrying out the research) in 1999 and 2000. A representative from NIH stated that the hexamethonium study was felt to be consistent with the original goals of the funded primary study and, thus, was not otherwise scientifically reviewed (Becker & Levy, 2001).

Questions Raised by the Death of Ellen Roche

- Why had the research team failed to find published manuscripts from the 1950s and 1970s that reported lung toxicity associated with the use of hexamethonium?
- Did the investigator(s) have sufficient experience with the agent?
- Did the institutional review board (IRB) do a thorough review of this study protocol?
- Was there any coercion involved in enrolling a subject who was an employee of the Asthma and Allergy Center?

Case #3: Nicole Wan

Nicole Wan was a 19-year-old sophomore pre-med student at the University of Rochester in 1996 when she volunteered for a study on the effects of environmental air quality. This pollution research project was funded by a Massachusetts Institute of Technology (MIT) grant from the National Institute of Environmental Health Sciences (NIEHS). Nicole Wan was one of 200 participants enrolled in an arm of the study at the University of Rochester Medical Center. Participants were paid $150 to undergo a bronchoscopy to examine and collect lung cells. A medical resident, who was functioning in the role of investigator, administered aerosolized lidocaine, a local anesthetic, to prevent Nicole from gagging and to allow for easier passage of the bronchoscope into the patient's lower airway. Because Nicole had discomfort during placement of the bronchoscope, additional lidocaine spray was administered. After completion of the study protocol, Nicole left the medical center and went to a friend's apartment, where she suffered a cardiac arrest 3 hours later. Although she was resuscitated by emergency personnel and admitted to an ICU at the medical center, she suffered irreversible pulmonary and neurological damage and died 2 days later. The county medical examiner ruled Nicole's death an accident due to acute lung toxicity. On autopsy, her serum levels of lidocaine were found to be four times the maximum levels (McGuire, 1996).

Questions Raised by the Death of Nicole Wan

- Is participation in a clinical trial appropriate for a 19-year-old college student? Should parents be notified?
- What is the "age of reason" for participation in a clinical trial that may carry risk?
- Why did a medical resident, rather than the principal investigator, administer the study protocol?
- Did the investigators fully explain the risks and benefits to study subjects?

These cases illustrate that ethical issues are not limited to historical settings. These and other examples make it imperative that the nurse researcher carefully consider all ethical concerns—and the potential for harm to subjects—in design and implementation of a study.

Research Integrity

These cases and numerous others point to the importance of conducting all types of research, but particularly those involving human subjects, under strict ethical guidelines. Research integrity involves more than meeting basic ethical principles for the treatment of human subjects. The researcher's work must demonstrate integrity in all phases of the research process—from design to analysis through reporting and follow-up.

A priori: Conceived or formulated before an investigation.

A well-designed study may be ethical by plan but manipulated during implementation. For this reason, most analysis decisions should be made *a priori*, meaning before data have been collected. Otherwise, it may be possible to manipulate the data to mislead the reader or to selectively report findings that are supportive of the researcher's point of view. This manipulation of data can be accomplished in statistical analysis by changing the significance level or making erroneous assumptions to make the results seem more conclusive. Data in graphs can be manipulated by changing the distance between the values on the axes to make the results appear more significant than they are. **FIGURE 3.1** demonstrates how the same data may be presented two different ways to mislead the reader. In these examples, the vertical axis and the legend on the charts have been altered to make it appear as if one hospital is making more money when, in fact, they have identical revenue figures.

Completing a training course in research protocol is one of the best ways to ensure that research is conducted under the most ethical guidelines. The National Institutes of Health requires ethics training for anyone involved with NIH grants or anyone who conducts research in NIH facilities. A few of the areas typically covered in this type of training include data acquisition and management, publication practices, research misconduct, and responsible authorship. Those new to the research process should par-

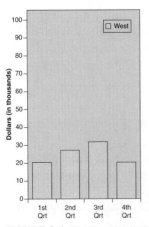
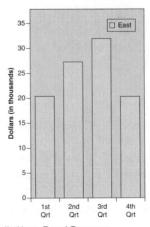

FIGURE 3.1 The Two Hospitals Actually Have Equal Revenue

ticipate in some type of training on the responsible conduct of research, whether or not the study is federally sponsored.

Legal and Regulatory Guidelines for Conducting Research

There is a strong link between ethics and law. It is much like a continuum. Obeying the law (the minimum standard) is at one end of the continuum, and acting ethically (above the expected minimum behavior) is at the opposite end. This duality of law and ethics also exists in research. The nurse researcher can think of the law as a minimum standard and ethics as a higher standard. Law can also be thought of as conflict resolution. Although most people do the right thing ethically, if they do not, the law is there to resolve the situation. The good researcher maximizes both the legal and ethical protections afforded to subjects in a study.

Brief Overview of Laws Related to Research

The four sources of law that may affect researchers are common law, administrative law, statutory law, and tort law. *Common law* is derived from judicial decisions made during a trial (case law) and often applies rules from early English common law. Medical malpractice lawsuits are an example of common law. *Administrative law* is formulated by the federal and state governments and other regulatory agencies and obtains its authority from Congress. An example of administrative law is the Health Insurance Portability and Accountability Act (HIPAA), which is a federal regulation governing the patient's right to privacy and confidentiality. Most laws that affect the clinical researcher are statutes or statutory laws. *Statutory laws* are enacted, amended, and repealed by the legislature.

A fourth category of legal issues has its roots in tort law. Torts are civil wrongs committed against individuals or their property. Examples of tort law include negligence, malpractice, assault, battery, false imprisonment, invasion of privacy, and invoking mental or emotional distress. Although these last allegations are unlikely in a clinical research project, they can happen and may subsequently motivate a malpractice claim. Most claims are brought when a subject believes he or she has been harmed due to negligence on the part of the researcher. Examples of negligence in clinical research include using an instrument known to be defective, using equipment that is not functioning properly, denying a patient reasonable treatment in order to obtain a control group, or not following a specified research protocol so that a patient's safety is compromised. All these circumstances may cause injury to the participant and result in a claim of negligence.

A researcher could be accused of defamation (a false and harmful oral statement) or libel (a false and harmful published statement) as a result of the way he or she presents information in the written account of the research. Truthful researchers need not fear either; both require the intent to distribute information that is known to be incorrect. Reporting the truth is the best defense against accusations of defamation and libel. To further protect the legal rights of subjects, the researcher should guard against referring to individuals' identity in

gray matter

Four categories of law
- Common
- Administrative
- Statutory
- Tort

any written research reports. Subjects should be described in terms so that an individual subject will not recognize him- or herself in the research. Patients often protest being referred to as "schizophrenic, obese, chronically ill," so it is best to use general terms when referring to subjects and to mask any individual descriptors.

The researcher must also guard against inflicting mental or emotional distress. In a research design that involves sensitive topics, the participant may experience painful emotions such as grief, despair, or shame. Most research protocols, therefore, include in the consent form statements such as "potential emotional distress may occur as a result of this research" so that the subject may make a fully informed decision about participation.

The right of privacy is the right to be left alone. Patients and research participants have a right to the confidentiality of their health records and the release of that information only to those whom they have authorized. The right to privacy covers the right both to physical privacy of the person's body and to the privacy of one's health information.

Privacy is also about human dignity and the privacy of one's own person. Accusations of invasion of privacy have been brought against personnel for uncovering patients' bodies unnecessarily or performing examinations in front of others. Data collectors may leave doors and privacy curtains open, exposing the patient to the stares of others and personal embarrassment. This may be particularly problematic when the research protocol calls for multiple data collectors to check inter-rater reliability.

Right of privacy: A person's right to have his or her health information kept confidential and released only to authorized individuals and his or her body shielded from public view.

Invasion of privacy may also involve the written word. Patients have a right to privacy of health information throughout the research process, whether they disclose it verbally or it is retrieved from an electronic or written record. In the field of clinical research, breaches of this right invoke HIPAA. In cases of breaches of confidentiality or invasion of privacy, the patient or participant need not prove damages, making it easier for the patient or subject to initiate a lawsuit.

To avoid accusations of discrimination in the population under study, researchers must be careful when choosing the populations to exclude from the research. Valid reasons to exclude a particular population, such as pregnant women, certain age groups, or certain diagnoses, must be specifically documented. These exclusion criteria are necessary both for good design and to ensure that subjects are selected without bias. Proper selection of the research population is a primary consideration when researchers are studying potentially life-saving treatments.

The key to avoiding any of these accusations is the accurate documentation of all research steps in addition to following the ethical principles discussed earlier in this chapter. Following these guidelines will minimize the threat of any legal action by a research participant and reassure the researcher that he or she is doing the right thing.

Legal Issues Surrounding Informed Consent

Signing a consent to participate in research carries the same purpose and value as does the consent for treatment signed by patients in healthcare facilities. Requirements governing what should be included on an informed consent form are the same for legal

Table 3.4

Participant Authorization for Release of Information

Full Name: _____ Record Identifier: _____
Date of Birth: _____
Address:_____
City, State, Zip
Code: _____
Other Contact
Information: _____

Select One Option Below:
1. _____ I authorize the following person(s) or agencies access to my personal health
   information for a period not to exceed 90 days from the date of signature below.
2. _____ I decline authorization for any and all requests for release of my personal health
   information.

_____   _____
     Patient/Participant/Date   Researcher/Agency/Date

purposes and for ethical purposes. However, legal issues are raised about who can provide consent for participation in a research study. If the individual cannot legally consent to participating in the research (for example, the individual is a minor, has been judged incompetent, or is a member of a vulnerable population), the researcher must ensure that the person's interests are protected. Consent must be obtained from the subject, if possible, as well as from the legal guardian. In some cases, formal consent is obtained from the legal guardian, and simultaneously assent is provided by the participant. For example, a child should agree that he or she is willing to participate in a study (assent) even though the legal consent is required from the parents.

If the research involves human subject participation, in addition to consent, the researcher should obtain an authorization that allows the researcher access to the participant's medical information. This authorization for access to medical information may be incorporated into the consent form. **Table 3.4** provides an example of an authorization for release of information.

Research that involves human subjects in some way—as opposed to retrieving data from records or databases—requires a higher level of oversight. This oversight is provided by legal entities that also are charged with maintaining ethical standards in research. These entities, called institutional review boards (IRBs), are required by law in any organization that allows the conduct of research involving people.

> **Institutional review board (IRB):** The board required in research institutions that reviews and oversees all research involving human subjects and ensures studies meet all federal regulation criteria, including ethical standards.

Institutional Review Boards

The National Commission for the Protection of Human Subjects of Biomedical and Behavioral Research was established in 1974. This commission advised the U.S. Department of Health and Human Services on policies related to research. The commission was instrumental in the adoption of the recommendations of the Belmont Report of 1978.

The U.S. Department of Health and Human Services then developed new regulations governing research and human subjects of research under the Code of Federal Regulations (CFR). These new regulations called for the creation of institutional review boards (IRBs), also known as human subjects committees, as safeguards against the inhumane treatment of individuals that had, in the past, been inflicted in the name of science. Part 46 of CFR 45 requires that any research conducted on human subjects be approved by an IRB. According to requirements in Part 46, the mission of the IRB is "to ensure that research is ethically acceptable and that the welfare and rights of research participants are protected."

The federal regulations dictate the composition of the IRB. It must have at least five members with varied backgrounds to be able to review research activities commonly conducted in the facility. The members should be qualified through experience and education and reflect an appropriate mix of diversity including age, race, and gender. Each IRB committee should include one member with experience in scientific areas, one member with experience in nonscientific areas, and one member not affiliated with the institution where the research is conducted. Most organizations that conduct healthcare research have at least a physician, nurse, research expert, and community member on the IRB. In some instances, the IRB may include or invite nonvoting consultative members with specific competence in an area deemed necessary to make a decision about a particular study or a study of a complex nature.

The Review Process

Research studies that involve human subjects must be reviewed by the IRB. After the researcher has outlined the proposal and data collection methods in detail, the final step before beginning the research is to gain the necessary approvals at the organizations that will either sponsor the research or give access to subjects. Organizational access must be granted by the appropriate administrative group to recruit subjects. The IRB helps the researcher determine if there is a potential for a legal or ethical breach and ensures safeguards are in place to avoid it. The IRB is also the organization's assurance that basic quality, ethical, and legal requirements have been met by the research study as proposed. Approvals for all research are granted by the facility's IRB or, in some cases, a privacy committee.

The size of the organization may dictate the level of the review process, but in most cases, an IRB submission is mandatory, particularly if human subjects are used and if the research is intended for publication.

There are three categories of research review by an IRB:

1. Exempt review
2. Expedited review
3. Full review

An exempt review covers proposals that do not require review by the IRB. (The IRB determines whether a study is exempt; this is not the researcher's decision.) This category is limited to studies that pose no risk for the subjects. It is common when the researcher employs surveys, noninvasive procedures, secondary data or documents, or other methods where it would be impossible to identify any research subject individually. To be exempt from IRB review, the proposed study must meet a number of criteria. FIGURE 3.2 depicts a checklist used by the IRB at one hospital system to determine whether a project is exempt. The exemption only refers to the fact that the IRB does not need to review the study proposal; it does not exempt the researcher from the same ethical principles that govern all research.

Expedited review is used for research that poses only minimal risk to the participants or for those studies that use drugs that do not require Federal Drug Administration (FDA) approval. Minimal risk means that the probability and/or magnitude of discomfort anticipated in the research is not greater than what is ordinarily encountered in daily life. It may also be considered no more risky than what would be encountered during the performance of routine physical or psychological examinations or tests. Expedited review research studies are usually reviewed by one or two members of the IRB who may consult with others as necessary.

A full review is used for all research that poses more than minimal risk to the subjects and for research that does not qualify for exempt status. These studies are reviewed by the full committee with particular attention to the methods, consent process, and selection of the subjects. Studies that require direct access to participants, use personally identifiable medical information, and involve more than minimal risk are subject to full review by the committee. Additional review by a privacy board may be required if personal health information (PHI) is needed for the study. This committee may or may not be part of an IRB and will determine whether patient authorization is required, a disclosure notice is required, or if a waiver can be issued to the researcher that exempts him or her from the consent process. A waiver means the research can be conducted using the methods described in the research protocol and that patient authorizations and disclosures documenting record access are not required. Disclosure forms will be discussed in more detail later in this chapter.

Researchers should not make assumptions based on these descriptions that their research may be exempt or expedited. No aspect of the study should commence without approval from the appropriate committee or review board. It is the IRB that tells the researcher whether a study is exempt or qualifies for expedited review, not the other way around.

Quality improvement studies are exempt from IRB review. Quality improvement studies are typically conducted for the purpose of internal organizational improvement, and there is no expectation of publication or generalization to larger groups. However, some quality improvement is conducted with the idea of publication; in this case, IRB oversight is appropriate. FIGURE 3.3 lists a set of questions that can help a study designer determine whether a proposed project is purely quality improvement—requiring no IRB oversight—or research.

> **Exempt review:** A review of study proposals that pose no risk to subjects; the full IRB is not required to participate.
> **Expedited review:** A review of study proposals that pose minimal risk to subjects; one or two IRB members participate.
> **Full review:** A review of study proposals that pose more than minimal risk to subjects, that do not qualify for exempt status, and in which the full IRB committee participates.

POUDRE VALLEY HEALTH SYSTEM

POUDRE VALLEY HEALTH SYSTEM
CHECK LIST TO DETERMINE
EXEMPT STATUS

In order to qualify as exempt, the research must fall under **one** *of the following categories [45 CFR 46.101(b).]*
NOTE: *Studies which qualify as exempt are subject to the same ethical principles governing all research at this institution.*

*If marked with an *, study does not qualify for Exempt.

1. **WHICH OF THE FOLLOWING CATEGORIES DESCRIBES THE RESEARCH?**
    A. ☐ **Research conducted in established or commonly accepted educational settings, involving normal educational practices such as:**
        ➤   Research on regular and special educational instructional strategies; or
        ➤   Research on the effectiveness of or the comparison among instructional techniques, curricula, or classroom management methods.

    B.1 ☐ **Research involving the use of educational tests (cognitive diagnostic, aptitude, and achievement), survey procedures, interview procedures, or observation of public behavior. It does not contain the following:**
        ➤   Information obtained is recorded in such a manner that human subjects can be identified, directly or through identifiers linked to the subjects;
                                                                                                            ☐ *Yes   ☐ No
        ➤   Any disclosure of the human subjects' responses outside the research could reasonably place the subjects at risk of criminal or civil liability or be damaging to the subjects' financial standing, employability, or reputation.   ☐ *Yes   ☐ No

    B.2 ☐ **Research involving the use of educational tests (cognitive, diagnostic, aptitude, achievement), survey procedures, interview procedures, or observation of public behavior that is not exempt under paragraph above and <u>does not have</u>:**
        ➤   The Human subjects elected or appointed as public officials or candidates for public office;
        ➤   (Federal statue(s) require without exception that the confidentiality of their personally identifiable information will be maintained throughout the research and thereafter.)

    C. ☐ **Research involving the collection or study of <u>existing</u> data, documents, records, pathological specimens or diagnostic specimens if these sources are publicly available or the information is recorded by the investigator in such a manner that the subjects <u>cannot be identified</u>, directly or through identifiers linked to the subjects.**

    D. ☐ **Research designed to evaluate public benefit or service programs** *(Medicare, Social Security).*

    E. ☐ **Taste and food evaluation without additives using ingredients found safe by FDA, EPA or USDA.**

2. **DOES THE RESEARCH INVOLVE ANY OF THE FOLLOWING POPULATIONS?**
    Prisoners ☐ Yes ☐ No   Pregnant Women   ☐ Yes ☐ No
    Fetuses   ☐ Yes ☐ No   In Vitro Fertilization? ☐ Yes ☐ No
    Children   ☐ *Yes ☐ No
    ➤   If yes, does the research involve the observation of public behavior?   ☐ Yes ☐ No
    ➤   If yes, will the investigator be a participant in the activities being observed? ☐ *Yes ☐ No

3. **IS A WAIVER OF AUTHORIZATION REQUESTED?**   ☐ **YES**   ☐ **NO**
    In order to access protected health information under a waiver of authorization for research, the IRB must make the following three findings:

    a) The disclosure involves no more than minimal risk to the privacy for the individual based on a plan to (i) protect patient identifier from improper use and disclosure; (ii) destroy patient identifiers at the earliest opportunity unless there is health or research justification for retaining identifiers or is required by law; and (iii) adequate written assurances that protected health information will not be reused or disclosed to others except as required by law, for oversight of the research, or for other research that would be permitted by HIPAA;
    b) The research could not be practically conducted without the waiver; and
    c) The research could not be practically conducted without access to protected health information.

    Exemption request: Approved ☐   Denied ☐

    _____
    Reviewed (IRB Staff)   Date

    KWM/lw 5-2006

FIGURE 3.2 Checklist to Determine IRB Exempt Status for a Study
Source: Used with permission of Poudre Valley Health System, Institutional Review Board, Fort Collins, CO, 2006.

Contact the IRB coordinator (ext. 7333) if your activity involves patients, employees, and/or lab specimens (from human subjects), **and** you answer yes/unsure to any of the following:	Yes/Unsure	No
1. It **does** assign people or lab specimens to groups for simultaneous comparison		
2. It **is** being conducted in hopes of contributing to generalizable knowledge in the area of study (and **not** for the sole purpose of improving PVHS processes)		
3. The initial intent **is** to publish the results*		
4. It **does** involve patients/subjects undergoing procedures that normally would not be done for their disease/problem (i.e., beyond the normal standard of care or for employees—their work day)		
5. It **does** involve increased risk or burden to the participants (e.g., additional blood draws, fatigue, embarrassment, or giving personal information)		
6. It **does** involve interactions or observations that don't routinely occur in patient care (for patients) or everyday life		
7. It **does** involve releasing protected health information (PHI) or personal information to individuals/entities other than for regulatory/accreditation purposes		

*If the initial intent was not to publish results, but it is later determined that the results will be published, then the IRB coordinator needs to be contacted.

FIGURE 3.3 Checklist to Differentiate Research from Quality Improvement Studies
Source: Used with permission of Poudre Valley Health System, Institutional Review Board, Fort Collins, CO, 2006.

When preparing the IRB/Human Subjects Approval Form, the researcher must clearly describe the following eight required elements (CFR 45, Part 46):

1. The research project, the subjects, and how they will be selected and informed
2. The methods and procedures to be used; the subjects should understand their level of participation, what is required, and for how long
3. Risks to the participants, particularly if drugs or treatments are used
4. Benefits to participants
5. How confidentiality and anonymity will be maintained
6. Contact information for questions of participants
7. Explanation of any compensation
8. Statement about voluntary participation

The IRB is more than a safety net for subjects. It has the capacity to advise, mentor, and develop new researchers. A tremendous amount of research expertise is available to the researcher via the members of the IRB. Consulting with them early and often in a study can help strengthen the study design. Although much is made of the regulatory authority of the IRB, much can also be said for its capacity to provide an additional critical evaluation of the research as it is designed. The IRB is another safeguard available to help the researcher design a strong, ethical, and legal research study. Doing the right thing from the beginning of a study is the best way to avoid legal and ethical accusations.

Research Misconduct

Obtaining the necessary approvals of the IRB and privacy committee does not guarantee that the researcher is then free from accusations of battery, negligence, or invasion of privacy. It is up to the researcher to carry out the research in an ethical, legal, and moral manner and to document the procedures and results accurately.

Research misconduct, as defined by the federal government, includes fabrication, falsification, and plagiarism. Fabrication is the intentional misrepresentation or "making up" of data or results by the researcher. Falsification occurs if the researcher falsifies or manipulates the results, changes the procedures, omits data, or accepts subjects into the study who were not in the original inclusion criteria. Plagiarism usually arises from the written account of the research when ideas, statements, results, or words are not attributed to the appropriate person but are represented as the writer's own work.

Research misconduct affects the cost of research overall by increasing the oversight required and by diminishing the confidence and respect of the public regarding the results of scientific research. The public may begin to grow skeptical of research results if such behaviors become commonplace.

The factor determining if research misconduct took place is whether the researcher intentionally misrepresented the data. Research misconduct has not occurred if a researcher made honest mistakes. Misconduct has not occurred if researchers simply have differences of opinion. This is an important distinction. Good researchers take calculated and controlled risks. As long as the researcher takes the time to carefully plan a strong study, gains the approval of involved IRB and privacy committees, and maintains inflexible ethical standards during the implementation of the study, the researcher has fulfilled his or her obligation as an accountable steward of the study.

The HIPAA Privacy Rule

What I may see or hear in the course of the treatment or even outside of the treatment in regard to the life of men, which on no account one must spread abroad, I will keep to myself, holding such things shameful to be spoken about.

—Hippocratic Oath (Edelstein, 1943)

HIPAA: Health Insurance Portability and Accountability Act passed by Congress in 1996 that protects the privacy of personal health information.

Since April 14, 2003, the effective date of the privacy rule, otherwise known as HIPAA, organizations have more tightly scrutinized research proposals, especially those that involve the use of patient data and human subjects.

Reacting to the increasing accessibility of electronic data available about an individual, Congress passed the Health Insurance Portability and Accountability Act (HIPAA) in 1996. Aimed mostly at electronic health record (EHR) initiatives, one of HIPAA's main elements is a requirement for the protection of personal health information. The rule protects all elements considered protected health information.

Table 3.5

Identifiable Personal Health Information (PHI)

- Name
- Geographic subdivisions smaller than a state, including street address, city, county, precinct, zip code, and the equivalent international address codes, except for the initial three digits of a zip code in certain situations
- All elements of date (except year) for dates directly related to an individual, including birth date, discharge date, date of death, all ages over 89, and all elements of dates indicative of such age except that such ages and elements may be aggregated into a single category of age 90 or older
- Telephone numbers
- Fax number
- E-mail address
- Social security number
- Medical record number
- Health plan beneficiary number
- Account number
- Certificate/license number
- Vehicle identification number
- Medical device identifier
- Web uniform resource locators (URLs)
- Internet Protocol (IP) address
- Biometric identifiers, including finger and voice print
- Full-face photographic images and any comparable image
- Any other unique identifying number, characteristic, or code

This covers a broad range of information from telephone numbers to diagnoses. **Table 3.5** lists the information that is considered identifiable personal health information.

The privacy rule changed the way hospitals traditionally handled patients and their information. Healthcare workers are only given access to PHI that is necessary to perform the assigned work at hand. For example, those personnel working in ancillary departments receive only a diagnosis that enables them to process the tests or bills. Therefore, the researcher cannot automatically assume that access to all the information required to complete research will be provided, even if the researcher is employed by the facility.

Recent revisions to the rule, Public Law 111-5 (American Recovery and Reinvestment Act, 2009), strengthened and revised the initial law. The newest version of the regulation implies that an organization must be able to account for all uses of PHI, even internal uses. Researchers may be required to include contact information and notices in patient records when data have been collected from them. Researchers could be held liable for any breaches of PHI data that occur as a result of data collection or analysis.

Failing to comply with the rule can be very costly to the researcher and the organization. The privacy rule specifically states that any employee who fails to comply with

Table 3.6

Sample Disclosure Statement for Research Records

Disclosure for Research Purposes

Date: _____   IRB/Approval # _____

Patient Name: _____   Medical Record# _____

Researcher: _____

The above-named patient's record was accessed by the researcher for purposes of data collection in a research study approved by this organization.

Information used from this record will not disclose any individually identifiable health information and will be kept confidential as described in the research protocol on file with the organization's research review board.

the privacy policy will be subject to corrective action, termination of employment, and possibly prosecution by the Office of Civil Rights. Heavy fines accompany proven violations of the rule. Additionally, new revisions to the rule allow individual fines applicable to the person who disclosed the information. Those fines can be anywhere from $100 per occurrence up to $250,000. These and other revisions to the rule have given organizations pause when requests for access to PHI are sought.

Therefore, researchers must not assume that because they work in a healthcare facility they will have ready access to that facility's patient data, databases, or diagnostic information or even limited data sets. The provisions of the privacy rule provide additional safeguards for the participants, which can make it difficult, though not impossible, to do research in healthcare facilities. The researcher should plan well in advance of the start of the study as to whether access to certain data elements and health information can be obtained and how.

If the researcher requires access to the medical records of the patient or participant, consent forms should be obtained authorizing the researcher to access the information. The research consent should include an authorization for access to records. If it is not included, the researcher must document how access to the information will be obtained. Retrospective studies that involve the use of patient data from electronic sources or the medical record may require the researcher to supply a disclosure statement to document access. Alternatively, the IRB may grant a waiver that exempts the researcher from obtaining authorization, although disclosure statements may still be required. See **Table 3.6** for an example of a disclosure statement.

Reading Research for Evidence-Based Practice

Most studies will not explicitly describe the ethical or legal issues they faced unless they were unusual or difficult to resolve. This is not a weakness but reflects the reality that ethical and legal compliance are a given when planning any research study. Ethical and

Checklist for Evaluating the Ethical Issues in a Study

✔ Adequate protections are in place to protect subjects from any potential harm.

✔ The authors document approval from the institutional review board.

✔ It clearly indicated that subjects underwent informed consent.

✔ If vulnerable populations were involved, special consideration was given to informed consent and study procedures.

✔ Steps were taken to protect the anonymity, confidentiality, and privacy of subjects.

✔ There was no evidence of any type of coercion (implied or otherwise) to motivate participants to agree to the study.

✔ The researchers provided full disclosure to potential subjects. If deception was necessary to achieve the goals of the study, participants were debriefed about the experience.

✔ The benefits of the study outweighed the risks for individual subjects; a risk/benefit assessment was considered.

✔ Subjects were recruited, selected, and assigned to groups in an equitable way.

regulatory guidelines are not negotiable, and so it may be simply stated that the study underwent IRB review. If so, then it is safe to assume the study was reviewed by an objective panel and met basic ethical and legal requirements.

If explicit reference to the IRB is not made, then the nurse reader will need to scrutinize the methods section to determine if a potential breach of ethical or legal requirements occurred. Particular attention should be paid to the method for selecting the sample, obtaining informed consent, assigning subjects to treatment groups, and accessing their medical data. All of these procedures should reflect a fundamental respect for the ethical principles described in this chapter. The reader should be especially concerned if there were significant risks associated with the study, or if data were collected from medical records without a description of how privacy was protected. However, the absence of any mention of procedures to safeguard subjects does not mean these safeguards were not in place.

Using Research in Nursing Practice

The nurse should be hesitant to use the results of research in practice if he or she suspects the study was conducted unethically or in some way breached the legal protections of subjects. The nurse should be aware that research misconduct can occur, and that studies that are the result of such misconduct cannot be trusted. Ethical and legal constraints also help ensure research quality and validity of findings; results that were generated through deception or duress will likely not represent the population well. In other words, if the researcher cannot be trusted, then the research findings cannot be trusted either.

Creating Evidence for Practice

The nurse researcher can best deal with the potential ethical and legal issues in a research study by focusing on strong designs that answer the research question with a minimum of disruption in subjects' lives. If the nurse researcher focuses on doing the right thing, it is rare that an ethical or legal issue will arise.

The researcher must keep in mind, however, that compliance with ethical and regulatory issues is not confined to the design period. Some problems arise during the implementation of a research study. The principles that guide the legal and ethical treatment of subjects—whether in preparation for an IRB review or for actual data collection—are ongoing throughout the study. Inadvertent problems and unforeseen issues happen during research. The careful researcher considers these fundamental guidelines as a basis for decisions about the entire research process, not just the IRB application.

Research contributes knowledge to a field. The public relies on this knowledge to determine future courses of action, whether it is to decide on a course of medical treatment or merely to keep abreast of trends and current data. All research, then, must always be conducted with integrity, honesty, and respect for all parties involved, and with the utmost attention to ethical guidelines and regulatory limits.

Summary of Key Concepts

- When humans participate as subjects in research studies, care must be taken to preserve their rights.
- Subjects have the right to be informed of the study processes and potential risks, to be treated in a fair manner, and to withdraw from the study at any time.

For More Depth and Detail

For a more in-depth look at the concepts in this chapter, try these references:

Alt-White, A., & Pranulis, M. (2006). Addressing nurses' ethical concerns about research in critical care settings. *Nursing Administration Quarterly, 30*(1), 67–75.

Byerly, W. (2009). Working with the institutional review board. *American Journal of Health-System Pharmacists, 66,* 176–184.

Hill, G. (2006). Professional issues associated with the role of the research nurse. *Nursing Standard, 29*(39), 41–47.

Kaiser, K. (2009). Protecting respondent confidentiality in qualitative research. *Qualitative Health Research, 19*(11), 1632–1641.

Nosowsky, R., & Giordano, T. (2006). The Health Insurance Portability and Accountability Act of 1996 (HIPAA) privacy rule: Implications for clinical research. *Annual Review of Medicine, 57*(1), 575–590.

Oberle, W. (2005). Issues in clinical nursing research: Clinical trials with complementary therapies. *Western Journal of Nursing Research, 27*(2), 232–239.

Pozgar, G. (2009). *Legal and ethical issues for health care professionals.* Sudbury, MA: Jones & Bartlett.

Shalowitz, D., & Wendler, D. (2006). Informed consent for research and authorization under the Health Insurance Portability and Accountability Act Privacy Rule: An integrated approach. *Annals of Internal Medicine, 144*(9), 685–688.

- The Nuremberg Code and the Declaration of Helsinki are international guidelines for the conduct of ethical research; the United States also has the Belmont Report to guide behavior.

- Therapeutic research, in which the subject can be expected to receive a potentially beneficial treatment, is different from nontherapeutic research, which contributes to the body of knowledge but not to an individual's health.

- The foundational ethical principles that guide researchers in the treatment of human subjects are respect for persons, beneficence, and justice.

- Vulnerable populations include those groups with limited autonomy or capacity to make decisions. These populations have special protections to ensure they are not exploited.

- Informed consent is a process of information exchange that begins with subject recruitment. Full disclosure of risks and benefits and the provision of understandable information needed to make a participation decision are hallmarks of a strong informed consent process.

- Deception or incomplete disclosure should be avoided in research. When it is necessary, there should be a strong rationale and subjects must be fully debriefed after the experience.

- Informed consent documents should be prepared in the most comprehensible way possible so subjects are fully aware of the particulars of the study.

- Research integrity extends beyond subject rights to the way data are collected, analyzed, and reported.

 CRITICAL APPRAISAL **EXERCISE**

Retrieve the following full text article from the Cumulative Index to Nursing and Allied Health Literature or similar search database:

   Hornor, G., Scribano, P., Curran, S., Stevens, J., & Roda, D. (2009). Emotional response to the ano-genital examination of suspected sexual abuse. *Journal of Forensic Nursing, 5,* 124–130.

   Review the article, looking for evidence of any ethical or legal issues that arose in the study and how the researchers dealt with them. Consider the following appraisal questions in your critical review of this research article:

1. In what ways are the subjects in this study vulnerable? What protections should be put in place to protect these subjects from harm?
2. Identify the potential risks inherent in this study for the subjects. What should specifically be included in the informed consent for this study?
3. What evidence is provided by the authors that the study was reviewed by the IRB and that appropriate informed consent was obtained?
4. What potential legal issues are inherent in this study? How do the authors protect the legal rights of the subjects?
5. How do the researchers address the following issues:
   a. Respect for persons
   b. Beneficence

- The nurse researcher advocates for the participants in research studies and must protect their autonomy and confidentiality at all times.
- IRB requirements have their origin in federal regulations and require varying levels of involvement in the approval process, depending on whether they are expedited, exempt, or full board review.
- The IRB was established in response to the inhumane treatment of subjects, and the protection of individuals who are asked to participate in research remains their primary concern. The IRB is also a helpful group in providing critical feedback that can improve the design and strength of a study.
- HIPAA provides another layer of protection by guaranteeing the subject's right to protection of private health information. The researcher must plan carefully to ensure that all legal requirements are met, particularly because violations can carry with them serious consequences.

For a full suite of assignments and additional learning activities, use the access code located in the front of your book to visit this exclusive website: http://go.jblearning .com/houser. If you do not have an access code, you can obtain one at the site.

References

American Recovery and Reinvestment Act of 2009. Pub.L. No. 111-5. § 13402–13424.

Becker, K., & Levy, M. (2001). Ensuring patient safety in clinical trials for treatment of acute stroke. *Journal of the American Medical Association, 286*(21), 2718–2719.

Edelstein, L. (Trans.). (1943). *The Hippocratic oath: Text, translation and interpretation.* Baltimore: Johns Hopkins University Press.

Flesch, R. (1948). A new readability yardstick. *Journal of Applied Psychology, 32,* 221–223.

Kapp, M. (2007). Patient autonomy in the age of consumer-driven health care: Informed consent and informed choice. *Journal of Legal Medicine, 28*(1), 91–117.

Kincaid, J. P., Fishburne, R. P., Rogers, R. L., & Chisson, B. S. (1975). *Derivation of new readability formulas (Automated Readability Index, Fog Count and Flesch Reading Ease Formula) for Navy enlisted personnel.* Research Branch Report 8-75. Millington, TN: Naval Technical Training, U.S. Naval Air Station, Memphis, TN.

Layman, E. (2009). Human experimentation: Historical perspective of breaches of ethics in U.S. healthcare. *Health Care Manager, 28*(4), 354–374.

Mayo, A., & Wallhagen, M. (2009). Considerations of informed consent and decision-making competence in older adults with cognitive impairment. *Research in Gerontological Nursing, 2*(2), 103–111.

McGuire, D. (1996, April 9). Rochester death halts MIT-funded study. *The Tech.* Retrieved May 29, 2006, from http://www-tech.mit.edu/V116/N17/rochester.17n.html

Mehlman, M., & Berg, J., (2008). Human subjects protections in biomedical enhancement research: Assessing risk and benefit and obtaining informed consent. *Journal of Law, Medicine and Ethics, 36*(3), 546–559.

National Academy of Sciences. (1995). *On being a scientist: Responsible conduct in research* (2nd ed.). Washington, DC: National Academies Press.

Oberle, K. (2006). Ethical considerations for nurses in clinical trials. *Nursing Ethics, 13*(2), 180–186.

Stolberg, S. K. (1999). The biotech death of Jesse Gelsinger. Retrieved May 29, 2006, from http://www.gene.ch/gentech/1999/Dec/msg00005.html

U.S. Department of Health and Human Services. (2005, June 23). CFR 45, Public Health. Part 46, Protection of human subjects. Retrieved February 1, 2011, from http://privacyruleandresearch.nih.gov/pdf/ocr_publichealth.pdf

U.S. Department of Health, Education, and Welfare. (1978). The Belmont report. Ethical principles and guidelines for the protection of human subjects of research. DHEW Publication Number (OS) 78-0012.

part II

Planning for Research

chapter 4

Finding Problems and Writing Questions

CHAPTER OBJECTIVES

The study of this chapter will help the learner to

- Discuss strategies for identifying research problems.
- Describe the process for narrowing a research problem down to a researchable question.
- Define and contrast problem statements and purpose statements.
- Develop and articulate problem statements and purpose statements.
- Perform a critical analysis of the problem statement and purpose statement from a research article.

KEY TERMS

Analytic question	Hypothesis	Prospective studies
Concepts	Inductive	Purpose statements
Correlation studies	Nondirectional hypothesis	Replication studies
Deductive	Null hypothesis	Research question
Directional hypothesis	Problem statements	Retrospective study

Introduction

The best research starts with two words: "I wonder." A sense of curiosity is all that is needed to begin the research process. Observations about a problem become questions, and these questions lead to nursing research.

Finding and developing significant problems for nursing research are critical to improving processes and outcomes for patients, nursing staff, and organizations. The

81

The idea for this research study actually had its beginnings when we took a class on critically reading research. We work on a medical–surgical unit, and we decided that we would like to try to do a small project. So we decided to do some observation and find a question to study, even though it is a really busy unit.

About that time, we had a physician who began doing more bariatric surgery. The standing orders for these patients were to have physical and occupational therapy evaluate the patient and get them up and walking. We had always interpreted that as the next morning, because the therapies were generally not available in the evenings when these patients were in shape to start moving. We had patients who wanted to get up and walking the first evening, though, and so we would help them walk. We noticed that these patients seemed to get less nausea. Nausea and retching are important in these patients because we cannot get their intravenous line out until they are not vomiting, and retching is very painful for them. They get their pain meds through the IV, and if they are vomiting we cannot switch to oral meds and pull their IV lines. So if the patient had to wait until the second day to walk, it seemed they had more nausea and vomiting, and it just backlogged everything. It usually meant their discharge was delayed until the evening of the second day. So we wondered if maybe it was the earlier walking that was helping with the nausea.

So we started with a literature search. Originally, we planned to find a study and replicate it; we really never thought we could do a study of our own. We just wanted to duplicate what someone else had done. But there were no studies to be found. We found lots of studies of the effects of ambulation in the postoperative period, but nothing with this specific group of patients, and none of the studies measured nausea as the outcome measure. So we thought, "Maybe we need to do a study." We were going to do something very simple, not even go through the institutional review board (IRB), more like a quality study. We were nervous about having to go to the IRB; we thought that would be way too deep for us. We thought a little study would be a good way, a really simple way for the staff to be involved in research, and we thought it was doable.

We had an opportunity to consult a researcher through our evidence-based practice council. The researcher told us, "This is a good study; this is publishable," and that was a turning point for us. We realized that this was as important as what other nurse researchers studied, and that we had an opportunity to make a contribution to practice.

What started as a simple little question—does walking affect nausea?—has evolved into something more complicated. Our research question is now based on time—in other words, how soon does the patient have to walk to get a benefit? The process kind of forced us to produce criteria for when a patient is ready to walk, and that was a conversation that the whole staff participated in. We introduced another element after consulting with physical therapy. We now have one group that will use a bedside pedaler and one that will walk, and we will see if there is an advantage of one over the other. That would be helpful to know, because when we have really chaotic days, we may not have a lot of time to stop and walk someone. If we can find that the pedaler does get that gut waking up faster, then we can use it, because it takes much less time.

When the people on the unit realized that our goal was publication, then they were on board. We have learned to appreciate the nurses we work with who have stayed in medical–surgical nursing. One of the driving things behind this is to gain some respect for the fact that we are a highly qualified group of nurses who care deeply about patient care and doing the right thing for patients. Taking our nursing practice to the next level, this could be a real source of pride for the staff. And we think that is why they are so behind it.

It has helped us to look at our whole nursing practice and realize it is not insignificant, that this is something someone would want to read. Now that we have finished the IRB process, we've realized, yeah, we really can do that.

Maureen Wentzel, RN

Ginnie Ferraro, RN

evolution of a research problem from a general topic of interest to the articulation of a problem statement and a purpose statement serves to narrow the focus of the research into a researchable question. This progression moves the research problem from the conceptual (abstract concepts) to the operational (measurable concepts or variables). FIGURE 4.1 depicts how the individual steps in translating a problem into a researchable question follow this continuum from conceptual to operational.

The traditional method for finding and developing research problems suggests a deductive, sequential process from a general interest to the development of a research question. FIGURE 4.2 demonstrates how the individual steps might look in the development of a specific researchable question.

In truth, the process for finding and developing research problems can be as chaotic as a busy parking lot. Some motorists drive their cars headfirst into the spaces, some motorists back their cars into the spaces, yet other motorists drive their cars into and out of the spaces until their cars are properly positioned. It is similar for research question development. Some researchers do, indeed, use a sequential set of steps to arrive at a specific and well-articulated question. But many nurse researchers also use nontraditional methods for finding and developing research problems. These processes may be more inductive, in which specific observations are the starting points, leading to a general focus or interest. FIGURE 4.3 demonstrates a nontraditional example of finding and developing a research problem. Still other methods may begin somewhere in the middle of the traditional process by recognizing a gap, and proceed to identify the big picture as well as the specific research question.

Regardless of the approach—deductive, inductive, or somewhere in between—finding and developing research problems may be a process best characterized as a work in progress, with the potential for false starts, rethinking, and ongoing refinement as researchers strive to meet the rigors of traditional research methods. In any case, the goal is to narrow the focus of the research problem so that a feasible research question emerges.

Deductive: A process of reasoning from a general theory to a specific and well-articulated question.

Inductive: A process of reasoning from specific observations to broader generalizations and theories.

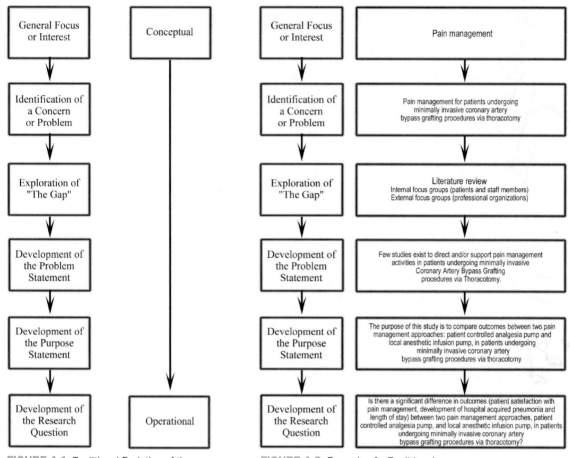

FIGURE 4.1 Traditional Evolution of the Research Process

FIGURE 4.2 Example of a Traditional Evolution of the Problem

Concepts: Abstract ideas or topics of interest that must be narrowed to researchable questions to be investigated.

The importance of narrowing the focus of the research cannot be overstressed. Research problems that have not been narrowed generate too many concepts and relationships to test.

Subjects or topics that are too broad become problematic for researchers because methodological complexities increase, expert methodologists are required, and resource demands (for example, money, people, and time) increase. With every additional concept and/or associated relationship examined, the feasibility of the study may be affected. The primary objective of nursing research is to increase knowledge to improve nursing practice. This will only be accomplished if the research is actually completed! Some researchers spend a lifetime studying a single concept; others spend their careers completing multiple, small studies. There is no shame in starting, or staying, small. Narrow questions are far easier for the novice researcher to address and may help the nurse learn skills that contribute to larger, more complex

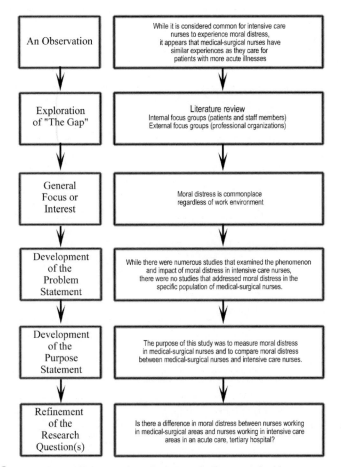

FIGURE 4.3 Nontraditional Example of the Evolution of a Research Problem

studies. **Table 4.1** demonstrates the narrowing of a research problem from the broad topic of "failure to rescue" to some narrower, researchable concepts associated with "rapid response teams."

As the research problem moves from a broad topic of interest to a narrowed, researchable question, measurable variables and outcomes become evident. It is paramount that consideration be given to the type of concept under investigation. Concepts may represent many things; however, they roughly fall into three categories: patient sensitive, staff member sensitive, or organizationally sensitive. Categorizing a concept is directly related to the type of process or outcome measured. Concepts studied by nurses, especially novice nurse researchers, should be limited to concepts within the nursing span of control. For example, a nurse interested in the development and severity of hematomas at arterial access sites after diagnostic or interventional coronary arteriography would be better suited to ask research questions about positioning and turning the patient, rather than questions about the method of arterial access used for the procedure. The first research question identifies nurse-sensitive concepts (repositioning and/or turning)

Table 4.1

Researchable Concepts for Failure to Rescue

Criteria
- Acute renal failure
- Acute ulcer: gastrointestinal hemorrhage
- Cardiac arrest
- Deep vein thrombosis
- Pneumonia
- Pulmonary embolism
- Sepsis
- Shock

Factors
- Patient characteristics
- Staffing effects
- Organizational resources

Process
- Bed management and patient placement
- Rapid response teams

Cardiopulmonary Events
- Impact on total number
- Impact on number on the medical–surgical patient care areas
- Impact on number on the intensive care units
- Impact on survivability to discharge

Table 4.2

Examples of Patient, Nursing, and Organizationally Sensitive Concepts

Patient-Sensitive Concepts	Nurse-Sensitive Concepts	Organizationally Sensitive Concepts
Anxiety	Burnout	Cost
Depression	Immobility-related injuries	Length of stay
Functional independence	Medication errors	Readmission
Blood glucose	Pain management	Resource utilization
Blood pressure	Patient falls	Satisfaction with nursing care
Quality of life	Restraint prevalence	
Satisfaction with nursing care		

whereas the second research question identifies medically sensitive concepts (arterial access methods). Table 4.2 provides examples of each of these kinds of concepts. This is not to say that nurses should not participate in research that examines concepts outside the traditional nursing domain; however, if the main purpose of nursing research is to increase the body of nursing knowledge, it is logical to study concepts as they relate to nurse-sensitive topics.

Finding and Developing Research Problems

Often, research problems find the nurse rather than the other way around. Frustrations with ineffective procedures, the search for a "better way," or the need to help a single patient may motivate the nurse to seek research-based evidence to improve patient care. The search for research problems is one of the easiest parts of the research process; researchable problems virtually surround the contemporary nurse in practice.

Sources of Research Problems

Researchable problems can come from a virtually unlimited number of sources (Burns & Grove, 2008; Polit & Beck, 2009). The following are some sources for researchable problems:

- Clinical practice observations
- Educational experiences
- Patient feedback
- Theoretical models and frameworks
- Professional literature
- Performance improvement studies
- Research reports and priorities
- Social issues

Clinical Practice

Research problems may be generated from active, passive, or other organizational activities. Active methods include experiences with direct patient care and discussion with other members of the health-care team through formal (interdisciplinary work teams) or informal (shift report) communications. Patient problems, ineffective clinical procedures, or changes in protocols all present opportunities for research. Passive methods for identifying problems include medical record review and observation. Other methods include data collection activities such as those performed for quality improvement or risk management.

> **gray matter**
>
> Three categories of nursing research concepts are those that are
> - Patient sensitive
> - Staff member sensitive
> - Organizationally sensitive

Educational Experience

Research problems may be generated from educational experiences. Nursing students taking research courses are required to develop problem, purpose, and research statements from required and/or self-determined topics. Educational institutions that are research-focused may have specified research activities examining interests such as age-specific care, the effects of caring, or nursing shortage outcomes. Within the assignments and disciplined inquiry that occur during the educational experience, particularly graduate study, nursing students and their mentors generate many researchable problems.

Consumer Feedback

Research problems may be generated from the results of activities aimed at soliciting patient feedback. Feedback may be solicited from the following sources:

- Patients and customers of the institution, both external and internal
- Leaders that represent the interests of specific services (for example, cardiac care)
- Departments (for example, the coronary care unit) and service lines (for example, cardiac services) within an organizational structure
- Advisory boards and other consumer input organizations
- Members of general or specialty professional organizations (for example, the American Nurses Association or the American Association of Critical Care Nurses)

The feedback that is garnered from these groups may generate problem statements, purpose statements, and research questions, as well as priorities for performance improvement or other research activities. Feedback may be solicited via survey, from formal and informal meetings, and at conferences and workshops, or it may be received electronically.

Theoretical Models and Frameworks

Research problems may be generated from the development and testing of concepts and their associated relationships within conceptual models and theoretical frameworks. Basic research focuses on the testing of theories, and models involve the testing of relationships, effects, and interactions. Models and frameworks may be originated by the researcher or retrieved from the literature for further study.

Professional Literature

Research problems may be generated from the results of professional literature reviews. Sources of professional literature review include clinical and nonclinical works, databases, and letters and opinions. Clinical works include books and journals representing nursing and medical topics, both general and specialty. Nonclinical works include books and journals representing nonnursing and nonmedical topics from other fields of study that may be generalized into an appropriate, researchable problem to expand nursing knowledge. Many databases, clinical and nonclinical, are capable of provoking inquiry. Examples of these databases include those that hold data from previous studies (clinical) and census data (nonclinical). Many research problems have been developed by using the data collected by other researchers and taking a unique approach to the analysis. Published letters and opinions are an interesting source of research problems. Letters and opinions written by nurses and other medical professionals often express concern, as well as directives, about researchable problems, gaps in current knowledge, limitations of available research, and recommendations for future research.

Performance Improvement Activities

Performance improvement activities, also known as quality improvement activities, are used to improve processes and outcomes and to meet regulatory requirements. Tools and techniques specific to performance improvement do not meet the requirements of traditional research methods. Performance improvement studies are often characterized by methodological limitations, a lack of control over extraneous variables, violation of assumptions for statistical testing, and small sample sizes in a single setting; all affect the generalizability of the findings. However, the results of performance improvement activities may be used as a springboard into formal research activities. Researchable problems may start as performance improvement activities and expand into formal research projects with alterations in methodological approach, sampling strategy, and informed consent procedures.

Research Reports and Priorities

Research problems may be generated from the outcomes of other research studies and evidence-based practice reviews. Previous research may directly or indirectly influence the generation of research problems. A conventional part of a research report is a section on "suggestions for future research," which outlines ways to extend and expand on the currently available research. Researchers may directly influence the generation of subsequent research problems by explicitly stating remaining problems, gaps, and questions. A common form of direct influence is the type of research known as the replication study. Replication studies may be used to validate findings and knowledge, increase generalizability (population and setting), and/or eliminate or minimize limitations (methodology). Replication studies are good exercises because they are a means of increasing the knowledge of inexperienced researchers. Research also may indirectly influence the generation of a problem when the reader identifies a problem with the written report (discrepancy, gap, inconsistency, or unidentified limitation) or disagrees with the methodology and/or results of the original investigator.

> **Replication studies:** Studies generated from previous research studies in which the research is reproduced to validate findings, increase generalizability, and/or eliminate or minimize limitations.

Research problems may also be generated from the directives and recommendations of individuals and organizations. Because of expertise, individuals (educators and researchers) and organizations (clinical, educational, funding, and regulatory) have identified problems and gaps in current knowledge. Some of these experts have developed problem statements and research questions to prioritize future research.

Social Issues

Research problems may be generated from social issues. Social issues include, but are not limited to, the effects of age, culture, education, gender, income, race, religion, and sexual preference. Social issues may be examined in the context of current events, the environment, and health policy. Social issues may also be examined as they affect local, state, national, or international populations.

This list of sources for research problems is not exhaustive nor is it mutually exclusive. Research problems are often the product of both internal and external driving forces; they are seldom generated from a single source. Any process or outcome associated with patient care, staff member work environment, or organizational success may become the basis for study. The potential nurse researcher can scrutinize the current practices and ask the following questions:

- Why are we doing it this way?
- Is there a better way of doing it?
- Should we be doing it at all?

All these questions may give rise to researchable problems, the solutions to which may add valuable evidence to the effective practice of nursing.

Articulation of Research Problem Statements

Problem statements: Statements of the disparity between what is known and what needs to be known and addressed by the research.

Research problem statements are declarations of disparity: the difference (gap) between what is known and what needs to be known about a topic. They articulate a discrepancy that is to be addressed by the research process. The disparity, whether a small gap or a large chasm, defines the area(s) of concern and focuses the research methods (Burns & Grove, 2008; Polit & Beck, 2009). Most problem statements are explicitly stated; however, some problem statements may be inferred. The inferred research problem statement may describe the importance and/or potential consequences of the disparity as it pertains to clinical practice.

Problem statements, explicitly stated or inferred, are usually located at the beginning of a research report, in the introduction, and/or in the review of literature, and may be repeated throughout the written report. The idea of a single problem statement is misleading; problem statements may resemble problem paragraphs, and often can be several sentences long. Problem statements are written as questions or statements, and well-written ones contain clear, concise, and well-defined components. An example of a well-written problem statement from a published article follows:

> Literature about adaptation to caesarean birthing is rooted in the experiences of women in the last three decades of the 20th century and may not inform care of contemporary caesarean-delivered women. Research findings document both normal and negative psychological outcomes. Although most research has focused on unplanned caesarean birth, elective planned caesarean is increasing in popularity. Postpartum care studies are limited to needs during hospitalization. Evidence about the needs of women in the immediate post-hospitalization period is lacking. (Weiss, Fawcett, & Aber, 2009)

Development of Research Purpose Statements

Purpose statements: Declarative and objective statements that indicate the general goal of the study and often describe the direction of the inquiry.

Whereas research problem statements identify a gap in knowledge that requires disciplined study, research purpose statements are declarations of intent. Purpose statements indicate the general goal of the study and often describe the direction of inquiry (Burns & Grove, 2008; Polit & Beck, 2009). The purpose of the research should be clearly stated. Purpose statements are written as objective statements. They are easily identified in reports because of words such as *aim*, *goal*, *intent*, *objective*, or *purpose*. They contain clear, concise, and well-defined components including key variables to be studied, their possible interrelationships, and the nature of the population of interest. An example follows of a purpose statement from a published study:

> The purpose of this study is to address gaps in knowledge about adaptation to planned and unplanned cesarean birth. The study will identify post-discharge needs and relevant nursing interventions. (Weiss et al., 2009)

This purpose statement indicated the methods used to examine the concepts (descriptive study), the variable of interest (adaptations, needs, and interventions), and the specific population (mothers experiencing cesarean birth).

Although many of these processes have been reviewed for quantitative studies, problem and purpose statements are not limited to research based on empirical measurement. Qualitative studies use subjective means to describe and examine concepts and their meanings but will still have an identifiable problem focus and purpose statement. The problem and purpose statements of qualitative studies may be more vague and less prescriptive than those for quantitative studies. This is primarily due to the emergent nature of research design in qualitative research. Although an overall problem is generally identified for a qualitative study, the purpose may be broader and less detailed than that of a quantitative study because the particulars of the study may only be clear after data collection has commenced. Quantitative studies, by nature, are more prescriptive and use objective measures to describe and examine concepts and the relationships between concepts. The problem and purpose statements for quantitative studies should be detailed and objective. **Table 4.3** outlines the most common components of research problem and purpose statements.

Researcher bias is a limitation that may cause readers to question the validity of research processes and outcomes. When developing purpose statements, researchers should use unbiased verbs such as *compare, describe, develop, discover, explore, test,* and *understand* and avoid biased verbs such as *demonstrate, prove,* and *show.*

Research Methods and Examples of Purpose Statement Verbs

Qualitative Methods	Quantitative Methods
Ethnographic	Correlation
▪ Assess	▪ Determine
▪ Describe	▪ Examine
▪ Examine	▪ Identify
▪ Understand	▪ Understand
Grounded Theory	Descriptive
▪ Develop	▪ Compare
▪ Extend	▪ Contrast
▪ Identify	▪ Describe
▪ Validate	▪ Identify
Phenomenological	Experimental
▪ Describe	▪ Determine
▪ Develop	▪ Examine
▪ Generate	▪ Investigate
▪ Understand	▪ Measure

> **Table 4.3**

Problem Statement and Purpose Statement Components

Problem Statement Components	Purpose Statement Components
▪ Description of the disparity or gap in knowledge	▪ Design of the study
▪ Concepts that are part of the problem	▪ Variables to be studied
	▪ Population to be included
	▪ Setting of the study

- *Example of using an unbiased verb:* The purpose of the study was to explore the effects of music therapy on speech recovery in adult stroke patients in a rehabilitation facility.
- *Example of using a biased verb:* The purpose of the study was to prove that music therapy improves speech recovery in adult stroke patients in a rehabilitation facility.

Carefully writing the purpose statement is the first step in demonstrating its appropriateness for study. Thoughtful inspection of the purpose statement for its feasibility and fit with the researcher's needs is worth the time. Although a purpose statement is relatively easy to compose, completing a study is a time-intensive, arduous process. It should be undertaken only when the researcher has a reasonable expectation of successfully achieving the purpose as stated.

Feasibility of the Purpose Statement

Purpose statements serve to refine the scope of the research, support problem statements, and clarify the significance of the research for the reader. They should be feasible to study, however, within the interests, resources, and capabilities of the nurse researcher (Burns & Grove, 2008; Polit & Beck, 2009). One way to analyze feasibility is to conduct a SWOT analysis. SWOT stands for strengths, weaknesses, opportunities, and threats, and it can serve as a systematic way to assess the overall practical feasibility of the purpose statement. A SWOT analysis is performed by evaluating the following considerations:

- Required resources in terms of time, money, equipment, and people
- Ethical considerations of the design
- Specific variables to be studied
- Availability of the population of interest
- Potential access to the setting of the research study

Performing a SWOT analysis will indicate whether the research study is feasible as articulated by the purpose statement. Research purpose statements that fail SWOT analysis and are determined to be nonresearchable because of resource or ethical issues require the researcher to either revise the statement or look at the research problem in a different way.

Fit of the Purpose Statement

Research purpose statements indicate how variables will be studied within specific populations and settings. There should be a good fit between the design suggested in the purpose statement and the methods used in the research study (Burns & Grove, 2008; Polit & Beck, 2009). Two examples follow of potential purpose statements for a quantitative, correlation design:

- The purpose of the study was to determine the direction and strength of the relationship between depression and functional independence in patients at an urban rehabilitation center.
- The purpose of the study was to measure the effects of depression on functional independence in patients at an urban rehabilitation center.

The purpose statement in the first example exemplifies a good fit between the purpose statement and the study methods. Correlation methods measure the direction and strength of a relationship; they are not appropriate for assessing cause and effect. The purpose statement in the second example does not have a good fit with this method because this statement indicates the researchers intend to determine a causal relationship between the variables. Example 2 would be better served with a quantitative, experimental design.

Differentiating Research Problem Statements and Research Purpose Statements

Research problem statements are declarations of disparity (why); research purpose statements are declarations of intent (what). Although problem statements and purpose statements clarify and support each other, they represent different levels of the deductive process, the process of moving from a general focus or interest to the development of a specific research question. As researchers identify problems, explore disparities or gaps, and develop problem and purpose statements, the focus of the research narrows, increasing feasibility.

Although problem and purpose statements for quantitative and qualitative research have many characteristics in common, they have some dissimilarity as well. Quantitative problem and purpose statements are generally detailed, based in previous literature, and outline the variables, populations, and settings to be studied (Burns & Grove, 2008; Polit & Beck, 2009). Qualitative problem and purpose statements are more general and allow for the flexibility that is characteristic of an emergent design (Burns & Grove, 2008; Polit & Beck, 2009). It remains important for a clear problem to be identified and a purpose statement to be articulated before research design begins. Tables 4.4 and 4.5 provide examples of problem and purpose statements for selected qualitative and quantitative research designs.

Developing the Research Question

The problem statement is a general review of why a particular research study is necessary; the purpose statement gives an overview of the intent of the study. Neither of these is

Table 4.4

Problem and Purpose Statements from Qualitative Research Studies

Design	General Focus or Interest	Problem and Purpose Statements
Ethnography	▪ Culture ▪ Empirical research report ▪ Experiences ▪ Nursing ▪ Patient-centered care ▪ Patients ▪ Trauma	**Title:** Professional Nursing Culture on a Trauma Unit: Experiences of Patients and Staff (Tutton, Seers, & Langstaff, 2008) **Problem Statement:** "For many patients, a traumatic event that leads to hospitalization has a major effect on their lives. . . . Hospitalization, although only a small part of recovery, has the potential to lay the foundations for future health and well-being. Therefore, it is important to understand the processes that facilitate or hamper patients' progress towards recovery" (p. 146). **Purpose Statement:** "The aim of the study was to explore patient and staff experiences of being on a trauma unit" (p. 146).
Grounded theory	▪ Community ▪ District nursing ▪ Dying patients ▪ Emotional support ▪ Palliative care	**Title:** Bridging Worlds: Meeting the Emotional Needs of Dying Patients (Law, 2009) **Problem Statement:** "In this study, it is acknowledged that nurses do provide supportive interventions but few studies have examined specifically the emotional aspects of nursing care" (p. 2632). **Purpose Statement:** "The aim of this study was to develop a grounded theory to explain how district nurses meet the emotional needs of dying patients in the community" (p. 2632).
Phenomenological	▪ Access to health care ▪ Homeless health care ▪ Qualitative study	**Title:** Experiences of Homeless People in the Health Care Delivery System: A Descriptive Phenomenological Study (Martins, 2008) **Problem Statement:** "This qualitative literature review shows growing data about the health problems of homeless people and issues of access to care; little is known about the experience of being ill while homeless and the experience of receiving health care services from the perspective of homeless people, particularly in the United States" (p. 432). **Purpose Statement:** "This qualitative study looked at the health care experience through the eyes of the homeless person using descriptive phenomenology, a valuable method for nursing research" (p. 432).

Research question: A question that outlines the primary components that will be studied and guides the design and methodology of the study.

prescriptive enough to give specific guidance to the design and methodology of the study. For this, a focused research question is necessary. The research question is the final step prior to beginning research design, and it outlines the primary components that will be studied. In some cases, the research question is analogous to the purpose statement, but constructed as a question instead of a statement. Questions that are clear, simple, and straightforward provide direction for subsequent design decisions and enable the researcher to focus the research process. Examples follow of research questions from a published study:

1. What are the learning needs of women with cesarean birth in the two weeks following hospital discharge?

Table 4.5

Problem and Purpose Statements from Quantitative Research Studies

Design	General Focus or Interest	Problem and Purpose Statements
Correlation	▪ Self-esteem ▪ Stress ▪ Coping ▪ Eating behavior ▪ Depressive mood ▪ Adolescent	**Title:** The Relationships Among Self-Esteem, Stress, Coping, Eating Behavior, and Depressive Mood in Adolescents (Martyn-Nemeth, Penckofer, Gulanick, Velsor-Friedrich, & Bryant, 2009) **Problem Statement:** "The relationships among self-esteem, stress, social support, coping, eating behavior, and depressive mood have not been examined simultaneously, nor has coping been examined as a mediator of this process" (p. 97). **Purpose Statement:** "The purpose of this study was to investigate relationships among self-esteem, stress, social support, and coping, and to test a model of their effects on unhealthy eating behavior and depressive mood in adolescents" (p. 97).
Descriptive	▪ Clinical effectiveness ▪ Evidence-based practice ▪ Institutional culture ▪ Management ▪ Nursing ▪ Organizational context ▪ Questionnaire	**Title:** Nurses' Perceptions of Evidence-Based Nursing Practice (Koehn & Lehman, 2008) **Problem Statement:** "Recent literature has reported substantial gaps between research and nursing practice . . . and has identified barriers that prevent the translation of evidence to clinical practice. . . . Only a few studies have examined the impact of organizational culture or context on the process of implementing EBP. . . . As there is also limited research on appropriate strategies for implementing EBP . . . it is best to consider using an active approach with multiple methods. Thus, it would be prudent to consider the characteristics and perceptions of nurses within an organization prior to developing an implementation plan" (p. 210). **Purpose Statement:** "The aim of this study was to investigate Registered Nurses' (RNs') perceptions, attitudes, and knowledge/skills associated with EBP" (p. 210).
Experimental	▪ Nursing practice ▪ Nursing practice environment ▪ Patient comfort rounds ▪ Patient satisfaction ▪ Pilot study	**Title:** Measuring the Effect of Patient Comfort Rounds on Practice Environment and Patient Satisfaction: A Pilot Study (Gardner, Woollett, Daly, & Richardson, 2009) **Problem Statement:** "Interventions involving 1- or 2-hourly nursing care rounds have been tested in pilot studies and larger studies and have been found to reduce call bell usage and improve patient safety and reported satisfaction. The specific concept of patient comfort rounds . . . has not been systematically trialed" (p. 288). **Purpose Statement:** "The aim of this pilot study was to test the effect of a model of practice that optimized the role of the assistant in nursing (AIN) in skill mix" (p. 288).

2. What are the physical needs of women with cesarean birth in the two weeks following discharge?

3. What nursing interventions can help mothers attain optimal health in the post-discharge period after cesarean birth? (Weiss et al., 2009, p. 2941)

As questions are refined, they should be critiqued continuously. The simple act of writing the question down and asking for input from colleagues may help to focus and refine the question. Does it make sense? Is it logical? Is this question important for clinical care? Could there be practical benefits from this research? This kind of feedback can help the nurse researcher generate a strong research question that provides guidance for subsequent research design and methodology. The time invested in carefully constructing the final research question is well worth the effort; it provides a foundation for the remaining decisions that must be made about the research process.

The Elements of a Good Research Question

Two guides are helpful in developing a good research question. One of them is described by the acronym *PICO*, which outlines the elements of a good quantitative question. PICO stands for population, intervention, comparison, and outcome. Using preoperative education for short-stay patients undergoing prostatectomy as an example, a research question based on PICO might look like this:

- *Population:* In radical prostatectomy patients staying in the hospital one day after surgery . . .
- *Intervention:* Does customized preoperative teaching . . .
- *Comparison:* Compared to standard preoperative teaching . . .
- *Outcomes:* Lead to better pain control as measured by a visual analog scale?

The qualitative research question is less prescriptive and outlines, in a general way, the phenomenon to be studied and the people who can best inform the question. The researcher defines the general boundaries of the inquiry, but even these are subject to change. The study is begun with a general question in mind, but the researcher is flexible enough to change the particulars of the question if the information that is gathered makes it relevant to do so. Measurements, interventions, and comparison groups are irrelevant in qualitative research, and so are not parts of the qualitative question. Specification of outcomes may be incorporated into the qualitative question, but are not necessary elements. Qualitative questions may actually evolve over the course of the study, and so are reported in detail only after the study is complete.

It can be seen that the elements of the research question are very similar to those in the purpose statement. The primary distinction is in format—a purpose statement is a statement, whereas a research question is stated as a question. In addition, the research question often spells out the outcome in a statement such as "as measured by the Wong Faces Pain Scale," and so gives more specificity to what is to be measured.

Another acronym—the FINER model—gives guidance in the appraisal of a question. It gives the nurse researcher a framework for evaluating the desirable characteristics of a good question:

- *Feasible:* Adequate subjects, technical expertise, time, and money are available; the scope is narrow enough for study.
- *Interesting:* The question is interesting to the investigator.

- *Novel:* The study confirms or refutes previous finding, or provides new findings.
- *Ethical:* The study cannot cause unacceptable risk to participants and does not invade privacy.
- *Relevant:* The question is relevant to scientific knowledge, clinical and health policy, or future research directions.

Once the question is carefully defined, then the link to design elements often becomes obvious. If not, then the question may require more specificity about the population, intervention, or outcomes. These three elements of the question will later provide guidance in the selection of a sample, the procedures, and the measurements.

The Link Between Questions and Design

As the research question is focused, it will guide how the question will be answered. The question will lead to a sampling strategy (Who is the patient population?), an intervention protocol (What treatment is being tested?), and the outcomes measured (How will effect be demonstrated?) There are also direct links between the kind of words used in the question and the design that is used to answer it.

Descriptive Questions

Descriptive questions ask simple questions about what is happening in a defined population or situation. For example, a descriptive question is, "What are the characteristics of surgical patients reporting high satisfaction with pain management during their hospitalization?" Sometimes a descriptive study is called a hypothesis-generating study, as opposed to hypothesis-testing studies. Three general research questions are best answered with descriptive studies:

1. Studies that investigate resource allocation
2. Studies that identify areas for further research
3. Studies that provide informal diagnostic information

Most qualitative questions are answered with descriptive studies because qualitative study is generally descriptive of a single sample. The broad nature of a qualitative research question lends itself to a variety of methods, from interviews to focus groups to observation. The specific verbiage used in the qualitative question may guide design, but in general, the design emerges from the nature of the phenomenon under study, not the particular way in which the research question is written.

Analytic Questions

Analytic studies compare one or more interventions to specific outcomes. For example, the questions "What is the effectiveness of individual or group educational sessions for hip surgery patients?" and "Is breast cancer associated with high fat intake?" are answered with quantitative analysis. The objective of an analytic study is to see if there is a causal relationship between variables, so the research question reflects study of the effect of an intervention on one or more outcomes. Statistical procedures are used to see if a relationship would likely have occurred by chance alone. Analytic studies usually compare two or more groups.

Analytic question: A type of research question that is posed to compare one or more interventions to specific outcomes.
Correlation studies: Research designed to quantify the strength and the direction of the relationship of two variables in a single subject or the relationship between a single variable in two samples.
Prospective studies: Studies planned by the researcher for collection of primary data for the specific research and implemented in the future.
Retrospective study: A study conducted using data that have already been collected about events that have already happened. These secondary data were originally collected for a purpose other than the current research.

Analytic questions are not limited to prospective studies, however. Comparison studies—sometimes called contemporary comparison, causal comparison, or retrospective studies—investigate the differences between groups that are formed based on the presence or absence of a shared characteristic. A question that reflects studying two groups for similarities or differences in specified characteristics is answered with comparison studies. The question "What are the differences in symptoms of myocardial infarction between men and women?" is answered with a comparison study. Comparison studies are needed when the research question is focused on a variable that cannot be practically or ethically manipulated, such as exposure to a risk factor or the diagnosis of a specific disease.

Questions that focus on associations or relationships are generally answered with correlation studies. Technically classified as descriptive studies, correlation studies focus on the relationships between two variables in the same population (for example, height and weight) or between the same variable in two populations (for example, the height of fathers and sons). Research questions focused on predicting one variable given the presence of another (for example, Can the height of the son be predicted if we know the height of the father?) are answered with a type of correlation study called a regression analysis.

Questions that are written in future tense will be answered with prospective studies. Interventions, data collection, and outcomes happen after subjects are enrolled. Examples of prospective studies are clinical trials and cohort studies. Prospective studies are indicated by research questions that focus on conditions that occur often and with relatively short follow-up periods. These two criteria are necessary so that sufficient numbers of eligible individuals can be followed for a reasonable period of time.

If a research question is written in past tense, it will be a retrospective study. All events of interest have already occurred and data are generated from records of the past (secondary data) or by asking subjects to recall events. Retrospective studies are less expensive than

---

Some Well-Done Questions

Zayac and Finch (2009) had several questions they wanted to answer in their review of the literature regarding adaptations required of recipients of implanted cardioverter-defibrillators (ICDs). Instead of constructing a complex, multi-concept question, they relied on simpler questions that were direct and descriptive: Do recipients of ICDs experience physical adaptation stress? Do recipients of ICDs experience psychological adaptation stress? Do themes expressed indicate a need for interventions that could facilitate postimplantation adjustment? Note that these authors made explicit the phenomenon of interest (adaptation) and the population (patients with ICDs).

Source: Zayac, S., & Finch, N. (2009). Recipients of implanted cardioverter-defibrillators actual and perceived adaptation: A review of the literature. *Journal of the American Academy of Nurse Practitioners, 21*(10), 549–556.

prospective studies and are often good starting points for exploratory research questions. Retrospective studies are far more effective when the research question involves a rare event because patient records of rare events are generally available even when there are few subjects to recruit.

Analytic studies are logical for questions answered with numbers or with measurements. These quantitative studies involve testing research questions using statistical analysis. Although research questions are not directly testable with numbers, their transformed version—the hypothesis—is subject to numerical analysis. It is important, then, to translate quantitative research questions into hypothesis statements that lend themselves to statistical analysis.

From Question to Hypothesis

Just as the research question guides the design of a study, the hypothesis guides the statistical analysis. The way a hypothesis is written will determine what tests are run, what outcome is expected, and how conservative the results are. A hypothesis is a restatement of the research question in a form that can be analyzed statistically for significance. For example, the research question "What is the association of environmental factors and reactive airway disease in otherwise healthy adults?" can be rewritten as a hypothesis as "There is no association between environmental factors and reactive airway disease in otherwise healthy adults." Although stating there is no expected relationship might seem a counterintuitive way to start a research analysis, it is, in fact, the only way that statistical significance can be measured. Although we cannot ever be sure that a relationship exists, we can calculate the probability it does not. Testing a null hypothesis in effect tells us how much uncertainty there is in the statistical conclusions, so the researcher can judge if it is within an acceptable range.

> **Hypothesis:** A restatement of the research question in a form that can be analyzed statistically for significance.

> **gray matter**
>
> Two essential aspects of a good hypothesis are
> - A statement of an expected relationship (or lack of one)
> - An identification of a direction of interest

There are two aspects that make a good hypothesis: the statement of an expected relationship (or, the lack of a relationship) and an identified direction of interest. A null hypothesis states there is no difference between groups whereas an alternative hypothesis would specify an expected difference between groups. In either case, the relationship between variables is defined. A second consideration is directionality. A nondirectional hypothesis is one that means the researcher is interested in a change in any direction, good or bad. In other words, a positive or negative association would be of interest. If we were testing a drug for hypertension, a nondirectional hypothesis would indicate we were interested in reductions in blood pressure, but we would also be interested in whether a rise in blood pressure occurred. Sometimes called two-sided hypotheses, these are appropriate for exploratory research questions or randomized trials of interventions. These are more rigorous tests than directional hypotheses.

Directional hypotheses, or one-sided tests, are interested only in one direction of change. These are appropriate for research questions in which there is a great

> **Null hypothesis:** A statement of the research question that declares there is no difference between groups.
> **Nondirectional hypothesis:** A two-sided statement of the research question that is interested in change in any direction.
> **Directional hypothesis:** A one-sided statement of the research question that is interested in only one direction of change.

Table 4.6

Examples of Hypotheses

Research Question	Null Hypotheses	Alternative, Nondirectional Hypotheses	Alternative, Directional Hypotheses
Do mean minutes of exercise per week differ between cardiac rehabilitation patients who have exercise equipment at home and patients who go to a gym to exercise?	H_0: There will be no difference in mean minutes of exercise per week between cardiac rehabilitation patients who have exercise equipment at home and patients who must travel to the rehabilitation center to exercise.	H_0: The mean minutes of exercise per week will be different for cardiac rehabilitation patients who have exercise equipment at home and patients who must travel to the rehabilitation center to exercise.	H_0: Cardiac rehabilitation patients who have exercise equipment at home will exercise more minutes per week than patients who have to go to the rehabilitation center to exercise.
	H_0: $\mu_1 = \mu_2$	H_0: $\mu_1 \neq \mu_2$	H_0: $\mu_1 > \mu_2$
Does the introduction of bar coding on a patient care unit result in lower medication error rates when compared to patient care units without bar coding?	H_0: There will be no difference in the medication error rate between units that do and do not have bar coding.	H_0: There will be a difference in the medication error rate between units that do and do not have bar coding.	H_0: Units with bar coding will have a lower medication error rate than units without bar coding.
	H_0: $\pi_1 = \pi_2$	H_0: $\pi_1 \neq \pi_2$	H_0: $\pi_1 < \pi_2$

deal of literature or empirical support for an existing relationship. Directional hypothesis tests are more liberal than nondirectional ones. Examples of null, alternative, directional, and nondirectional research hypotheses appear in Table 4.6.

Reading Research for Evidence-Based Practice

The primary reason for critically reading problem statements is to identify concerns or problems and to understand the disparities or gaps between what is known and what still needs to be known about concepts. A secondary reason is to determine the significance of the concerns or problems. The primary reason for critically reading purpose statements is to identify the variables and study design within the context and scope of specific populations and settings. A secondary reason is to determine feasibility and fit.

Problem and purpose statements, as well as research questions, should be stated early in a research report. The problem statement may be inferred and incorporated into the introduction and review of the need for the study. Often the context of the problem appears in the literature review. The purpose statement should be explicit and near the beginning of the study. It may be alternatively called "objectives," "aims," or "goals." The research question itself should be specific and clear early in the study. The study may or may not report hypotheses, even if it is clearly quantitative and experimental in design. If they are reported, hypotheses often appear in the results section with their associated statistical conclusion.

Using Research in Evidence-Based Practice

By understanding problems, their related concepts or variables, the definition of the population, and the context for a research study, the nurse may be able to generalize the findings to his or her specific nursing practice. The best evidence may then be used to design changes to improve processes and outcomes.

Literature searches may produce hundreds or even thousands of applicable and non-applicable results. To easily and quickly identify applicable studies look for the problem statements and the purpose statements. Problem statements and purpose statements provide readers with the focused context and scope required to generalize research findings to their own nursing practice and establish and support evidenced-based practice within their organizations.

Creating Evidence for Practice

Finding and developing research problems begins with a general concern or focus about a subject or topic. Subjects and topics consist of broad categories and may include examples such as hospital-acquired infections, pain management, patient falls, physiological monitoring, and pressure ulcer prevention. As the process evolves, a problem is identified.

Checklist for Critically Reading Problem Statements

Development
✔ Deductive narrowing from general focus or interest

Articulation
✔ Stated or inferred?
✔ Placement in written report (helpful and logical)
✔ Sentence structure (question or statement)
✔ Concern (disparity or gap)

Significance
✔ Develops, expands, or validates nursing knowledge
✔ Develops, expands, or validates conceptual models or theoretical frameworks
✔ Improves patient care, staff member, and/or organizational processes and/or outcomes

Checklist for Critically Reading Purpose Statements

Development

✔ Deductive narrowing from problem statement

Articulation

✔ Stated or inferred
✔ Placement in written report (helpful and logical)
✔ Sentence structure (statement)
✔ Verb (biased or unbiased)
✔ Design described
✔ Variables described
✔ Population defined
✔ Setting specified

Feasibility

✔ Required resources (people, time, money, equipment, materials, and facilities)
✔ Ethical issues (people and facilities)

Fit

✔ Between purpose statement and design
✔ Between purpose statement and conceptual models or theoretical frameworks

Research problems consist of narrower categories and may include examples such as ventilator-associated pneumonia, patient-controlled analgesia, blood pressure monitoring, and use of specialty beds to prevent skin breakdown.

Once a problem is identified, the gap between what is known about the problem and what remains to be known about the problem is examined. Special consideration should be given to exploring the gap within the context and scope (population and setting) of the problem. This gap examination occurs primarily through a literature review. Research activities should be focused on narrowing or filling in the gaps. After the gap has been identified, the problem statement(s), purpose statement(s), and research question(s) are developed. The problem statement indicates the focus or interest of the study and raises concerns and questions (disparities and gaps) about general concepts. The purpose statement indicates why the study is being conducted and suggests methods for examining the concepts or variables, and the relationships between them, within a specific population and setting. The research question is a rewording of the purpose statement into a question that suggests methods for examining the concepts or variables and the relationships between them.

Actions that are necessary to create a good research study include a thorough examination of the process traditionally associated with identifying and developing research problems:

- A general focus or interest
- Identification of a concern or problem

Where to Look

Where to look for information about the research question or hypothesis:

- The research question may be explicitly stated in the research abstract but is commonly only implied by the title of the article, purpose statement, or objectives for the study.
- Ideally, the question is discussed at the beginning of the article, often at the end of the introduction. When it is stated early, it is followed by evidence from the literature review to support why this question is important to investigate further. It may be written as a statement instead of a question. If not at the beginning, look for the question at the end of the literature review.
- The null and alternate hypotheses are often found in the methods section where statistical methods are discussed, along with the rationale for the statistical tests used to test the hypotheses. Hypotheses are typically easy to find and are explicitly identified as such.
- Sometimes a separate section is created for a formal statement of the problem, the purpose of the study, and the research question. It may be labeled "Purpose," "Aims," or "Objectives." The research question may similarly have its own heading.
- If the researcher used any inferential statistical tests, which most quantitative studies do, then there were hypotheses, whether they are stated or not. Sometimes the reader is left to infer what the hypotheses were based on the tests that were reported.

SKILL Builder | Write Stronger Research Questions

The most important part of the research process is getting the question right. How the problem is stated determines what measures will be used, what data will be collected, the kind of analysis that will be used, and the conclusions that can be drawn. It is worth the time, then, to carefully consider how this element of the research study is developed. A thoughtful process does not necessarily mean a complicated process, however. Here are some simple suggestions for creating strong research questions:

- Answer the "why" question first. With a solid understanding of the reason for the study, the specifics of the research question are easier to identify.
- Review the literature before finalizing the question. Do not hesitate to replicate the question of a research study that accomplishes similar goals. It is flattering to a researcher—even established, well-known ones—to have their work replicated. Be sure to give credit where credit is due.
- Focus, focus, focus. Refine the research question, mull it over for a bit, and then refine it again. The effort spent to get the question just right will be worth it, because there will be less confusion later as to how to answer the question.
- That said, do not wait until the question is perfect to begin the design of the study. The question is, to some extent, a work in progress as the specifics of the research unfold. The question can, and likely will, be revised as new information, resources, and constraints come to light.
- Keep the research questions focused; do not include more than one major concept per question. Compound questions are hard to study and make it harder to isolate the effects of a single independent variable. Multiple research questions should be used instead of multiple parts of a single question.

For More Depth and Detail

For a more in-depth look at the concepts in this chapter, try these references:

Beckman, L., & Earthman, C. (2010). Developing the research question and study design. *Support Line, 32*(1), 3–7.

Biau, D., Jolles, B., & Porcher. R. (2010). P value and the theory of hypothesis testing: An explanation for new researchers. *Clinical Orthopaedics and Related Research, 468*(3), 885–892.

Burns, N., & Grove, S. (2008). *The practice of nursing research: Appraisal, synthesis, and generation of evidence* (6th ed.). St. Louis: Elsevier.

Campo, M., & Lichtman, S. (2008). Interpretation of research in physical therapy: Limitations of null hypothesis significance testing. *Journal of Physical Therapy Education, 229*(1), 43–48.

Harvey, B., & Lang, T. (2010). Hypothesis testing, study power, and sample size. *Chest, 138*(3), 734–737.

Lehman, E., & Romano, J. (2010). *Testing statistical hypotheses.* Philadelphia: Springer.

Lipowski, E. (2008). Developing great research questions. *American Journal of Health-System Pharmacy, 65*(17), 1667–1670.

Mantzoukas, S. (2008). Facilitating research students in formulating qualitative research questions. *Nurse Education Today, 28*(3), 371–377.

Pereira, S., & Leslie, G. (2009). Hypothesis testing. *Australian Critical Care, 22*(4), 187–191.

Weber, R., & Cobaugh, D. (2008). Developing and executing an effective research plan. *American Journal of Health System Pharmacy, 65*(21), 2058–2065.

Wood, M., & Ross-Kerr, B. (2010). *Basic steps in planning nursing research: From question to proposal* (7th ed.). Sudbury, MA: Jones & Bartlett.

- Exploration of the disparity or gap between what is known and what still needs to be known
- Development of the problem statement
- Development of the purpose statement
- Development of the research question

Summary of Key Concepts

- Finding and developing significant problems for research are critical to improving processes and outcomes for patients, staff members, and organizations. For both the researcher and the reader, problem statements, purpose statements, and research questions serve to guide and direct research activities.
- The evolution of a research problem from a general topic of interest to the articulation of a problem statement and a purpose statement serves to narrow the focus of the research into a researchable question.

CRITICAL APPRAISAL **EXERCISE**

Retrieve the following full text article from the Cumulative Index to Nursing and Allied Health Literature or similar search database:

Halcomb, E., Griffiths, R., & Fernandez, R. (2008). The role of patient isolation and compliance with isolation practices in the control of nosocomial MRSA in acute care. *International Journal of Evidence-Based Healthcare, 6*(2), 206–224.

Review the article, looking for information about the problem and purpose statements and the research question. Consider the following appraisal questions in your critical review of these elements of the research article:

1. Is there evidence of deductive narrowing (from general focus to a question) or inductive thinking (from an observation to an overall purpose)? Is it an appropriate approach?
2. Is the problem statement clearly articulated? Is it a question or a statement?
3. Does the problem meet the FINER criteria?
4. Does the research question have all of the PICO elements present?
5. Discuss whether and how this study will contribute to nursing practice.
6. Evaluate what type of research design would answer this question.

- Subjects or topics that are too broad become problematic for researchers because methodological complexities increase, experienced researchers or consultants are required, and resource demands (for example, money, people, and time) increase.
- Sources for researchable problems include clinical practice, educational institutions, focus groups, frameworks and models, professional literature review, performance improvement activities, research, research priorities, and social issues.
- Research problem statements are declarations of disparity: the difference (gap) between what is known and what needs to be known about a topic. They are written as questions or statements and contain clear, concise, and well-defined components (disparities or gaps and concepts).
- Research purpose statements are declarations of intent: what is going to be studied, how it is going to be studied, who is going to be studied, and the context for the study. They are written as declarative, objective statements and contain clear, concise, and well-defined components (design, variables, population, and setting).
- Feasibility is determined by analyzing the strengths, weaknesses, opportunities, and threats (SWOT) of the purpose statement components. Performing the SWOT analysis will indicate if the research study is researchable or nonresearchable.
- There should be a good fit between the design suggested in the purpose statement and the methods used in the research study. There should also be a good fit between the research question and the specifics of the research design, sampling strategy, and measurement.
- Qualitative problem and purpose statements, as well as research questions, are generally broader, more vague, and less prescriptive than those created for quantitative studies. This is because qualitative designs are emergent and may be revised frequently as the study unfolds.

- Research questions for quantitative studies can be developed using the PICO guide by specifying population, intervention, comparison, and outcome. All elements will not necessarily be in every question, because PICO guidelines are most appropriate for experimental designs.
- The FINER criteria—feasible, interesting, novel, ethical, and relevant—serve as a good basis for analysis of the quality of a researchable question. The research question should have an identifiable link to the research design.

For a full suite of assignments and additional learning activities, use the access code located in the front of your book to visit this exclusive website: http://go.jblearning.com/houser. If you do not have an access code, you can obtain one at the site.

References

Burns, N., & Grove, S. (2008). *The practice of nursing research: Appraisal, synthesis, and generation of evidence* (6th ed.). St. Louis: Elsevier.

Gardner, G., Woollett, K., Daly, N., & Richardson, B. (2009). Measuring the effect of patient comfort rounds on practice environment and patient satisfaction: A pilot study. *International Journal of Nursing Practice, 15*(4), 287–293.

Halcomb, E., Griffiths, R., & Fernandez, R. (2008). The role of patient isolation and compliance with isolation practices in the control of nosocomial MRSA in acute care. *International Journal of Evidence-Based Healthcare, 6*(2), 206–224.

Koehn, M., & Lehman, K. (2008). Nurses' perceptions of evidence-based nursing practice. *Journal of Advanced Nursing, 62*(2), 209–215.

Law, R. (2009). Bridging worlds: Meeting the emotional needs of dying patients. *Journal of Advanced Nursing, 65*(12), 2630–2641.

Martins, D. (2008). Experiences of homeless people in the health care delivery system: A descriptive phenomenological study. *Public Health Nursing, 25*(5), 420–430.

Martyn-Nemeth, P., Penckofer, S., Gulanick, M., Velsor-Friedrich, B., & Bryant, F. (2009). The relationships among self-esteem, stress, coping, eating behavior, and depressive mood in adolescents. *Research in Nursing and Health, 32*(1), 96–109.

Polit, D., & Beck, C. (2009). *Essentials of nursing research: Appraising evidence for nursing practice* (7th ed.). Philadelphia: Lippincott Williams & Wilkins.

Tutton, E., Seers, K., & Langstaff, D. (2008). Professional nursing culture on a trauma unit: Experiences of patients and staff. *Journal of Advanced Nursing, 61*(2), 145–153.

Weiss, M., Fawcett, J., & Aber, C. (2009). Adaptation, postpartum concerns, and learning needs in the first two weeks after caesarean birth. *Journal of Clinical Nursing, 18*(21), 2938–2948.

Zayac, S., & Finch, N. (2009). Recipients of implanted cardioverter-defibrillators actual and perceived adaptation: A review of the literature. *Journal of the American Academy of Nurse Practitioners, 21*(10), 549–556.

chapter 5

The Successful Literature Review

 CHAPTER OBJECTIVES

The study of this chapter will help the learner to

- Discuss the rationale for conducting a thorough search of the literature.
- Describe the types of literature that are used as support for a research study.
- Relate the steps of a systematic search strategy for a research problem.
- Compare the literature search for a qualitative study to that of a quantitative study.
- Contrast the literature search for research to that of a practice guideline.
- Critically appraise the literature review section of a research article.
- Reflect on the ways that research literature can be used as evidence for nursing practice.

 KEY TERMS

Citation analysis

Concept map

Database (bibliographic database)

Empirical literature

Information literacy

Journal impact factor

Literature review

Open access

Primary sources

Search strategy

Search terms

Secondary sources

Seminal work

Theoretical literature

An Introduction to the Literature Review

The literature review is a critical component of the research process. It provides an in-depth analysis of recently published research findings in specifically identified areas of interest. Today's nursing professionals must function in an atmosphere that produces best practices when rendering patient care. To provide for best practice, researchers must build a foundation of the

> **Literature review:** A critical component of the research process that provides an in-depth analysis of recently published research findings in specifically identified areas of interest. The review informs the research question and guides development of the research plan.

Voices from the Field

My interest in examining hypothermia as part of a protocol to treat traumatic brain injuries (TBI) in children began because of a conference presentation and some journal articles I had read. These articles focused on using hypothermia in the treatment of adult traumatic head injuries, but I thought it might apply in kids. When I did a more thorough review of the literature, I found several excellent randomized controlled trials (RCTs) in adults that yielded promising results. However, as I focused the search on children, I discovered only observational studies and no randomized trials to evaluate if hypothermia could really help children with TBI.

The children's hospital where I was doing my Pediatric Intensive Care Medicine Fellowship was a Level 1 Trauma Center, so children throughout the region who had traumatic head injuries were admitted on a regular basis. Although our mortality outcomes were good, and our morbidity outcomes were similar to those experienced in similar centers nationwide, my neurosurgery colleagues and I felt there were things we could do to help improve our morbidity outcomes. TBI initiates several metabolic processes that can injure the brain further if not held in check. We knew that one possible way was to minimize adverse brain metabolic processes triggered by the brain injury during the first 48 hours after the brain injury. The literature on adults showed evidence that hypothermia may limit some of these devastating metabolic responses.

My first goal was to determine a research design that would answer my question, "Does a course of moderate hypothermia (32 to 24°C) in pediatric patients, within the first 48 hours after a TBI, result in decreased severity and duration of intracranial hypertension?" As I searched the literature, I realized we needed to design a hypothermia protocol for children that had some similarities to the adult TBI hypothermia studies. This protocol would also need to be safe for children and address their unique needs. I realized that in order to truly understand the impact of hypothermia on morbidity, we would need to collect data beyond the ICU stay, possibly up to a year after the injury.

I wanted to build on existing research study designs so others could compare their outcomes with mine. This helped me build on what was known instead of starting from scratch. My intensivist colleagues and I made sure our existing practice was based on the highest level of evidence available.

There were challenging aspects of the literature review. It took a lot of time and it was sometimes tough to get to full text articles. I also realized that it was good to get colleagues from other organizations involved, including primary investigators of other similar studies. They helped point me to key articles and shared valuable experiences from their ongoing studies that were not yet published.

Our resulting RCT answered the questions we asked, with a total of 21 patients enrolled in the study, 11 in the normothermia group and 10 in the hypothermia group. Hypothermia is safe to use in pediatric TBI patients and it does decrease cerebral hypertension.

Abhik Biswas, MD
Pediatric Intensivist

best evidence—proof of what is and is not known on the topic under investigation. Once the challenge of identifying the research problem has been resolved, the researcher needs to ascertain the knowledge that has been established on the topic in question. Sources for this best evidence come from primary and secondary literature resources. We are in a time of unprecedented access to information. As a result, researchers have a plethora of sources to search—print materials, electronic databases, symposia proceedings, and the Internet. The volume of accessible information does not ensure its quality, however. It is essential that nurses acquire the skills to retrieve and evaluate relevant, high quality information that can answer their practice and research questions.

The Rationale for the Literature Review

Literature reviews add credence to the researcher's assertions of the importance of the topic proposed for investigation. It is the responsibility of the researcher to determine what other researchers have discovered on the same topic. A solid research plan is substantiated by the findings of others. A thorough literature review may turn up studies that can be replicated, instruments that have been standardized and tested for research use, or procedures that can be adapted to the proposed study. The literature often reveals an appropriate theoretical framework and, at a minimum, helps the researcher understand what is already known about the topic under study.

The literature review enhances the body of knowledge on a particular issue or may establish that there is a paucity of knowledge on the subject in question. Although many researchers are discouraged by a lack of published findings on a specific topic, this may in fact be a good sign. A gap in the knowledge of a professional issue is an area that is ripe for exploratory and interventional study and could signal that the nurse is pioneering a new issue for investigations. It also increases the likelihood of publication and can serve as the basis for advanced academic study. Either way, the literature review is the first step in evaluating the importance of a research question and potential methods for its study.

gray matter

A literature review serves the following purposes:

- Adding credence to the importance of the topic proposed for investigation
- Providing studies that can be replicated, instruments that have been standardized and tested, or procedures that can be adapted
- Revealing appropriate theoretical frameworks
- Enhancing the body of knowledge or establishing the lack of published findings on a subject

The Purpose, Importance, and Scope of the Literature Review

The appropriate literature search provides a rich basis for establishing the importance of the study, verifies that the study has not already been performed by other researchers, clarifies the issues that are directly related to the research question, and reveals an appropriate theoretical framework. A synthesis of the existing literature is important because, otherwise, the study will not contribute to the overall body of knowledge related to the phenomenon of interest. It is critical to frame a study within its historical and clinical context to establish the uniqueness of the current study and to encourage efficiency in study design.

Although the researcher needs to provide substantial literature support that directly relates to the problem, the temptation to include everything must be resisted. Researchers can find themselves in a state of "analysis paralysis" when they fail to proceed to action planning for fear that they may miss one last piece of literature. A researcher must choose when to stop searching. This point may be obvious: The researcher may consciously note that nothing new is being revealed, or literature sources may simply be exhausted. If too many articles are found, the researcher may want to establish criteria for inclusion and/or methodological soundness and review only those articles that meet the criteria. The scope of a scholarly research literature review will obviously be more in-depth than one for a small bedside science project. Likewise, a study for a practice journal may have fewer references than one intended for a research journal. The type of study, the expectations of the readers, and the level of scholarly sophistication required will drive the scope of the literature review.

Types of Literature Used in the Review

Theoretical literature: Published conceptual models, frameworks, and theories that provide a basis for the researcher's belief system and for ways of thinking about the problem studied.

Empirical literature: Published works that demonstrate how theories apply to individual behavior or observed events.

Seminal work: A classic work of research literature that is more than 5 years old and is marked by its uniqueness and contribution to professional knowledge.

Multiple types of information are used to enhance the breadth and depth of the review. Two types of literature support research: theoretical and empirical. Theoretical literature includes published conceptual models, frameworks, and theories. The theoretical literature provides a basis for the researcher's belief system and a road map for ways to think about the problem under study. Empirical literature includes published works demonstrating how theories apply to individual behavior or observed events. Either type of literature may be accessible through multiple channels. Journal articles, books, conference proceedings, practice guidelines, and dissertations are some of the sources of theoretical and empirical literature.

Comprehensiveness in terms of both the time period reviewed and appropriate coverage of the subject matter is important. When a researcher investigates a new treatment protocol or medication efficacy, for example, he or she needs to delve into the literature to determine what other researchers have or have not discovered on the subject. This phase must determine if the planned study is an extension of previous research findings or if it will be groundbreaking. Rogers (2009) notes that it may take more than 10 years before evidence from research is incorporated into practice. This means research that is more than a few years old may refer to findings that are, in reality, much older. Researchers ponder how far back the literature review should delve; in general, 3 to 5 years is considered appropriate for a research review (LoBiondo-Wood & Haber, 2006).

gray matter

Scholarly literature includes the following sources:
- Periodicals
- Books
- Monographs
- Conference proceedings
- Practice guidelines
- Dissertations

There are exceptions to every rule. A seminal work in the research literature (one that is a classic in its field) may go back for many more years and is not bound by time. For example, the important findings of Marie Curie, Albert Einstein, Florence Nightingale, and Socrates are still referenced in the twenty-first century for their uniqueness and timeless knowledge. Trailblazers in the field of nursing theory will be remembered as seminal works in nursing. Likewise, literature supporting statistical treatments or measurement instruments may be from less recent sources, if one can ascertain that their relevance and desirable properties still exist.

A Review of the Evidence for a Research Problem

It is easy enough to say that the researcher should examine all sources of relevant information that are available to address the specific research question. The more difficult question is how to accomplish this search. In general, the literature review is guided by the research problem, the specific elements of the research question, and the researcher's experience. An explicit search strategy is helpful in ensuring that the literature search is comprehensive and unbiased. The search strategy involves deciding upon search terms and the specific sources of information (databases, journals, and books) that will be examined.

A solid literature search starts by identifying search terms that will serve as the foundation for the search strategy. These search terms may be words that are included in the problem statement, variables that appear in the research question, and the characteristics of the population of interest. Words from the PICO statement (population, intervention, comparison, outcome) can be used as a source of terms (Thabane, Thomas, Ye, & Paul, 2009). Boolean operators (AND, OR, and NOT) are then used to combine the search terms into a search statement. A detailed explanation of the use of Boolean operators appears later in this chapter. An example of a research question that has been broken down into search terms appears in **Table 5.1**. If a theoretical framework has been identified, then it will appear among the search terms as well.

> **Search strategy:** The identification of search terms and search statements that will be used in the literature review.
> **Search terms:** Words or phrases derived from elements in the problem statement, variables in the research question, characteristics of the population of interest, and the theoretical framework that are used to conduct the literature search.

Table 5.1

Search Terms Derived from Problem Statements and Research Questions

Problem Statement

Pediatric patients can have complications from the metabolic consequences of traumatic brain injury.

Relevant Search Terms

- Traumatic AND "brain injury"
- "Metabolic response" AND trauma
- Pediatric AND "brain injury"
- "Brain injury" AND children
- Hypothermia AND "brain injury"
- Hypothermia AND pediatric

Research Question

Do patients who use a bedside pedaler after bariatric surgery have the same postoperative length of stay as patients who ambulate?

Relevant Search Terms

- "Bariatric surgery" AND exercise
- Effects AND postoperative AND exercise
- Exercise AND "length of stay"
- Ambulation AND "length of stay"

The next step is to compile a list of all electronic databases that will be searched, a list of relevant books published on the subject, and a list of the most important journals that the researcher intends to hand search. These hand searches may seem unnecessary at a time when electronic databases are available to nearly every nurse, but the truth is that even experienced database searchers may have gaps in what they find (Hopewell, Clarke, Lefebvre, & Scherer, 2009). By examining the tables of contents from key journals over a 1- or 2-year period, researchers can be more certain that they have located the most recent, relevant sources of information on which to base a study.

These two elements—identifying search terms and sources of information—are determined up front (called *a priori*) to avoid researcher bias. This kind of bias may be completely unconscious, but it may lead a researcher to examine only those articles that support his or her point of view. Identifying a search strategy before the search begins can ensure that all the relevant literature—whether it supports or refutes the researcher's viewpoint—will be examined.

Concept map: A plan for literature review that identifies all relevant concepts that are pertinent to an individual topic or question.

A tool that the researcher can use to plan a literature review is called a **concept map**. Borrowed from the field of marketing, the concept map entails the identification of all the relevant concepts that are pertinent to an individual topic or question. An example of a concept map appears in **FIGURE 5.1**.

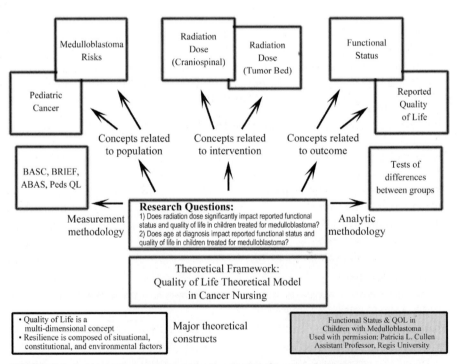

FIGURE 5.1 An Example of a Concept Map Used to Design a Search Strategy
Source: Functional Status and QOL in Children with Medulloblastoma. Used with permission: Patricia L. Cullen, Associate Professor, Regis University.

Primary sources are reports of original research authored by the researcher and published in a peer-reviewed research journal or scholarly book. Secondary sources include comments on and summaries of multiple research studies on one topic (for example, systematic reviews, meta-analyses, and meta-syntheses). Secondary sources may be based on the secondary author's interpretation of the primary work; it is necessary, then, to review primary sources whenever possible to ensure accuracy. Table 5.2 defines primary and secondary sources with examples and sources of each.

A Note About Open Access

Many databases and sources of literature are proprietary, meaning that the nurse or an organization must pay a fee to gain access to the database search engine or to full text articles online. Through the Internet, the latest information can be disseminated rapidly and relatively inexpensively to a worldwide audience. This technology has prompted a debate regarding open access to research results published in peer-reviewed journals, especially research that has been funded by governments using taxpayers' dollars. "Open-access (OA) literature is digital, online, free of charge, and free of most copyright and licensing restrictions" (Suber, 2007, para 1).

Researchers, authors, healthcare professions, scientists, and members of the public have been urging publishers of research to provide it freely on the public Internet and to permit any use of it (for example, reading, downloading, copying, distributing, printing, or passing articles as data to software). The Budapest Open Access Initiative (www.soros.org/openaccess/) met in 2001 to discuss ways in which the international community could accelerate and sustain open access. In the United States, the National Institutes of Health (NIH) Public Access Policy requires that peer-reviewed articles that are the result of research partially or fully funded by NIH (in other words, by taxpayers) must be submitted for electronic publication in the open access PubMed Central database within 12 months of the publication date of the article (U.S. Department of Health and Human Services, 2009). The Federal Research Public Access Act (FRPAA), which was introduced in 2009, would take this a step further, requiring open access within 6 months of publication in a peer-reviewed journal for research funded by any U.S. government agency with an extramural research budget of $100,000 or more (U.S. Library of Congress, 2009). The European Research Council (ERC) has adopted a similar policy (Lenzer, 2008). Updates on current public access issues may be found on the web site of the Alliance for Taxpayer Access (www.taxpayeraccess.org).

Although complete open access to research results is not yet here, there are sources that nurses and other healthcare professionals can use to access free evidence for practice. The National Institutes of Health operates a web site (www.guidelines.gov) that publishes a broad range of practice guidelines. Many universities and organizations are in the process of creating digital repositories of research, theses, and dissertations produced by their

Primary sources: Reports of original research authored by the researcher and published in a scholarly source such as a peer-reviewed research journal or scholarly book.

Secondary sources: Comments and summaries of multiple research studies on one topic such as systematic reviews, meta-analyses, and meta-syntheses, which are based on the secondary author's interpretation of the primary work.

Open access: Publication of material in a form that allows anyone to have free access to it.

Table 5.2

Primary and Secondary Sources of Information Retrieval

Primary

Definition

Resources that publish the findings of original research and other types of studies in their first and original form

Examples

- Journals
- Books
- Monographs
- Dissertations/theses

Potential Search Tools and Sources

- CINAHL
- MEDLINE
- PsychINFO
- Cochrane Library (Clinical Trials)
- National Guideline Clearinghouse (AHRQ)
- FIRSTConsult
- DISEASEDEX

Secondary

Definition

Resources that synthesize, summarize, or comment on original research

Examples

- Systematic reviews
- Meta-analyses
- Integrative reviews
- Qualitative synthesis
- Reviews of individual articles
- Clinical practice guidelines

Potential Search Tools and Sources

- CINAHL
- MEDLINE
- PsycINFO
- Cochrane Library (Cochrane Reviews)
- Guidelines.gov
- Professional association databases of practice guidelines
- Specialized databases containing secondary sources of literature

faculty and students (Goodfellow, 2009). Open access resources include the following web sites, which provide free access to many professional journals:

Journal Articles:

BioMed Central: www.biomedcentral.com

Directory of Open Access Journals (DOAJ): www.doaj.org

Public Library of Science (PLOS): www.plos.org

PubMed Central: www.pubmed.gov

Dissertations and Theses:

Networked Digital Library of Theses and Dissertations: www.ndltd.org

Although it may be difficult for a nurse to conduct a thorough, comprehensive literature review without access to proprietary databases, free research databases, including PubMed, Google Scholar, and the Cochrane Collaboration Reviews, are available and can serve as a basis to begin exploration of a topic. Using open access sources first may limit the amount of time the nurse researcher must spend at a library to access more expensive sources for database searches.

The Importance of Peer Review

One of the hallmarks of research is peer review. Scholarly works are those that have been subjected to the critical review provided by objective reviewers who are unaware of the author's name, credentials, or professional status. This ensures a thorough review of the research using objective standards without being influenced by the status of the researcher.

When a researcher submits his or her manuscript to a peer-reviewed (sometimes called refereed) professional journal, it is understood that it will be critically appraised by a team of reviewers who are experienced in the content and methodology reflected in the manuscript. This rigorous review process adds legitimacy to the findings reported in the study.

The peer review process itself, however, may not be a standard process. Quantitative research studies are generally submitted to a thorough review that focuses on potential sources of bias and error and that applies strict standards to the evaluation of methodology and design. Qualitative research, on the other hand, lends itself more appropriately to peer review that focuses on the efforts the author has made to ensure credibility and trustworthiness.

Researchers may prefer their research to be published in journals with a high impact factor. Citation analysis and journal impact factor are "quantitative metrics that are gaining increasing attention, perhaps because they are viewed as the easiest and most objective way to measure quality and impact of research. They can also be used to provide numeric data that can be used to rank researchers and the institutions in which those researchers work" (Cheek, Garnham, & Quan, 2006, p. 424). Citation analysis relies on the establishment of how often a researcher's articles are referred to in another researcher's research. Researchers gain status

Citation analysis: A way to measure quality and impact of research by noting how often a researcher's articles are referred to in another researcher's work.

Journal impact factor: A way to measure quality and impact of research by calculating a ratio of current citations of the journal to all the citations in the same time period.

when their work has been cited many times. Journal impact factor is defined as a ratio of the number of these current citations to all citations in the same publication period; some use this as a measure of journal quality.

Competencies for Information Literacy

Information literacy: The competencies necessary to access, retrieve, and analyze research evidence for application to nursing practice.

It is clearly important that nurses and nurse researchers alike possess the competencies necessary to access, retrieve, and analyze research evidence for their practice throughout their career. Information literacy is important for nurses to acquire because they must decipher the vast expanse of knowledge that is generated through healthcare research. As a result of cost-cutting measures, a number of organizations have closed their medical libraries, which makes it even more imperative that nursing students be proficient in locating and evaluating information that supports evidence-based practice before they leave school for the workplace. These skills can be mastered through repeated practice and application throughout the curriculum with feedback and instruction from the nursing faculty in partnership with the healthcare librarian (Leasure, Delise, Clifton, & Pascucci, 2009). When students graduate, they bring their information literacy skills to their organizations. Nurses are required to make patient care decisions on a daily basis, so they must be able to incorporate evidence-based research into their clinical nursing practice. Competent nurses today must possess lifelong learning and information literacy skills that include the following:

- Identifying and succinctly stating the question or problem to be researched
- Using the appropriate Internet databases, web sites of professional organizations, and other reliable resources for the retrieval of scholarly research and the best evidence
- Creating effective search strategies that yield relevant, current, research-based results
- Skill in critical thinking and analysis of problems, issues, and the evidence
- The ability to integrate evidence into practice
- Competency with computers and the Internet, word processing, spreadsheet analysis, databases, and new applications that are relevant to the job
- Motivation for lifelong learning

gray matter

A literature search for evidence-based nursing practice should be
- Focused on a clinical question.
- Limited to a time frame so the evidence is current.
- Applicable directly to nursing practice.

Searching the literature as support for a research project involves focusing on a research problem and identifying literature that forms a theoretical and conceptual basis for the planned project. Although the literature is focused on a single question, the search itself may be broad ranging and may involve research that is both directly and indirectly related to the research question. The goal of the search is to provide support and a context for the specific question under study.

Searching the literature specifically for evidence-based nursing practice is a process focused on a clinical question that is limited in

Table 5.3

Contrast of Literature Review for Research and for Practice Guideline Development

	For a Research Study	For Practice Guidelines
Conceptual basis	• Provides background and context for the particular study that is planned • Incorporates a theoretical framework • Specific to the research question	• Provides evidence that can be applied to a clinical problem • Focuses on application of research to practice • Specific to the clinical question
Type of evidence appraised	• Scholarly works that are published in peer-reviewed journals • Research reported in other peer-reviewed venues such as symposia, dissertations, and monographs	• Scientific works that are published in peer-reviewed journals • Systematic reviews, meta-analyses, and integrative reviews published in journals, professional associations, or other organizations • Opinions presented by expert panels or task forces
Critical appraisal skills used	• Critical appraisal of single-focused research reports	• Critical appraisal of single studies and aggregate research reports

time frame so the evidence is current and directly applicable to nursing practice. **Table 5.3** depicts some of the differences between a literature review for a research study and a literature review for the development of practice guidelines.

Reading the Literature Review Section

The literature review section of a research study provides rich information about the quality of the study and its potential for use as evidence for practice. Studies based on thoroughly searched and synthesized literature produce evidence that is more standard, easily aggregated, and likely to be valid. A well-done literature review section will support the hypothesis that the question is worth answering and provide implications for practice. It may provide a link to the theoretical basis of the question and provide support for the methods and procedures. The literature review should provide a logical argument, in essence, that builds a case for the importance of the study and its particular design.

The literature reviews for qualitative and quantitative research designs may be quite different. The biggest difference between the two is the timing of the literature review. Quantitative researchers conduct the literature review after the research question has been determined but before finalizing the research methods and design. On the other hand, qualitative researchers often conduct the literature review after the study has begun

Where to Look

A review of literature often appears throughout a published research article. Citations generally first appear in the introduction and provide information about the scope of the research problem, the importance of the problem, and why the problem is worthy of study.

The bulk of the literature review will be cited in the literature section. It usually follows the introduction, purpose, and research question and may be labeled straightforwardly as such. It may also be called "background" or "context of the problem." On occasion it might not be a separate section but may be embedded into the introductory paragraphs.

Literature may also be cited to support the measurements that were used, the intervention protocol, or the data analysis procedures. The literature is often referred to during discussion and conclusions; it is here that the authors compare their findings to the findings of previous studies. In discussing the findings of the study, the researcher should identify results that confirm previous studies, clear up contradictions, or highlight inconsistencies with the findings of other studies. Each citation in the text should be linked to an entry in the reference list.

The use and placement of the literature review is standard for most quantitative studies. Qualitative studies may refer to and cite the literature in various ways. Some qualitative researchers believe the researcher should not have preconceived notions about a study and so should complete the literature search only after completing the study. Others use a fairly traditional approach. The literature review for qualitative studies often appears throughout the sections noted above but may also appear in the results section, supporting the themes recorded, and in the words of informants.

to check their findings with those of others. This approach helps researchers avoid preconceived ideas about what they may find. Many qualitative researchers, however, use the same approach to the literature review as quantitative researchers by scanning the literature before beginning the study to support the importance of the question and the design of the study.

Checklist for Evaluating a Literature Review

✔ The literature review relies primarily on studies conducted in the last 5 years.
✔ The relationship of the research problem to the previous research is made clear.
✔ All or most of the major studies related to the topic of interest are included.
✔ The review can be linked directly and indirectly to the research question.
✔ The theoretical or conceptual framework is described.
✔ The review provides support for the importance of the study.
✔ The authors have used primary, rather than secondary, sources.
✔ Studies are critically examined and reported objectively.
✔ The review is unbiased and includes findings that are conclusive and those that have inconsistencies.
✔ The author's opinion is virtually undetectable.
✔ The review is organized so that a logical unfolding of ideas is apparent that supports the need for the research.
✔ The review ends with a summary of the most important knowledge on the topic.

The literature review should include a variety of sources of data; these sources should be sorted and analyzed for usefulness to the study. The literature review can be arranged in chronological order or by subject matter. This review should be unbiased; that is, there should be a mix of previous studies related to the research question—some that support the author's viewpoint and some that do not. Contradictory results from the literature should be reported because one goal of nursing research is to clarify previous confusing results.

The references should be dated within the past 5 years, unless the work is a seminal one or a theoretical selection. Each citation in the text should be clearly linked to an entry in the reference list, and the reference should be complete. The reader should be able to retrieve the reference based on the information provided by the author.

Using a Literature Review in Nursing Practice

Nurses use literature reviews for a variety of reasons. Students will use a literature search to compose scholarly papers and to design research studies. For practicing nurses, the literature may supply a specific answer to a particular patient problem. For the profession, articles may be combined to arrive at practice guidelines. Each of these requires competency in retrieving and using the literature appropriately.

Undergraduate and graduate nursing students must conduct a literature search to provide a basis for their scholarly work. Students often are expected to both retrieve and critique research articles as a basis for their own conclusions. The evolution of evidence-based practice in nursing has changed the way learners use research. Systematic searching skills, the ability to appraise the quality of studies, and a capacity to synthesize findings are critical competencies for students. Table 5.4 demonstrates how nurses are expected to use the literature in education and in practice. Just as the research skill of a nurse is expected to become more complex and skilled as he or she acquires education and experience, the literature search skills of a nurse evolve as well.

Practicing nurses use literature reviews to enhance, support, or refute what is already known on a particular clinical issue. Using evidence that exists in the literature leads to better clinical decisions and, ultimately, enhanced outcomes for patients. Some of the ways practicing nurses may use literature reviews include:

- Resolving clinical practice issues and answering questions
- Developing generic and unit-specific practice guidelines
- Establishing standards for nursing practice
- Providing a basis for outcome measurements
- Describing optimal procedures, interventions, and protocols
- Designing performance improvement projects

Table 5.5 provides a review of some of the ways that research literature is integrated into clinical practice at the individual and the organizational levels.

The wise practicing nurse will forge a strong bond with a health services librarian. Health services librarians are specialists in gathering information and whose library

Table 5.4	

Expectations for Use of Literature in Education and Practice

Baccalaureate

Conduct literature reviews on a clinical subject they are studying

Critically appraise the data retrieved

Synthesize summaries of literature reviewed

Apply research findings to clinical practice

Write academic papers

Prepare academic presentations

Graduate

The BSN skills plus the following:

Test the efficacy of nursing interventions yielding evidence for "best practices"

Develop research and/or evidence-based proposals

Develop research and/or evidence-based protocols

Develop research and/or evidence-based scholarly projects

Postgraduate

The BSN and graduate skills plus the following:

Conduct the research on proposals

Publish research and/or evidence-based findings from own research

Develop systematic reviews

Collaborate with other nursing colleagues to develop future studies

Clinical

Conduct literature reviews on a clinical subject being studied

Critically appraise the data retrieved

Synthesize summaries of the literature reviewed

Apply research findings to clinical practice

Develop research and/or evidence-based proposals

Develop research and/or evidence-based protocols

Develop research and/or evidence-based scholarly projects

science training is enhanced by knowledge of the health sciences. In an era of sophisticated information technology, students and nurses alike must access comprehensive literature about clinical problems. The health services librarians are experts in this field and can offer a wealth of knowledge and support to the literature retrieval process.

The profession of nursing benefits from literature review. Each unique study contributes another piece of information about what is effective and ineffective in caring for patients. One of the hallmarks of a profession is a foundation in scholarly work; literature reviews help demonstrate that nursing practice is, indeed, founded on rigorously conducted research.

Table 5.5

Integration of Literature Review into Clinical Practice

	Definition	Application to Clinical Practice
Independent reading	Personal reading for enrichment and professional knowledge.	▪ Improvement of patient care ▪ Improvement of professional self
Journal clubs	Assist clinicians who want to improve the application of research into their practices. Group discussions regarding clinical issues and the scientific evidence that addresses them via critical appraisal of selected journal articles.	▪ Improvement of patient care ▪ Improvement of professional self ▪ Increase in new knowledge of clinical issues with associated evidence ▪ Learning research methodologies ▪ Learning new clinical practice techniques ▪ Discussing professional nursing issues
Research conferences	Professional meetings focusing on research findings.	▪ Improvement of patient care ▪ Improvement of professional self ▪ Increase in new knowledge of clinical issues with associated evidence ▪ Learning research methodologies ▪ Learning new clinical practice techniques ▪ Discussing professional nursing issues
Nursing practice councils/ committees	A forum to research, craft, and revise nursing practice standards.	▪ Learning about EBP ▪ Development of professional practice guidelines: standards of care, procedures, protocols, and practice changes ▪ Identification of "best practices"
Performance improvement councils/ committees	A forum that focuses on analysis and improvement of care.	▪ Evidence-based measurement outcomes: nurse-sensitive indicators ▪ Use of the Plan-Do-Check-Act (PDCA) or PICO assessment form for quality management
Peer reviews	Processes wherein nurses review the practice of other nurses and compare actual practice to evidence-based professional standards.	▪ Promotes excellence in professional practice ▪ Identifies the need for safety and quality interventions

Source: Levin, R.F., & Feldman, H.R. (2006). *Teaching evidence-based nursing.* New York, NY: Springer.

Creating a Strong Literature Review

To successfully create a literature review, an organized approach must be used to address the clinical problem and research question. A seven-step process for creating a strong literature review appears in Table 5.6.

Table 5.6

A Seven-Step Literature Search Strategy

1. IDENTIFY the research problem and review the research question.
2. PLAN the information retrieval process.
3. CARRY OUT the search strategy.
4. SCREEN the initial list of citations and abstracts for relevance and date.
5. RETRIEVE full text of the relevant studies for evaluation.
6. CRITICALLY APPRAISE the study quality and findings.
7. SUMMARIZE and synthesize the findings.

Identify the Research Problem and Review the Research Question

This will be the source of the basic search terms that are used for the literature review search process. Identify the variables that are inherent in the problem statement and research question, the relevant populations, and the expected relationships between variables. Each of these will provide a basic search term that later will be used for searching electronic databases. Consider using the PICO approach (population/patient, intervention, comparison, outcome) to help in the selection of search terms.

Plan the Information Retrieval Process

Based on the concepts reflected in the research problem and question, the next step is to develop a plan for retrieving evidence from multiple sources. These sources will include electronic and print media. This is where the advice of a health sciences librarian can be invaluable. A qualified librarian can help guide the nurse or student to the most appropriate databases and information sources for the problem and question under study. A librarian can also help the researcher develop an effective search strategy that results in the retrieval of a greater number of relevant and fewer irrelevant articles.

The plan should consider the amount of information needed for the study under consideration. The amount of information required depends on the reason for the study, the potential audience for the research, and the eventual communication process. The literature review for a school project will likely be less intensive than one for a doctoral dissertation. Typically, undergraduate and graduate literature reviews are comprehensive in that they cover a broad range of studies related to the topic. Doctoral literature reviews are exhaustive, meaning that the search for literature is so complete that no additional literature support can be found.

Reviews for the development of practice guidelines are focused on intervention research that is application-oriented; scholarly reviews may focus on theoretical and conceptual works in addition to research studies. A literature review intended for a research publication may be more in-depth than one intended for a performance improvement project. The goals of the study will determine the amount of information retrieved.

Carry Out the Search Strategy

A **bibliographic database** is typically an electronic index of journal article citations, abstracts, subject headings, and possibly full text articles that is searchable by keywords, subjects, authors, journals, and other relevant categories. It is wise to carry out the search strategy in several databases because this increases the likelihood of covering the literature more thoroughly. The CINAHL database searches for articles in nursing and allied health journals. MEDLINE, which is part of the free government database, PubMed, allows the user to search for articles from a huge index of medical journals. The Cochrane Database of Systematic Reviews, a database in the Cochrane Library, is considered to be the gold standard for evidence-based practice. An interesting development in recent years has been the inclusion of Google Scholar (scholar.google.com) as a database utilized for literature reviews for scholarly research. Google Scholar complements the other databases because it searches journals and other sources in a variety of disciplines and may indicate more recent articles that have cited a previously published article on the topic. Unlike Google .com, it is primarily restricted to scholarly journal articles and books. On the other hand, Google Scholar lacks a number of useful tools, such as subject headings and certain limiters, found in MEDLINE and CINAHL, which can help narrow results (Shultz, 2007). Each database has its strengths and weaknesses. By searching several databases, a more complete search is achieved and it is less likely that an important article will be missed.

> **Database (bibliographic database):** An electronic index of journal article citations, abstracts, subject headings, and possibly full text articles that is searchable by keywords, subjects, authors, journals, and other relevant categories.

Libraries purchase subscriptions to MEDLINE, CINAHL, the Cochrane Library, and other databases through various vendors such as Ovid, EBSCOhost, and Thomson Gale. Some of the full text journal articles may be included in the database. PubMed is provided free by the federal government and contains links to the full text of open access journals, although the selection of open access journals is not vast. Summaries of abstracts from the Cochrane Database of Systematic Reviews are searchable and provided free by the Cochrane Collaboration, although a subscription is required for access to the complete full text reviews.

Databases contain the citations to articles. An abstract or synopsis of the article may be included. A citation is composed of the author, article title, journal name, volume number, issue number, publication date, and page numbers. If the full text of the journal article (or a link to it) is not included in the database, it is then necessary to locate the journal in print form or in a different online database that contains the full text article. The fees for access to major medical databases can be quite expensive, and so these may require access through an academic institution or medical center. If the library or institution does not have access to a journal article that is needed, it may be possible for the library to request a copy of the article from another library through their Interlibrary Loan Department.

Databases can be searched in a variety of ways. It is possible to retrieve results using a keyword search, similar to a search in Google. Most databases offer a variety of options such as searching by fields (for example, author, journal title, or publication type), combining search fields, and searching by subject headings.

SKILL Builder | Conduct Strong Literature Searches

It is easy to see the literature search as a task that has to be done to get at the "real" work of research. But if it is done well, a thorough review of previous work can actually save the researcher time in the long run. The literature search can help focus the research question, develop the details of a study design, and put the study in a larger context. Doing a literature search requires time and a bit of frustration tolerance—but there are ways to get the most from this critical step.

- Involve a medical librarian in the literature search early in the process. Searching the literature is a methodical science, and the expertise a librarian brings can be invaluable. A medical librarian can help locate databases and assist in developing a search strategy, both of which can improve the chances of a successful search.
- Go from general to specific in the search strategy. Look for studies on the overall topic first, and then search for research that is more specific to the unique question.
- Select references to review from the lists of the most relevant studies.
- Resist the urge to look only at full text databases. Valuable studies may be missed, and the research may end up with an incomplete literature review if the focus is exclusively on easily accessible articles.
- Use a broad range of sources, including "gray literature" such as conference proceedings and dissertation abstracts. Though time-consuming, hand searches of the tables of contents of the most relevant journals may reveal studies that were missed in the electronic search.
- Rely on primary sources—in other words, the original studies—instead of quotes or summaries from other articles. Studies may be misquoted and findings reported incorrectly, so the primary source must be evaluated to ensure the findings are reported correctly.

It is important to carefully choose the terms to narrow a search. Although many researchers are concerned they will be unable to find any supportive literature, the opposite problem is more often the case. A poorly focused search strategy may result in a return of thousands of citations, most of which may be irrelevant to the topic under consideration.

Most databases and search engines use a system referred to as Boolean logic, named for the mathematician who invented it. Boolean logic uses the operators AND, OR, and NOT to refine or broaden a search. Use AND between terms (a phrase, keyword, or subject heading) to retrieve articles containing both of the terms (for example, *smoking* AND *cancer*). The Boolean operator OR is used to retrieve articles containing either word (for example, *cancer* OR *neoplasms*). NOT is used to eliminate articles containing a specific word (*nursing* NOT *homes*). Quotation marks can be used around more than one word to create a phrase search. For example, if looking for research on care of an infant's umbilical cord, the researcher might enter the terms *infant* AND *"skin care"*. The results from this search would likely include many items that are not directly relevant to cord care, but rather to the generic care of an infant's skin. If the number of returned results is too large, then Boolean operators may be used to limit the results even more, for example, *infant* AND *"skin care"* AND *"umbilical cord"*. If the result list included too many articles that did not apply directly to cord care, Boolean logic could also be used to eliminate subjects that are not of interest. For example, the final search statement could be *infant* AND *"skin care"* AND *"umbilical cord"* NOT *bathing*. The judicious use of Boolean operators can help limit the results of a literature search to a carefully focused group of citations that are more likely to be relevant to the research study. The PubMed web site (www.pubmed.gov) has animated online tutorials demonstrating how to perform searches in PubMed.

Using well-chosen search terms gives a search sensitivity and specificity. Sensitivity of a search means it is able to identify articles that are directly relevant to the topic under study. Specificity means a search does not yield articles that are unrelated to the topic (Hoogendam, De Vries Robbé, Stalenhoef, & Overbeke, 2009). The use of the correct fields and Boolean operators can increase the chance that a search will be both sensitive and specific. If the return is still too large, various limiters and tags are available on most major databases. For example, a search can be limited to a publication type, a particular age group, a span of years, or a single language. Limiters can help focus a search and reduce the number of irrelevant results. It is important to record the search strategies and the databases that were used for future reference and to avoid duplication of searches. This information can be recorded on a sheet of paper, in a computer document, or in the database. CINAHL, MEDLINE, and PubMed have a "save search" feature that can be used to save search histories (the terms and search strategies that were used).

Internet information retrieval must be used with caution. Not every web site, database, or other Internet source is supported by a reputable provider. The reader in general has little assurance that information on Internet sources is peer-reviewed. Researchers must secure information from bona fide, established, and reputable sources. The Medical Library Association (2009) has developed guidelines for evaluating web sites:

- *Sponsor:* Can you identify the organization or person responsible for the site? The web address can provide clues about the web site.
  - U.S. government sites have the extension .gov.
  - Universities and colleges use .edu.
  - Professional organizations often have .org, but that extension is not restricted to organizations.
  - The extension .com refers to a commercial site. (The site may be selling something.)
- *Date:* Is the web site up-to-date? The date that the web site was most recently updated should be indicated.
- *Fact-based:* Can the information be confirmed in scholarly sources or links to other web sites? Does the site indicate whether the information is opinion or fact? Is the viewpoint biased?
- *Audience:* Is the web site geared for healthcare professionals or consumers?

Common databases and associated web sites used in nursing research and evidence-based practice appear in **Table 5.7**. Some common professional journals that focus on

Table 5.7

Databases and Web Sites Used for Nursing Literature Searches

Databases	Location
Academic Search Premier	Available at some academic, medical, or public libraries
Business Source Premier	Available at some academic, medical, or public libraries
CINAHL	Available at some academic, medical, or public libraries
Cochrane Database of Systematic Reviews	www.cochrane.org (free, except for complete full text of systematic reviews; must pay or access at a library)
Educational Resources Information Center (ERIC)	Available at some academic, medical, or public libraries
EMBASE (Excerpta Medica Online)	Available at some academic or medical libraries
Google Scholar	scholar.google.com (free on the web)
MEDLINE/PubMed	www.pubmed.gov (free; libraries may have links/subscriptions to a number of the full text journals)
PsycINFO	Available at some academic, medical, or public libraries

Web Sites	URL
Academic Center for Evidence-Based Practice	www.acestar.uthscsa.edu
American Association of Critical-Care Nurses	www.aacn.org
American Nurses Association	www.nursingworld.org
Hartford Institute for Geriatric Nursing	www.hartfordign.org
HRSA Bureau of Health Professions, Division of Nursing	http://bhpr.hrsa.gov/nursing
HRSA Evidence-Based Practice Centers	www.ahrq.gov/clinic/epc/
Joanna Briggs Institute for Evidence-Based Nursing and Midwifery	www.joannabriggs.edu.au
MEDSCAPE Nurses	www.medscape.com/nurseshome
National Institute of Nursing Research (NINR)	www.ninr.nih.gov
National Guidelines Clearinghouse	www.guideline.gov
National Library of Medicine	www.nlm.nih.gov
National Network of Libraries of Medicine (NN/LM)	www.nnlm.gov
Oncology Nursing Society	www.ons.org
PDQ, National Cancer Institute's Comprehensive Cancer Database	www.cancer.gov/cancer_information/pdq

Table 5.8

Professional Nursing Research and Evidence-Based Practice Journals

Advances in Nursing Science
Applied Nursing Research
Biological Research for Nursing
Canadian Journal of Nursing Research
Clinical Nursing Research
Evidence-Based Nursing
Journal of Nursing Measurement
Journal of Nursing Scholarship
NT Research
Nurse Researcher
Nursing Research
Nursing Science Quarterly
Oncology Nursing Forum
Online Journal of Knowledge Synthesis
Research in Nursing and Health
Scholarly Inquiry for Nursing Practice
Western Journal of Nursing Research
WORLDviews on Evidence-Based Nursing

nursing research and evidence-based practice are listed in **Table 5.8**. Searching databases and journals with established research credentials and a history of trustworthiness is one of the most reliable ways of ensuring a quality literature search.

Screen the Initial List of Citations and Abstracts

The initial literature search will almost certainly return a list that includes both relevant and irrelevant citations. Rather than wasting time reading articles that are not appropriate, the researcher should start by screening the citations list for relevance. This process is supported if the researcher begins by developing a set of inclusion and exclusion criteria for the content and type of studies that are appropriate.

Inclusion criteria are most commonly based on an identification of the population of interest, the intervention being considered, and the outcomes of significance. The researcher may also limit the types of studies that are of interest. If the researcher is interested only in the effectiveness of an intervention, then citations may be retained only if they represent experimental or quasi-experimental designs. If the evidence that is needed relates to patient preferences, then the researcher may focus on qualitative studies. Using criteria related to topic and type of studies ensures that the researcher remains focused on the most relevant studies without being bogged down by literature that is only indirectly related to the topic.

Practical considerations dictate the need for a second screening of the remaining citations to determine if they are accessible to the researcher. Although full text versions of some citations may be available electronically, others may be available only as hard copy journals in a medical library, or the researcher may need to request the literature through interlibrary loan. Most medical libraries belong to consortia that enable the sharing of literature, and so it is likely that most of the citations in a review will be accessible in some way. The researcher must determine how much effort can be expended tracking down the literature in the final list of citations. The librarian's assistance can be very helpful in this process.

Retrieve Full Text of the Relevant Studies for Evaluation

When the researcher has retrieved the full text of each article, he or she then needs to evaluate the content and quality. Most researchers will find they need to organize the review of the full text articles so the summary is both complete and efficient. The research question, methods, findings, and conclusions of each study should be summarized. The review should focus on relevant results and the quality of the evidence. At this point, it is helpful to record any quotes the researcher may want to include in the write-up along with page numbers so the quote can be appropriately attributed. All of these elements can be recorded in software such as RefWorks, EndNote, or the free software Zotero (www .zotero.org). Other options include a spreadsheet or note cards. In general, it is helpful to record the following for any study that may end up in the literature review:

- Full article citations
- Purpose of study
- Research design
- Sample size
- Methodology and measurements
- Treatment(s)
- Results
- Findings
- Implications for the current research question
- Implications for nursing practice

Critically Appraise the Study Quality and Findings

Once the researcher has a final stack of relevant research articles, he or she should appraise the studies for quality of design and methodology. Studies that do not meet the methodological standards of the researcher should be discarded, and those that remain constitute the final literature review. It is best for the researcher to use preset criteria to evaluate the research studies so potential bias in study selection is minimized. Use of evaluation checklists such as those that appear in this text can help maintain an objective appraisal process. The final step in the critical appraisal is to record an assessment of the methodological quality of the study and a summary of its key results.

For More Depth and Detail

For a more in-depth look at the concepts in this chapter, try these references:

Boss, C., & Wurmser, T. (2009). Searching for evidence: Mission-critical tips. *Nursing Management, 40*(9), 12.

Klem, M., & Northcutt, T. (2008). Finding the best evidence, part 2: The basics of literature searches. *JEN: Journal of Emergency Nursing, 34*(2), 151–153.

Pickett, K. (2008). Reaching beyond MEDLINE: A beginner's overview of electronic biomedical resources. *Journal of Hospital Librarianship, 8*(4), 398–410.

Wilczynski, N., Marks, S., & Haynes, R. (2007). Search strategies for identifying qualitative studies in CINAHL. *Qualitative Health Research, 17*(5), 705–710.

Summarize and Synthesize the Findings

The final step of any literature review is to compose a synthesis of the key findings of the studies into a coherent summary. The summary should not be a simple reiteration of the studies that were reviewed, but rather a logical unfolding of the relationships discovered

 CRITICAL APPRAISAL EXERCISE

Retrieve the following full text article online from CINAHL, PubMed, or in print at a library. If it is not available, ask if the Interlibrary Loan service can obtain it:

Mok, L., & Fung-Kam Lee, I. (2008). Anxiety, depression and pain intensity in patients with low back pain who are admitted to acute care hospitals. *Journal of Clinical Nursing, 17*, 1471–1480.

Review the article, focusing on the way the authors use the literature to support the importance of the problem and provide a background and context for the study. Evaluate how the literature is used in the discussion and conclusions section. Consider the following appraisal questions in your critical review of this element of the research article:

1. How is the literature review used in the introduction to establish the importance of the problem and to point out gaps in knowledge related to this topic?

2. Describe the ways in which the literature in the introduction is related to the research problem and question.

3. How is the literature used to support subsequent sections of the research report, including the operational definitions, sampling strategies, data collection, and analysis?

4. Do the authors display any bias in the way the literature is retrieved and/or reported?

5. How do the authors use the literature in the discussion to relate the study findings to previous evidence?

6. Evaluate the reference list for currency, relevance, comprehensiveness, and variety.

in the research studies. The summary should emphasize the significance of the research that was reviewed and link it to the current research question.

The author should avoid a heavy reliance on direct quotations. The word *synthesis* means to produce something new from existing knowledge. A strong literature review will reflect the researcher's thinking based on the research studies that were evaluated. This does not mean the author's opinions are evident in the literature review; rather, the review should show a logical progression of ideas that are supported by the research literature and that leads the reader to the conclusion that the current study is well founded, important, and necessary.

A strong literature review will include studies that both support and refute the researcher's ideas. Any gaps, particular strengths, or evident weaknesses in the current evidence should be revealed. The goal of a literature review is to explore the support for a research project, not prove a point. The best literature reviews provide guidance to the researcher while reinforcing the need for specialized inquiry.

Summary of Key Concepts

- The literature review provides an in-depth analysis of recently published research findings in a specific area of interest.
- The two major sources of information to be searched are primary and secondary sources; the bulk of a literature review should focus on primary sources.
- Multiple types of information, including theoretical and empirical literature, are used to enhance the breadth and depth of a review.
- An explicit search strategy is helpful in ensuring that the literature search is comprehensive and unbiased.
- A search strategy involves identifying search terms, developing a search statement, performing the search, locating appropriate sources of literature, and appraising the studies for value and quality.
- Peer review is critical for ensuring the credibility and trustworthiness of research publications.
- Information literacy is a key competency for students and practicing nurses to ensure nursing practice is based on appropriate evidence.

For a full suite of assignments and additional learning activities, use the access code located in the front of your book to visit this exclusive website: http://go.jblearning .com/houser. If you do not have an access code, you can obtain one at the site.

References

Cheek, J., Garnham, B., & Quan, J. (2006). What's in a number? Issues in providing evidence of impact and quality of researcher(s). *Qualitative Health Research, 16*(3), 423–435.

Goodfellow, L. M. (2009). Electronic theses and dissertations: A review of this valuable resource for nurse scholars worldwide. *International Nursing Review, 56*(2), 159–165.

Hoogendam, A., De Vries Robbé, P., Stalenhoef, A., & Overbeke, A. (2009). Evaluation of PubMed filters used for evidence-based searching: Validation using relative recall. *Journal of the Medical Library Association, 97*(3), 186–193.

Hopewell, S., Clarke, M. J., Lefebvre, C., & Scherer, R. W. (2007). Hand searching versus electronic searching to identify reports of randomized trials. *Cochrane Database of Systematic Reviews, 2*, MR000001.

Leasure, A., Delise, D., Clifton, S., & Pascucci, M. (2009). Health information literacy: Hardwiring behavior through multilevels of instruction and application. *Dimensions of Critical Care Nursing, 28*(6), 276–282.

Lenzer, J. (2008). US Congress and European Research Council insist on open access to research results. *BMJ (Clinical Research Ed.), 336*(7637), 176–177.

LoBiondo-Wood, G., & Haber, J. (2006). *Nursing research: Methods and critical appraisal for evidence-based practice.* St. Louis: Mosby Elsevier.

Medical Library Association. (2009). A user's guide to finding and evaluation of health information on the web. Retrieved February 2, 2011, from http://mlanet.org/resources/userguide.html

Rogers, J. (2009). Transferring research into practice: An integrative review. *Clinical Nurse Specialist: The Journal for Advanced Nursing Practice, 23*(4), 192–199.

Shultz, M. (2007). Comparing test searches in PubMed and Google Scholar. *Journal of the Medical Library Association, 95*(4), 442–445.

Suber, P. (2007). Open access overview: Focusing on open access to peer-reviewed research articles and their preprints. Retrieved February 2, 2011, from http://earlham.edu/~peters/fos/overview.htm

Thabane, L., Thomas, T., Ye, C., & Paul, J. (2009). Posing the research question: Not so simple. *Canadian Journal of Anaesthesia, 56*(1), 71–79.

U.S. Department of Health and Human Services. (2009). NIH public access policy details. Retrieved January 30, 2010, from http://publicaccess.nih.gov/policy.htm

U.S. Library of Congress. Federal Research Public Access Act 2009. Retrieved January 31, 2010, from http://thomas.loc.gov/cgi-bin/query/z?c111:S.1373:

chapter 6

Theoretical Frameworks

CHAPTER OBJECTIVES

The study of this chapter will help the learner to

- Explain current terminology relative to theoretical and conceptual frameworks.
- Evaluate the identifying characteristics of theoretical and conceptual frameworks.
- Analyze various frameworks currently in use in nursing practice and research.
- Explore emerging complexity and linear and nonlinear frameworks for generalizability in nursing applications.
- Discuss the use of a particular theoretical framework for application in nursing.

KEY TERMS

Borrowed theories	Construct	Relational statements
Concept	Grand theories	Shared theories
Conceptual definitions	Microtheories	Theoretical frameworks
Conceptual model	Middle-range theories	Theory

Introduction

If the research question is the beginning of a research study, and the literature review is a historical view, then the theoretical and conceptual framework is the road map for the researcher. **Theoretical frameworks** are the foundations of a research design. A well-done framework is often considered a plan or a guide for the actual research. Studies that are not based on a sound foundation may lack direction and subsequently target populations,

> **Theoretical frameworks:** Collections of interrelated concepts that depict a piece of theory that is to be examined as the basis for research studies. These are the foundations that guide the research.

❝❝ *Voices from the Field* ❞❞

I wouldn't call myself a researcher; I'm a staff nurse in an ICU. So when I think of research, I want it to be applicable to what I do. I really did not have much interest in theoretical research studies, although I was exposed to nursing theories in graduate school. When I read my journals, I tended toward clinical studies, stuff I could use. I didn't give much thought to how theories might apply in practice.

About 2 years ago, the nurses on my unit and I began talking about designing a small study, something specific to the problems we face, but designed well so it could have broader appeal. In the past, scientific articles were my focus so I'm always thinking in terms of cause and effect. But I heard a speaker who said research was about "wondering," and so I started thinking a little broader about what I might want to study.

It started with an observation. I noticed that families in the waiting room seemed to bond together. Strangers became friends, and they were like one big support group. I saw, for example, people sharing food and space, taking messages when someone was out of the room; I even saw a guy taking a woman's blood pressure for her. When good news was delivered, everyone reacted to it. I've always believed that the patient gets better faster with a solid family support system, and so I started thinking about how we might support this process. But I didn't give it any attention in terms of research, mostly because it didn't seem like something that could be studied.

Then I ran across the web site of Jean Watson, a philosopher–nurse who developed the Theory of Human Caring (http://www2.uchsc.edu/son/caring/content/). She says that her theory is grounded in the study of relationships. The caring perspective has a worldview that is unified and connected. I thought, "This is what I was thinking about; the waiting room situation is about relationships that are based on a bigger view of the world." The people in the waiting room were consistent with Jean Watson's theory, and I could use her theory to help me design my study.

The web site started me on a search to understand the theory better, and to see how it might help me think about my research project. The theory can be tested in many ways—the author notes that even nontraditional inquiries, like poetry and music, might be used to explore what caring means. It got me thinking about how I could test the theory on a smaller scale, in our waiting room.

I've just really started on the design of my study. I know that I want it to be an observational study, describing what I see in terms of people building relationships. I'd like to know the nature of those relationships, and whether they can be supported by nursing actions. After that, I'd like to study how I might put nursing practices in place to support the way the groups come together, and then see if I can relate the amount of support in the waiting room to the patients' outcomes. I think that would be a great study.

So it turns out that I could apply theory in my practice. It actually has helped a lot in terms of trying to figure out how I think about my research problem, and how I try to address it. I guess it was the spark that lit the fire.

A. Nichole Duling, MSN, CCRN
ICU Advanced Practice Nurse

techniques, or designs that are inappropriate for the study. Once a theory or framework is selected to guide the research, the study can progress in a systematic and orderly fashion.

The presence of a theoretical or conceptual framework is crucial for credibility and to develop nursing knowledge. By building on previous knowledge, evidence for best practices is established. Well-done research has an associated framework. Some forms of research—particularly qualitative designs—may not start with theory but seek to develop and test it. This is referred to as inductive reasoning, or building general knowledge based on specific observations. Quantitative designs, however, have their beginnings in theory, because these designs are deductive, meaning they go from general theoretical ideas to testing specific ideas. The intent of the research will drive how a theoretical framework is used.

When reading research, the theoretical framework is assessed to determine the soundness of the study design, the applicability of the findings, and the potential value to practice. A research study that is undertaken without the proper framework limits the use of the results in practice and constrains the ability to build future research studies from the results. Creating an adequate framework requires that the nurse researcher select and define the basic ideas to be tested in a study, find and examine concepts and relationships between them, and determine the characteristics of relationships. Theory can help the nurse researcher refine the question, identify variables, pose cause-and-effect questions, and determine expected relationships. This requires a mix of inspiration, persistence, and disciplined inquiry, but it is critical to ensure that the results can be confidently applied as evidence for nursing practice.

> **gray matter**
>
> The theoretical framework is assessed when reading research to determine the soundness of the following components:
> - Study design
> - Applicability of the findings
> - Potential value to the practice

An Overview of Theory and Theoretical Frameworks

When a study's findings are soundly based on an appropriate framework, the use, application, and future directions of a body of research become clear. Thus, a good working knowledge of frameworks is essential for the nurse researcher. To understand theoretical and conceptual frameworks, the nurse researcher must first understand the terminology that is used in theory and in the conceptual language of nursing.

Exploring Terminology

In short, theory is an attempt to explain the world around us. Nurses become part of the world of health care through an understanding of theories about nursing, which attempt to explain why nurses do what they do. Nursing care is a complex process, and explanations of human actions and interactions can be complicated and difficult to understand without a road map. Theory is a method of mapping the complex processes of human action and interaction that affect nursing care.

The word *theory* comes from the Greek *theoria*, which means "vision." Nurse scientists use theories to explain their visions of reality. Theories are not facts; instead, they are methods of perceiving reality. Perceptions of reality may take

> **Theory:** A method of perceiving reality and mapping the complex processes of human action and interaction that affect nursing care.

a variety of forms—some of them quite abstract—and these perceptions can differ and change over time. According to numerous nursing scientists, employing precise and clear statements of theory is only one method of classifying theoretical science. Nursing theorists are reporting that more ambiguous and metaphorical statements are also useful in explanations of reality (Greenwood & Bonner, 2008). Just as there are many visions of reality, there are many explanations of that reality. Nurse scientists have created numerous and diverse theories as each theorist attempts to explain his or her vision of the reality of nursing.

Classifying Theories

Grand theories: The most abstract and complex theories, broadly defining concepts that are central to the nursing profession and linking them using the theorist's view of the discipline.

Middle-range theories: Those nursing theories located midway between abstract and concrete theories that are more limited in scope and address specific phenomena or concepts.

Microtheories: Precise theories that are very narrow in scope and usually related to a particular situation or set of circumstances in nursing practice.

Theories can be classified by their level of generality. For example, grand theories (or macrotheories) are considered the most abstract of theories because they attempt to explain what the discipline of nursing is all about. They broadly define concepts that are central to the nursing profession, such as "person" or "health." Grand theories are often, by necessity, macro views that may be complex to understand.

One example of a grand theory—Rogers's model of the science of unitary, irreducible human beings (1960, 1990)—uses concepts such as environment and energy field patterns to define an overall view of the purpose of nursing. This theory focuses on promoting maximum well-being through an understanding of the energy and interactions inherent in the practice of nursing. Other grand theories are more intuitive and easily grasped. For example, Watson's theory of human caring (1969) depicts nursing as a caring-healing profession and portrays the concept of health in various modes, such as "alignment of mindbodyspirit, wholeness, and unity of being" (Watson, 2002, p. 15).

There are also middle-range theories, which are so named because they come from the center of a continuum of theories stretching from most abstract to most concrete. As the name implies, middle-range theories are those theories located midway between abstract and concrete theories. They are more limited in scope and less abstract than grand theories, addressing specific phenomena or concepts. They are considered more testable and more readily generalizable to nursing practice than grand theories. Examples include Pender's theory of health promotion (1996), which provides a basis for investigative work about health behaviors, and Kolcaba's comfort theory (1994), which examines the intentional comforting actions of nurses.

Microtheories are precise theories that guide very specific aspects of nursing practice. These theoretical frameworks are concrete and narrow in scope. They are composed of concepts that are readily measurable, objective, and applicable to limited populations and/or practice settings. Microtheories describe, explain, or provide understanding of the patients' experiences of a specific phenomenon. For example, Im and Meleis (1999) adapted Schumaker and Meleis's mid-range transition theory (1994) into a situation-specific theory of menopausal transition in Korean women to give "more focused guidelines for clinical practice with this particular population of women" (p. 19). **FIGURE 6.1** depicts the relationship and scope of each level of theory in research.

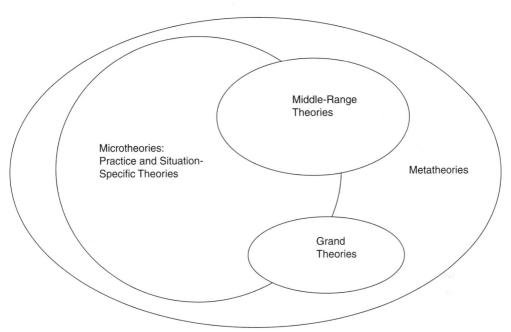

FIGURE 6.1 Theory Relationships
Source: Adapted from Im (2005). Development of situation-specific theories, *Advances in Nursing Science, 28*(2), 136–151.

Theories may also be classified as being specific to the discipline of nursing or arising from other disciplines. Nursing uses many borrowed theories. Borrowed theories are theories taken from other disciplines and used as frameworks or models for solving nursing problems. As noted in Kuhn (1960), disciplines that are undergoing scientific development can be influenced by a number of schools of thought. Nursing practice is enhanced through knowledge of psychology, epidemiology, sociology, and many other disciplines. Thus, nurses must be open to different types of theory for application in nursing science. Although borrowed theories are used in nursing quite often, some of the more frequently used examples include Parson's sick role theory (1951) and Becker's health belief model (1966).

There is much controversy over the use of borrowed theories in nursing. However, nursing is considered to be in a state of knowledge development, so it is very likely that nursing as a discipline will continue on its current path of conducting studies that use both nursing-specific and **borrowed theories**. Because of this, yet another classification of theory is emerging—the **shared theory**. These are theories that are borrowed, tested, and found to be empirically adequate in more than one discipline. Examples would include Lazarus and Folkman's theory of stress and coping (1984) and Melzack and Wall's gate control theory of pain (1965).

It is clear that the theories that are the foundation of nursing practice are diverse and include a broad range of classifications. These theories also guide the research

Borrowed theories: Theories taken from other disciplines and used as frameworks or models for nursing practice.
Shared theories: Theories that have been borrowed, tested, and found to be empirically adequate in more than one discipline.

that forms the evidence for nursing practice. Each theory has several components that can help the nurse researcher understand more clearly the phenomena of interest and design research that is conceptually sound.

Building Blocks of Theory

Nursing theories include the following building blocks:

- Concepts
- Constructs
- Conceptual definitions
- Relational statements
- Conceptual models

Concept: An abstract idea that is used to describe or identify phenomena.
Construct: A broad or high-level concept that is often complex and abstract.

These elements are used to help formulate the basis for nursing science and nursing research. A **concept** is considered to be an abstract idea that is used to describe or identify phenomena. Concepts generally represent broad categories or groupings that are not considered to be directly observable in the world. Two good examples of concepts are uncertainty, such as uncertainty in illness, and the concept of care, as in the care a nurse provides. However, both of these concepts have more than one definition or meaning and need to be defined within the context of their use to be understood.

Concepts are further subdivided into broad or narrow levels of abstraction. At a broad or high level of abstraction, a concept is known as a **construct**. "Care," therefore, would be a concept and the "continuum of care" would be a construct of that concept. Definitions of constructs are often complex and require the use of abstract terms for description. For example, the "continuum of care" as a construct is defined by McBryde-Foster and Allen (2005) as a "series of initiating, continuing and concluding care events that result when the patient seeks providers in one or more environments within the healthcare system" (p. 630).

gray matter

Theories may be classified by the following criteria:
- Level of generality (grand theories, middle-range theories, microtheories)
- Discipline/nondiscipline (nursing theories, borrowed theories, shared theories)

At a narrow or more concrete level, a concept is known as a variable. A variable is the measurable aspect of a concept. The concept of "care" was narrowed and made into a measurable variable in a study by Duffy et al. (2005). First, care factors were identified from a study involving a caring framework that described the essence of the concept in an abstract way (Duffy & Hoskins, 2003; Watson, 1985). Some of these factors included respect, sensitivity, and trust. Next, a comprehensive intervention was developed in which these care factors were added to enhance the intervention. When the care-enhanced intervention was used, it allowed for an examination and measurement of the effects of the variable "care" as part of nursing interventions performed for a specific population. At this concrete level, the concept of care was narrowed into a measurable variable.

Conceptual definitions: Clearly stated meanings of the abstract ideas or concepts used by a researcher in a study.

Concepts must be refined and described through research to allow for consistency in the way the terms are used. It is extremely important to use **conceptual** definitions that are clear, accurate, and explained at the outset of a study, even if the concepts seem to be very basic and uncomplicated. For example, it is not uncommon to find several different definitions for a concept, as noted by Morse et al. (1990) in their examination of the definitions of the concept of "caring" or Wagner (2006) in her examination of the concept of "organizational commitment." The definition that has been chosen by the researcher in a particular study must be clearly stated. It is desirable to use previously established definitions as often as possible to establish congruency of findings across research studies as well as to allow for comparison of evidence across research studies.

> **Relational statement:** A definition of the relationships between and among concepts in a theory that are its foundation.
> **Conceptual model:** A visualization of a grouping of phenomena involving more than one conceptual map in which interrelated phenomena are linked for broader interpretation.

Concepts that have been thoroughly defined form the building blocks of the theory. These concepts are then connected with statements about the expected relationships among them. **Relational statements** enable the theorist to state the expected relationships among the concepts. Relational statements can describe positive or negative relationships, direct or indirect effects, or linear or nonlinear associations. The result is a **conceptual model**, a careful description of the concepts and the relationships among them.

Models may be simple, representing only a small number of concepts and relationships, or they may be quite complex and multifaceted. FIGURE 6.2 depicts a model that proposed the relationship between characteristics of the nurses' work environment and perceived workload. This is a relatively simple model depicting linear relationships among concepts. There are both direct effects (teamwork on workload) and indirect effects (leadership on workload) hypothesized in the model (Houser, 2000).

FIGURE 6.3 depicts a complex, nonlinear model with direct and indirect effects. This model was developed to explain turnover using an innovative application of catastrophe theory (Wagner, 2009). In this model, turnover is expected to result from varying combinations of organizational commitment, job tension, and anticipated turnover intention. There may be a slow building of behavior to the point of exiting (Path B in the model) or an abrupt decision to leave in a catastrophic state (Path A). Both models demonstrate useful applications in actual nursing research and practice. Generally, these

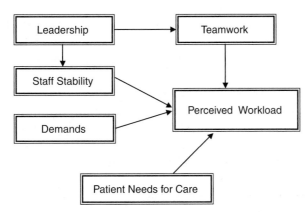

FIGURE 6.2 Linear Framework Model

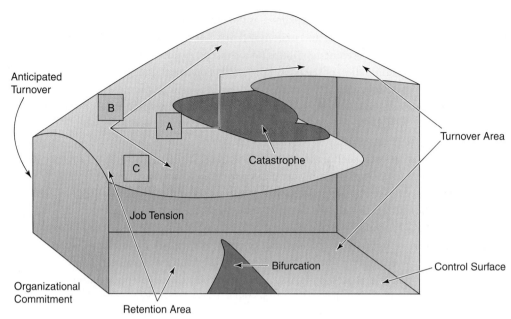

FIGURE 6.3 Nonlinear Framework Model
Source: Adapted with permission, *Wagner Cusp Catastrophe Nursing Turnover Model,* © Cheryl Wagner, 2009.

models demonstrate theoretical relationships, but they still require a written description of the theory before the reader readily grasps the relationships represented by the map.

One relatively new and innovative application of concept analysis pertains to the field of qualitatively derived theory (QDT) or concept development. Whereas concept *analysis* is considered to be the "study of an existing concept through integration of what is known at a particular point in time," concept *development* "pushes the boundaries of understanding towards synthesis of new insights and theory generation" (Finfgeld-Connett, 2006, p. 104). Through concept development, a union between similar concepts arises, forming broad yet highly useful theories. According to Finfgeld-Connett (2008), this methodology is a relatively unexplored area that can provide systematic examination and integration of nursing concepts.

Many nursing theorists insist that the use of concept development be incorporated into nursing education, stating "*If* our theories are to develop to a high level of abstraction, *if* they are to be broad in scope and useful, *then* these theories must be developed logically and rationally by integrating related concepts" (Morse, Hupcey, Penrod, & Mitcham, 2002, p. 6). These concept developments appear to be most applicable to middle-range theory, forming "models of interrelated concepts with overlapping attributes, rather like a 3-dimensional puzzle" as the concepts "intersect, parallel, converge, or diverge from one another within the developing theory" (Morse et al., 2006, p. 6). An example of this is found in Finfgeld-Connett's (2008) convergence study of the concepts of the art of nursing, presence, and caring. She established that nurses and patients "appear to take an active role in co-creating an intimate partnership" (2008, p. 533) during an interaction episode, leading to questions regarding the potential partnership formed for unconscious, belligerent, immature, or cognitively impaired patients.

Theoretical Frameworks

Theoretical frameworks are collections of concepts, concept maps, and/or conceptual models that depict a piece of a theory that is to be examined as the basis for a research study. In general, the theoretical framework is the basic structure of the ideas to be tested in a study. Not all studies are based on a published theory, but all studies should have an easily discernible framework that guides and directs the study. This is not always the case in reported research. There may only be an implied framework, with no formal acknowledgment of the basis or foundation of the study. Theory can never be completely proven, so the relationships depicted in a theoretical framework are hypothesized relationships. These ongoing tests become the basis for nursing research studies.

Reading the Theoretical Framework of a Research Study

Nurses need to read research with a critical eye to determine whether the theoretical foundation for the study is sound. Lack of an identifiable theoretical framework weakens a study and renders it less able to make a contribution to the overall body of nursing science. A necessary element of research critique involves searching for the presence or absence of an adequate theoretical framework that is the basis of the study. This is most important in quantitative research in which specific inquiry is designed as a result of deductive reflection on theory, but it is also important in qualitative study. Even when one is able to identify a framework, most critical analyses stop there and do not evaluate the soundness of the framework. However, because the design of a theoretical framework is critical for conveying its usefulness for research studies, examination and critique are needed to advance the science of nursing.

When analyzing a framework, one must remember that the ultimate goal is to determine whether the framework truly guides the research and is structurally sound. To do this, the framework should be scrutinized piece by piece. **Table 6.1** depicts a detailed process for evaluating the theoretical framework of a research study for appropriateness; however, a general critique can be accomplished with a simpler, three-step process.

1. Extract each concept from the framework and locate each concept definition within the study; these are examined for consistency. Each conceptual definition should have a validating reference from the literature.
2. Determine how the relationships between the concepts are described, analyzed, and validated; these should similarly be compared with the theorist's definition and references.
3. Examine the claims of the researcher in relation to the framework and determine whether the framework is adequate to explain the phenomena and relationships being examined in the research study. This review should give the nurse reader

Table 6.1	

Theory Critique Steps

Step	Description
1. Identify concepts/ constructs	Determine all the concepts, constructs, and operational definitions listed in a framework.
2. Examine definitions	Determine the definitions for each concept and construct and examine each for adequacy and literature citation support. A concept analysis may be indicated for multidimensional concepts.
3. Examine relationships	Determine the relationships between concepts and examine each for adequacy and support in the literature.
4. Examine variables	Determine all the variables listed in the study and determine if they adequately reflect the constructs or concepts identified in the study, as well as demonstrate adequate reliability and validity.
5. Examine the hypotheses	Determine whether the hypotheses, research questions, or objectives are logically linked to the proposed framework, and whether the framework is adequate to explain the phenomena.
6. Examine the methodology	Determine whether the design (including setting, subjects, sample size, and analyses methods) are appropriate.
7. Examine the findings	Determine if the findings are interpreted in terms of the framework, can be used to validate the framework, and are consistent with findings from other studies that use the same framework.

an idea of whether the theoretical framework has been used appropriately as a basis for the research study, represented accurately, and reported in a way that is consistent with the original theory.

Using Theory to Guide Nursing Practice and Research

Nurses pride themselves on providing the best possible care to patients, and one method of ensuring the best possible care delivery is to base the care on soundly developed nursing theory. Nurses can use theory that has been tested through research to guide their practice. By reflecting on the grand theories, the nurse can determine what he or she believes to be essential elements of the nursing process. Both grand and middle-range theories can be used to describe or explain phenomena of interest to nursing. Both of these groups of theories can be used to outline the framework for evidence-based practices. Practice guidelines are often developed based on middle-range, borrowed, shared, and microtheories.

For example, a nurse may use Orem's 1995 theory of self-care to guide the nursing process. Orem believed that the nurse's role is to facilitate an individual's efforts to achieve self-care. The nurse may support or supplant the patient's efforts to meet his or her needs, and so nursing practice is a series of actions intended to achieve this end. An evidence-based practice guideline based on Orem's theoretical framework would focus on helping the patient achieve the capacity for optimal self-care. Another grand theory

Where to Look

The theoretical or conceptual framework of a research study may be explicitly identified in the published report or not mentioned at all. Simply because the authors do not report a theoretical foundation does not necessarily mean there was none. Many times the reader is left to infer the theoretical model based on the concepts that are defined, the way the concepts are linked, and even the references that are used.

Authors who carry out quantitative studies based on theoretical models usually describe them fairly early in the report. Look for the theory to be described in the introduction or in the literature review section. Sometimes the theoretical framework may have its own section and be described in detail; other times it is mentioned only in passing or not at all. The section may be called "theoretical framework," "conceptual model," or "conceptual framework." When a theoretical framework is identified, it is usually described in enough depth that the reader can understand the context for the current study.

Finding the conceptual basis of a qualitative study may be more difficult. The theoretical underpinnings may be mentioned in the introduction, described in the results section, or referred to in the discussion section. In qualitative studies, the purpose may be to develop a theory, and so theory may be the outcome of the study instead of its foundation.

If the research design and the theory do not seem to fit, then the author may have used a backward approach to identify the theoretical framework. In other words, the researcher identified a research question and then looked for a theoretical justification for the study. This will be most obvious if some elements of the study—the question, design, variables, or analysis—do not fit with the identified theory. All these elements should flow from the theoretical foundation, so if they do not, the researcher may have identified a theoretical foundation only as an afterthought.

that can guide nursing practice is Roy's 1960 theory of adaptation. Sister Callista Roy believed that health was a result of the individual's interaction with the environment, and that nursing care is intended to help the patient adapt to the environment in an optimal way. If the nurse believed in Roy's theory, then the basis for most nursing care would be actions to help the patient adapt physiologically, psychosocially, and spiritually.

Checklist for Evaluating the Theoretical Framework

✔ The theoretical framework for the research is clearly identified early in the report.

✔ The theoretical basis for the research is described in sufficient depth that the context for the research design can be deduced.

✔ If no theoretical foundation is identified, the development of theory is an outcome of the study.

✔ The theoretical framework is consistent with the research question, design, variables, and interpretation of the study.

✔ Concepts, constructs, and operational definitions are listed in the framework.

✔ The definitions are adequate and supported by literature citations.

✔ The authors report the expected relationships between concepts, based on the theoretical framework.

✔ The research design logically flows from the theoretical foundation and the relationships that are expected.

✔ The authors refer to the theoretical framework when interpreting the outcome of the study.

Middle-range theories such as Kolcaba's 1994 theory of holistic comfort in nursing can be useful in the development of evidence-based practice guidelines. This theory is based on assumptions that human beings have holistic responses to complex stimuli and strive to meet basic comfort needs, and that nursing as a profession embraces comfort provision. Practice guidelines based on this theory would focus on assessing the patient's holistic needs and developing approaches to meet those needs that focus on the maintenance of comfort. Another middle-range theory that is helpful in nursing practice is the theory of transitions, developed and tested by Meleis et al. (2000). This theory advances the notion that changes in health and illness create a state of transition that is both "a result of and result in change in lives, health, relationships and environment" (p. 12). Transitions cause persons to be vulnerable, and the nurse's role is to help the patient transition away from vulnerability. Practice guidelines based on this theory would determine the patient's vulnerabilities—including those that are a result of illness, lifespan, and sociocultural changes—and plan interventions that help address those vulnerabilities.

These are only a few of the nursing theories that can be helpful in guiding evidence-based practice. Some theoretical frameworks lend themselves to study in a particular context or within a subset of nursing practice. Borrowed and shared theories are often useful in nursing research. Just as some theories are useful in guiding practice, others are useful in guiding research. There is no sharp demarcation, however. Theories that guide both practice and research may be used as a basis for inquiry; indeed, often nurses are involved in testing theories of nursing practice through nursing research.

Creating Research Based on a Theoretical Framework

In choosing a framework for a research study, the researcher starts with the building blocks of theory by choosing a concept of interest. Selecting a concept that has a particular significance or meaning for the researcher is best because examination of appropriate frameworks can be tedious if one does not have an interest in the subject. Perhaps the issue of adequate staffing is of interest to the researcher. An initial literature search is performed related to the topic. From this information, a further refinement of the idea occurs, which may lead the researcher to decide that nurse burnout due to inadequate staffing is of more interest. This modification of the initial idea leads the researcher to numerous published frameworks and models related to nurse burnout. The selected concepts are then defined based on the literature, using previously established definitions where possible, to build on prior research and keep a consistency in language. Areas of convergence are teased out of the set of selected concepts.

The concepts that have been established as the topics of interest are now linked in statements that describe the expected relationships, or they can be mapped diagrammatically. Relationships are generally found using the literature, which defines and describes the concepts; however, relationships may also need to be synthesized from what is discovered in the overall literature review, following the technique of concept development.

The researcher then selects a framework that best depicts the concept(s) and its relationship(s) as determined from the researcher's investigation. In this case, perhaps

For More Depth and Detail

For a more in-depth look at the concepts in this chapter, try these references:

Colley, S. (2005). Nursing theory: Its importance to practice. *Nursing Standard, 16*(46), 33–36.

Finfgeld-Connett, D. (2006). Qualitative concept development: Implications for nursing research and knowledge. *Nursing Forum, 41*(3), 103–112.

Finfgeld-Connett, D. (2008). Qualitative convergence of three nursing concepts: Art of nursing, presence and caring. *Journal of Advanced Nursing, 63*(5), 526–534.

Graff, D. (2006). The challenging process of selecting a conceptual framework. *Clinical Nurse Specialist: The Journal for Advanced Nursing Practice, 20*(2), 90–91.

Greenwood, J., & Bonner, A. (2008). The role of theory-constitutive metaphor in nursing science. *Nursing Philosophy, 9,* 154–168.

Marrs, J. (2006). Nursing theory and practice: Connecting the dots. *Nursing Science Quarterly, 19*(1), 44–50.

Morse, J.M., Hupcey, J.E., Penrod, J., & Mitcham, C. (2002). Integrating concepts for the development of qualitatively-derived theory. *Research and Theory for Nursing Practice, 16*(1), 5–18.

Penrod, J. (2005). Concept advancement: Extending science through concept-driven research. *Research and Theory for Nursing Practice, 19*(3), 231–241.

Reed, P. (2006). The force of nursing theory-guided practice. *Nursing Science Quarterly, 19*(3), 225.

Weaver, K. (2006). Understanding paradigms used for nursing research. *Journal of Advanced Nursing, 53*(4), 459–469.

Wiest, D. (2006). Impact of conceptual nursing models in a professional environment. *Topics in Emergency Medicine, 28*(2), 161–166.

the nursing worklife model of burnout (Leiter & Spence-Laschinger, 2006) is appropriate. When the researcher has selected the framework, he or she should then perform a literature review to search for studies detailing use of the framework, examine the resulting studies, and assess the conclusions for application to the nurse researcher's own study. Building a body of support for the selection of a framework is a necessary step in the process. Successful applications of the framework are noted as well as problems or adaptations that were required.

Once these steps have been completed and the framework continues to show promise for the purposes of the new research, the researcher can begin to apply the chosen framework as a road map to design the study. For example, the researcher might identify concepts that reflect nursing burnout, ways of measuring these concepts as variables, and expectations about how burnout and staffing are related. These may all translate into elements of the ultimate research design. If examination of the theoretical foundation was performed with diligence, most likely the framework will be appropriate in the new study applications.

Theoretical and conceptual frameworks are the necessary backbones of a research study. Using a well-founded and well-referenced framework lends credence to the study, but more importantly, allows for comparisons across studies as well as building from or between studies. Researchers need to be aware of the impact of their work, and they must determine before proceeding that the important groundwork has been done. Building a study on a sound theoretical framework is one of the essentials of a good research study.

Summary of Key Concepts

- Theoretical and conceptual frameworks are the necessary backbones of a research study.
- Theories are organizations or groupings of facts or concepts to clarify relationships among and between phenomena.
- Grand theories are considered the most abstract of theories and attempt to explain what the discipline of nursing is all about.
- Middle-range theories are located midway between the abstract and concrete theories. They are more limited in scope and less abstract than grand theories, addressing specific phenomena or concepts.

 CRITICAL APPRAISAL EXERCISE

Retrieve the following full text article from the Cumulative Index to Nursing and Allied Health Literature or similar search database:

Park, S., Weaver, T., & Romer, D. (2009). Predictors of the transition from experimental to daily smoking among adolescents in the United States. *Journal of Specialists in Pediatric Nursing, 14*(2), 102–111.

Review the article, focusing on the theoretical framework that is identified and how it is used to guide development and implementation of the study. Consider the following appraisal questions in your critical review of this research article:

1. Describe the theoretical framework for the study. Is it appropriate for this research question? Is it discussed in sufficient detail?
2. Would you classify this theory as a grand theory, middle-range theory, or microtheory? Explain the reasoning for your classification.
3. Does this theory appear to be a nursing theory, a borrowed theory, or a shared theory? Explain the reasoning for your classification.
4. Explain the ways that the authors describe the theoretical framework. Is the description sufficiently explicit to link the theoretical framework to the context of the study, specifically:
   - The research question
   - The research design
   - The selected variables to be tested
   - Interpretation of the outcome
5. Are study concepts identified adequately? How are definitions linked to both study concepts and study variables?
6. What relationships do these researchers expect? Are these relationships grounded in the theoretical framework?
7. How do the authors use the theoretical framework when reporting the results of the study, if at all? Is the theoretical framework integrated into the discussion of study implications?

- Microtheories (also known as situation-specific theories or practice theories) are specific theories usually related to a particular situation, population, or set of circumstances in nursing practice.
- Nursing uses many borrowed theories, taken from other disciplines and used as frameworks or models for nursing problems.
- Nursing theories are made up of building blocks that are called concepts, conceptual definitions, concept analyses, concept developments, relational statements, and conceptual maps and models.
- Developing a conceptual framework involves a series of steps that include selecting and defining concepts, examining concepts for relationships, determining all the characteristics of those relationships, and mapping out the concepts appropriately.
- New applications of concept development focus on providing increased union between similar concepts, forming broad yet highly useful middle-range theories.
- Theoretical frameworks are collections of concepts and/or concept maps that depict a theory piece or pieces that are to be examined in a research project or study.
- Critiquing a framework in a research study involves finding the major variables in a study, analyzing the levels of abstraction among the variables, identifying hypothesized relationships among variables, and connecting the theoretical basis of the study to the methodology.
- Theoretical frameworks can be used as evidence for nursing practice or as a basis for research inquiry.

References

Becker, M.H. (1966). *The health belief model and personal health behavior.* Thorofare, NJ: Slack.

Duffy, J.R., & Hoskins, L.M. (2003). The quality-caring model: Blending dual paradigms. *Advances in Nursing Science, 26*(1), 66–88.

Duffy, J.R., Hoskins, L.M., & Dudley-Brown, S. (2005). Development and testing of a caring based intervention for older adults with heart failure. *Journal of Cardiovascular Nursing, 20*(5), 325–333.

Finfgeld-Connett, D. (2006). Qualitative concept development: Implications for nursing research and knowledge. *Nursing Forum, 41*(3), 103–112.

Finfgeld-Connett, D. (2008). Qualitative convergence of three nursing concepts: Art of nursing, presence and caring. *Journal of Advanced Nursing, 63*(5), 526–534.

Greenwood, J., & Bonner, A. (2008). The role of theory-constitutive metaphor in nursing science. *Nursing Philosophy, 9,* 154–168.

Houser, J. (2000). Evaluation of a model of the context of nursing care delivery. *Journal of Nursing Administration, 49*(1), 36–45.

Im, E.O., & Meleis, A.I. (1999). Situation-specific theories: Philosophical roots, properties and approach. *Advances in Nursing Science, 22*(2), 11–24.

Kolcaba, K. (1994). A theory of holistic comfort for nursing. *Journal of Advanced Nursing, 19*(6), 1168–1184.

Kuhn, T. (1960). *The structure of scientific revolutions* (2nd ed.). New York: Holt, Rinehart, & Winston.

Lazarus, R.S., & Folkman, S. (1984). *Stress appraisal and coping.* New York: Springer.

Leiter, M.P., & Spence-Laschinger, H.K. (2006). Relationships of work and practice environment to professional burnout: Testing a causal model. *Nursing Research, 55*(2), 136–146.

McBryde-Foster, M., & Allen, T. (2005). The continuum of care: A concept development study. *Journal of Advanced Nursing, 50*(6), 624–632.

Meleis, A.I., Sawyer, L.M., Im, E.O., Hilfinger, D.K., & Schumaker, K. (2000). Experiencing transitions: An emerging middle-range theory. *Advances in Nursing Science, 23*(1), 12–28.

Melzack, R., & Wall, P.D. (1965). Pain mechanisms: A new theory. *Science, 150*(3699), 961–969.

Morse, J.M., Hupcey J.E., Penrod J., & Mitcham C. (2002). Integrating concepts for the development of qualitatively-derived theory. *Research in Theory and Nursing Practice, 16*(1), 5–18.

Morse, J.M., Solberg, S.M., Neander, W.L., Bottorff, J.L., & Johnson, J.L. (1990). Concepts of caring and caring as a concept. *Advances in Nursing Science, 13*(1), 1–14.

Orem, D. (1995). *Nursing: Concepts of practice.* St. Louis, MO: Mosby.

Parsons, T. (1951). *The social system.* Glencoe, IL: Free Press.

Pender, N.J. (1996). *Health promotion in nursing practice* (3rd ed.). Stanford, CT: Appleton & Lange.

Reilly, D. (1995). Research homeopathy, and therapeutic consultation. *Alternative Therapies in Health and Medicine, 1*(4), 64–73.

Rogers, M.E. (1960). *An introduction to the theoretical basis of nursing.* Philadelphia: F.A. Davis.

Rogers, M.E. (1990). Nursing: Science of irreducible unitary human beings: Update 1990. In E.A.M. Barrett (ed.), *Visions of Rogers' Science Based Nursing* (pp. 5–11). New York: National League for Nursing.

Roy, C. (1960). Adaptation: A conceptual framework for nursing. *Nursing Outlook, 18*(3), 42–45.

Schumaker, K.L., & Meleis, A.I. (1994). Transitions: A central concept in nursing. *Image: The Journal of Nursing Scholarship, 26*(2), 119–126.

Wagner, C.M. (2006). Organizational commitment as a predictor variable for nursing turnover. *Journal of Advanced Nursing, 60*(3), 235–246.

Wagner, C.M. (2009). The value of a nonlinear model in predicting nursing turnover. *Journal of Nursing Administration, 39*(5), 200–203.

Watson, J. (1969). *The philosophy and science of caring.* Boston, MA: Little, Brown.

Watson, J. (1985). *Nursing: Human science and human care.* New York: Appleton-Century-Crofts.

Watson, J. (2002). Intentionality and caring-healing consciousness: A practice of transpersonal nursing. *Holistic Nursing Practice, 16*(4), 12–19.

chapter 7

Selecting an Appropriate Research Design

 CHAPTER OBJECTIVES

The study of this chapter will help the learner to

- Establish the link between the research question and the study design.
- Evaluate the characteristics that are the basis for design decisions.
- Differentiate the kinds of questions that require quantitative, qualitative, and mixed method designs.
- Identify the types of variables that reflect the concepts in a research question.
- Review designs that describe populations, test relationships, or examine causality.

KEY TERMS

Bias	Descriptive studies	Independent variable
Confirmatory studies	Descriptive variables	Predictive research
Correlation research	Exploratory studies	Research design
Dependent variable	Extraneous variables	Variable

Introduction

In the best of all possible worlds, evidence would be the result of well-controlled, perfectly designed studies. But most nurses do not practice in the best of all possible worlds; nursing research is planned by making a series of decisions, each of which involves weighing alternatives and options in the search for knowledge. It is important, then, to understand

Voices from the Field

The Dance of the Call Bells study originated while I was involved in some research on the broader topic of patient satisfaction on an in-patient unit. Patient interviews revealed that patients were commenting about the lack of timely response to call bells. I also noticed that sometimes the call bell console at the nurse's station would be lit up and no one made a move to answer the bells, even when people were standing right by the console. This information suggested that call bell response might be an important aspect of patient satisfaction that should be studied. I began gathering information on call bells as part of a larger research project, and found that, yes, call bells were indeed a problem.

I then had to decide on a method. My decisions about methods to use for a research study are made based on the problem under study or the question being asked. I choose methods that will answer the question and address the problem, including methods that are qualitative or quantitative. My goal is to get the information. I employ mixed/multiple methods when possible to enable cross-checking of the data, so this is part of my thought process as I consider design.

My personal philosophy about research design is that, regardless of the approach, it should be as rigorous as possible. To me, this means that the research can be replicated and results can be validated through triangulation or cross-checking of findings. This ensures that the resulting paper will be "solid" and more likely to be accepted by peer-reviewed publications.

I also consider who will be collecting the data and the budget available for things such as transcription of interview tapes and measurement tools. This is important; if you have people collecting the data who are not trained, the results may not be reliable. Also, the data collected by novice researchers needs to be validated or cross-checked by a trained researcher to ensure accuracy. Thus, considerations such as the skill set of the people doing the research and the available budget are critical. Measurement tools can be expensive. Transcription of audio tapes of interviews or focus groups can be both costly and time consuming, but a critically important component of qualitative research. Thus, a limited budget or lack of resources might influence the type of research and the amount of data that can be collected.

A good researcher has to consider their own skills and abilities when deciding on a methodology. I am an applied medical anthropologist, and so I try to design projects that will provide information from a holistic perspective. I try to get information on both the internal and external perspectives, to be sure that a broad understanding of the issue is obtained. I think this makes for stronger research.

For the call bells project I used observations, mapping, photographs, and interviews to gather the information I needed to understand what was happening regarding the whole dynamic of call bells. This qualitative approach most closely matched the demands of the research question, the resources that were available, and my own particular strengths. It also yielded a much richer picture of what was happening than numbers alone may have been able to provide.

Lynn M. Deitrick, RN, PhD

each of the predominant research designs so a study can be planned that best answers the research question.

To call this process "design" may give the wrong impression. This singular word implies that it is an event that happens and then is complete. In reality, design may be a circuitous process, with each decision producing a variety of implications that require consideration and that may even require the researcher to revisit earlier decisions. The ultimate result of this process is a detailed plan for the ensuing research project, which addresses the research question with a minimum of bias. Bias may come from several sources in a research study—the researcher, the subjects, the measurements, the sampling procedures—and solid design is the way to control the threat that bias presents to the overall credibility of the results.

No design is perfect. The researcher can predict some threats that will require attention during design; others may arrive, unanticipated, in the midst of the study. The design process is a series of decisions, balancing research rigor with reality. If a researcher considers design options thoughtfully, makes decisions based on the goals of the study, and can provide a rationale for each decision, the final product will be valid.

What Is a Design?

A **research design** is an outline of the study, in both a macro and a micro sense. From a macro view, design refers to an overall approach to the study, grounded in a set of beliefs about knowledge and the question that must be answered. From this macro view, there are only a handful of research classifications. Each has specific characteristics that bring with them unique strengths and weaknesses in producing credible knowledge. These macro research approaches have specific kinds of questions that they best serve, and part of the researcher's job is to match the requirements of the question to the uniqueness of a study type.

> **Research design:** The overall approach to or outline of the study that details all the major components of the research.

Macro decisions are among the first to be made, but within each large classification of studies are numerous ways to conduct the study. This requires a more micro view of the research process, requiring decisions that will give the researcher specific guidance in implementing the study. This micro view is sometimes called research design. For quantitative studies, the design will detail how the subjects will be selected and assigned to groups, the way the intervention will be applied, a measurement strategy, and a plan for data analysis. The goal of design in a quantitative study is to minimize error, limit the potential for bias, and address clinical as well as statistical issues (Parfrey & Ravani, 2009). In qualitative studies, the design will describe the planned approach to data gathering, including the researcher's beliefs about the nature of the information to be generated. Criteria for selecting informants, general guides for data collection, and plans for data analysis may be explicit in a qualitative research design.

Both the macro and micro views of research design are focused on one outcome: answering the research question with the greatest level of credibility. Reflecting on this overriding purpose can guide the researcher in the decisions that must be made.

The Basis for Design Selection

Ultimately, the basis for selecting a design is the *demands of the research question*. If a research question has been carefully considered and purposefully constructed, then it can be matched to a specific design. This match between well-constructed question and best possible answer is the goal of the research design process (Weaver & Olson, 2006).

The *nature of the variables* of the study may keep the ethical researcher from manipulating the environment or the treatment situation. These ethical limitations are strong ones and may require a weaker design in exchange for subject protections. For example, it would be unethical to inflict a disease on a patient intentionally to test a treatment for it.

Other factors affecting design are the measurements, which often present a challenge. They may result in unreliable data, or the information could be difficult to collect accurately.

The *researcher* brings strengths and limitations to the study. The researcher may not possess the skill and competence to conduct a wide range of study types; researchers often focus on one tradition, or even one design, for most of the studies they conduct. Even when the researcher has the skill and competence to conduct the type of research needed, he or she may not have the resources to carry out a study in an ideal way. These resources range from measurement instruments to data collection forms to software, which are often expensive and difficult to obtain. Almost all research studies require funding for expenses; all of them require time. Both may be in short supply for the nurse researcher. Without the necessary *resources*, even a strong design may wind up with compromises during execution. Consideration of the available resources—people, money, and materials—should also be part of the research planning process.

The *time frame* is an important consideration in research design. The length of time available to the researcher from planning to implementation to write-up is a critical concern when finalizing design decisions (Endacott, 2007). It would be unrealistic to plan a longitudinal study of the development patterns of infants as they mature into toddlers, for example, if the researcher has only a year for study.

The *amount of control* the researcher needs in the study provides guidance in the design of the study. Studies that require a high level of control (for example, drug trials and intervention studies) will need a high level of structure. Threats to the validity of the results must be anticipated and dealt with *a priori*, or before the study begins. Quantitative studies are often concerned with managing threats to internal validity. The researcher can use three broad strategies for controlling these threats: Threats can be eliminated, controlled, or accounted for.

Some issues can be eliminated or controlled during the design process. For example, the effects of demographic variables can be eliminated by careful sampling. The effects of extraneous variables may not be eliminated, but effects can be controlled statistically. There are a host of design options that can deal with preconceived threats; however, threats are not always apparent before the study starts, and many will appear only during implementation. In this case, the ethical researcher accounts for them, describes attempts to deal with the threats, and admits to the effect they may have had.

Most threats to the trustworthiness of the results of the study—called *internal validity*—are controlled by the researcher through processes that

- Assign subjects to groups equitably.
- Document the equivalence of study groups.
- Control elements of the environment.
- Ensure the treatment is applied reliably.
- Provide consistent, accurate measurements.
- Control variables extraneous to the study.

In some studies, particularly qualitative or descriptive ones, control is not much of an issue. The qualitative paradigm is a naturalistic one, requiring only that the researcher have general direction prior to starting the study. The research design may be planned, but it is allowed to morph and emerge as the study progresses. These are described as emergent designs and are expected in qualitative research. Qualitative researchers are less concerned with the effects of extraneous variables because they are not measuring effects at all, but rather attempting to understand phenomena. This understanding requires using the subject's frame of reference, not the researcher's, as the guiding voice in the study. For these studies, very little may be prescribed *a priori*.

Finally, the researcher must consider the ultimate audience for the study results. Some clinical fields focus on specific designs; for example, the practice of pharmacy is based almost exclusively on evidence produced via randomized controlled trials. The profession of nursing uses a variety of research paradigms to answer questions about nursing care, and yet even within the profession some audiences expect specific types of research. Critical care nursing, with its focus on data-driven decision making and managing physiological responses, relies heavily on the scientific method to produce evidence. Mental health nursing, on the other hand, is often based on the results of qualitative studies. The expectations of the audience that will be reached with the study should be incorporated into the design decisions.

It is not always possible to control a research process as well as one might desire. A host of practical issues may affect design. Subjects are human beings and may behave in unpredictable ways. They may be difficult to recruit or to keep in a study. The researcher may have limited access to the subjects' information or may have to rely on secondary data. Subjects may be untruthful, behave unnaturally, or refuse treatment.

It is important to emphasize that all studies have strengths and weaknesses; no single study can be definitively and perfectly designed. It is the convergence of findings across studies that adds knowledge to a profession, not the perfection of a single design (DelBoca & Darkes, 2007). Although the researcher should strive to control extraneous variables and threats to validity as much as possible, every study will have its limitations. If the nurse researcher waits until the perfect design is achieved, research will never get accomplished.

The Design Decisions

Research design requires researchers to make a series of decisions. Although they can follow a general sequence when making these decisions, researchers may move back and forth among decisions until they hit on the right design to solve the research problem. These decisions become the plan that guides the researcher in implementation of the study.

Design decisions paint the study in broad strokes first and then focus at a more detailed level as the study is planned. Different decisions have a different relative weight depending on the amount of structure needed in the study. For example, sampling might be more important in a case–control study, where matching of cases and controls is essential. On the other hand, qualitative studies require more emphasis on the way information is elicited and checked with informants, and so willingness to communicate verbally may be a primary concern.

Design always involves tradeoffs. Some design flaws may have little impact; others may fatally affect the credibility of the results. The researcher's obligation is to clarify the purpose of the study and design the study to achieve this purpose in a trustworthy way.

There is no single best design. Even expert researchers often disagree on the merits of a particular design decision. Although some designs provide stronger levels of evidence for nursing practice, in reality, all good designs are rigorous and systematic. The nature of the data collected may vary substantially, but a focus on finding truth should be unwavering in good research design. A great deal of the credibility of a study is based not on a researcher making a single correct decision, but on the researcher making a sequence of defensible, rational decisions.

It is probably unrealistic to think of these decisions as occurring in a particular sequence. Researchers often move back and forth between decision levels that are interrelated, rather than mutually exclusive. In general, however, the decision-making process has three major phases. These phases start with a high-level, macro view of the problem and purpose of the study and focus on more detailed decisions as the design plan unfolds. Think of these phases as looking at the study with more and more powerful microscopes, focusing more tightly with each subsequent look. The three phases are

1. Identify assumptions about the knowledge to be gained from the study.
2. Select a design that serves the purpose of the study.
3. Develop detailed plans for implementation of the study.

Identify Assumptions About the Knowledge to Be Gained from the Study

When designing a research study, the researcher must reflect on any assumptions he or she has made regarding the nature of the knowledge needed to answer the question. These assumptions will guide the researcher to a quantitative or qualitative design or may reveal that a mix of both methods is required (Creswell, 2008).

Quantitative approaches to design are appropriate when the purpose of the study is to measure the effect of an intervention, test a theory about relationships, or describe a phenomenon with precision. Quantitative designs require measurement of some sort and so will ultimately involve the analysis of numbers. These studies require control of internal validity for trustworthiness and strong external validity for generalizability. Quantitative designs are appropriate when the results must reveal the true relationship between a cause and an effect or between two variables. Measurement gives the researcher a level of certainty about the relationship that is quantifiable, and the effects of error and random chance can be calculated (Hartung & Touchette, 2009). The control inherent in a quantitative design allows the researcher to rule out rival explanations for the results and quantify the amount of confidence the reader can place in the findings.

Qualitative approaches to design are appropriate when the purpose of the study is to understand the meaning of a phenomenon. The qualitative researcher has a goal of describing social reactions and interactions with such vividness that the reader can understand the meaning of the event, even if he or she has not experienced it. Qualitative research can also be used to develop theories, build models of relationships and interrelationships, and develop instrumentation (Speziale & Carpenter, 2006). Qualitative research places little emphasis on control. The context for the study is a natural one, and the study is allowed to unfold as information is gathered and analyzed. Often, a qualitative study follows twists and turns as the investigator strives to understand the phenomenon by exploring its meaning with informants. The design is an emergent one, with only general guidelines planned up front. This emergent design enables the qualitative researcher to follow leads provided by informants to understand the social context for behavior (Munhall, 2006).

A mixed method is appropriate when a combination of meaning and control is needed. Frequently, a mixed method is used when a qualitative approach is used to design an instrument or an intervention that is subsequently tested for effectiveness using quantitative methods. A mixed method may also be indicated for evaluation research, where effectiveness, efficiency, and satisfaction are important elements (Miller & Fredericks, 2006). The desirability of a treatment may be measured using qualitative measures, while the effectiveness of the treatment is documented quantitatively. Mixed methods seem attractive—it makes intuitive sense to consider the meaning of an event prior to testing its effectiveness—but they are complex, difficult designs to implement. The rigorous nature of both research traditions must be reflected in the design, and the researcher must be competent in both traditions.

Although these traditions may seem diametrically opposed, in actuality they have much in common. By nature, the characteristics of one may overlap with those of another. Both types of research are characterized by rigorous attention to the scholarly nature of the work. Both aim for reliability of results, confidence in the conclusions, and a focus on creating credible evidence. Both research traditions have a single goal—the establishment of truth. Although specific methods may be quite different, the goals of each are to produce quality results that answer the question in a trustworthy way. In that way, they are very much alike.

Select a Design That Serves the Purpose of the Study

Once assumptions of the study question have been determined, then the researcher selects an approach that will answer the research question and meet the goals of the study. This selection process is the result of a series of decisions based on reflection on the aim of the study, the concepts under study, and the nature of the research question. The researcher can make these decisions by answering a series of questions.

Exploratory studies: Research approaches designed to explore and describe a phenomenon of interest and generate new knowledge.

Confirmatory studies: Research approaches in which a relationship between variables has been posed and the study is designed to examine these hypotheses.

Is the Aim of the Study Exploratory or Confirmatory?

Exploratory studies are often qualitative or mixed methods studies, but they may also be quantitative if measurement is employed. Exploratory studies are classified as descriptive, even if they may describe relationships and associations. They explore and describe a given phenomenon. Survey methods are frequently used for exploratory studies; mixed methods are common as well in the initial exploration of a topic. For example, a study that explores the reasons that nurses choose a clinical specialty may determine the specific characteristics that the nurse was looking for, such as certifications required and work hours, but also explore the value-based reasons a particular selection was made. The former might be measured by a survey instrument, whereas the value-based information would be more appropriately gathered through an interview.

Confirmatory studies are those in which a relationship between variables has been posed, and the study is designed to test the relationship statistically while minimizing bias. In this case, some form of study to determine relationships or examine causality is required. Confirmatory studies are more structured and controlled than exploratory studies. These studies require careful definition of the variables and concepts of interest so they can be adequately measured and analyzed. Confirmatory studies are often "next steps" from exploratory studies. For example, an analysis of the results of a knowledge-based questionnaire for diabetic patients might be used to design a specific diabetic education program that is subsequently tested for effectiveness.

What Concepts Will Be Studied?

A clear definition of the concepts that will be studied guides the design of a study and the subsequent measurement strategy. In quantitative research, the concepts that are of interest are translated into measurable characteristics called **variables**. A variable is a characteristic, event, or response that represents the elements of the research question in a detectable way (Creswell, 2008). Variables are carefully described up front to guide the design of quantitative studies. There are several types of variables that may represent the intent of the research question. **Table 7.1** represents some research questions in terms of their respective variables and concepts.

Variable: Characteristic, event, or response that represents the elements of the research question in a detectable or measurable way.

Descriptive variables: Characteristics that describe the sample and provide a composite picture of the subjects of the study; they are not manipulated or controlled by the researcher.

Descriptive Variables

As the name implies, **descriptive variables** are those that describe the sample or some characteristic of the phenomenon under study. A descriptive variable may represent demographic data about the subjects (for example, age, gender, and ethnicity) or measurable characteristics (for example, blood pressure, weight, and hematocrit). The variables of interest may be perceptual, as in responses on a pain scale, or attitudinal, as in patient satisfaction. The primary characteristic of a descriptive variable is that it is used solely to provide a composite picture of the subjects of study. Descriptive variables are not considered part of a cause-and-effect equation, and although the researcher may look for associations between variables, no attempt is made to manipulate or control descriptive variables.

Research Variables

Research variables are introduced into a study explicitly to measure an expected effect. A research variable may be categorized as either independent or dependent. An **independent variable** is one that is applied to the experimental situation to measure its effects. The variable is independent of the naturally occurring situation and is introduced into the experiment so that its impact on a specified outcome can be quantified. In a true experiment, the independent variable is manipulated, meaning it is introduced by the researcher. It may also be called a treatment, experimental variable, or intervention. One can think of an independent variable as the "cause" in "cause and effect." For example, if a nurse is interested in studying the effects of therapeutic touch on postoperative pain, therapeutic touch is the independent variable. It is artificially inserted into a situation in order to measure its effects.

> **Independent variable:** A factor that is artificially introduced into a study explicitly to measure an expected effect. The "cause" of "cause and effect."

Some designs consider causal variables to be independent even if they are not manipulated; in these cases, the variable of interest is found in its naturally occurring state, and subjects with the specified characteristic are compared to those without it to understand its potential effects. For example, a researcher might be interested in studying the effects of breast cancer on body image. Although breast cancer is not manipulated, its effects are of interest in this study, and it may be referred to as an independent variable. Technically, independent variables are only those that are artificially introduced to subjects, but the term is used loosely to apply to other types of casual variables.

Table 7.1

Research Questions and Concepts/Variables

Research Question	Concepts/Variables
What is the perception of the effectiveness of complementary medicine among intensive care unit nurses?	Descriptive variable: perception of effectiveness
Is music therapy an effective treatment for patients who experience anxiety in the intensive care unit when compared to patients who receive no music therapy?	■ Research variables: independent—music therapy; dependent—anxiety ■ Extraneous variable: sound level in the ICU; preexisting anxiety disorder
What are the emotional and psychological reactions of patients who have been patients in the intensive care unit for more than 5 days?	Concepts: emotional and psychological reactions

A **dependent variable** is the outcome of interest. In an experiment, it is expected that an independent variable will have an effect on the dependent variable. In other words, the outcome is dependent on the independent variable having been introduced into the experiment. The dependent variable can be considered the "effect" in "cause and effect."

In a specific type of design that is focused on prediction, the independent variable is more accurately called a predictor variable, and the dependent variable is referred to as an outcome variable. Although the terms *independent* and *dependent* are commonly used to describe the predictive relationship, technically the terms are not accurate descriptions of these variables because the predictor variable is not manipulated. Predictive studies are classified as descriptive, and so these variables are more accurately referred to by their function, rather than by their dependent nature. For example, a nurse researcher may want to find the characteristics of patients who present to the emergency department who are at high risk for multiple visits. In this case, demographic variables such as age, diagnoses, socioeconomic status, and family support might be studied to determine if some of them are predictive of repeat admissions. In this example, age, diagnoses, socioeconomic status, and family support would accurately be described as predictor variables and repeat admissions identified as the outcome variable.

Extraneous Variables

A goal of design is to control external influences on a process so that rival explanations for the outcome can be ruled out. These rival explanations are considered **extraneous variables**, or variables that exert an effect on the outcome but that are not part of the planned experiment. Realistically, extraneous variables exist in every study, but they are most problematic in experiments. Extraneous variables can be controlled if they are expected and/or recognized when they occur. The most problematic extraneous variables are those that cannot be predicted, are difficult to control, or go unrecognized until the study is complete. Extraneous variables confuse the interpretation of the results and may render an experiment so flawed that the results cannot be used in practice. A primary goal of research design, particularly experimental designs, is the elimination or control of extraneous variables.

A specific type of extraneous variable is a confounder. Confounding occurs when the association between cause and effect is partially or entirely due to a third factor that is not part of the experiment. For example, a study might show that alcoholism is a causative factor in lung cancer, when in reality the relationship is due to a confounder—smoking. Because smoking rates are higher among alcoholics, this third factor confounds the true relationship between alcoholism and lung disease. For a variable to be a true confounder, it must be associated with the independent variable and a true cause of the dependent variable (Hartung & Touchette, 2009). When a confounder is suspected, the research design must be altered to control or account for its effects. The most common ways to control confounders are through random sampling, matching subjects, and statistical analysis of covariates.

Qualitative Concepts

The term *variable* is rarely used in qualitative research. This is because a variable, by definition, is something that is measurable, and measurement is not typical of qualitative designs. However, qualitative studies do have goals related to understanding a phenomenon, belief, perception, or set of values (Speziale & Carpenter, 2006). In the case of qualitative research, the design is driven by the nature of the information to be gained from the study, and this requires thoughtful consideration of the particular phenomenon of interest. Although it is unnecessary to develop operational definitions for qualitative phenomena, the researcher should be able to articulate the concepts, theories, or processes that are of interest. In the case of grounded theory—a specific type of qualitative research design—the researcher may also plan to study relationships between these phenomena.

Whether the researcher plans to measure variables or study phenomena, consideration of these characteristics will help determine the specifics of the research design. Sometimes it is necessary to incorporate elements of both types of study. It is important to keep in mind that the characteristics of concepts under study guide the selection of strategies to best examine nursing practices (Iversen & Petersson, 2006). Identifying the variables and concepts in a study is an important precursor to design. By clarifying the conceptual focus of the study, the researcher can begin to implement the research question in a way that lends itself to study.

What Is the Nature of the Research Question?

Once the conceptual basis of the study is articulated, the research question becomes the focus of more specific design decisions. The nature of the research question is the foundation for the next set of decisions: classification of the specific research study design. Most research questions can be classified into one of three categories:

1. Questions that seek to describe a phenomenon or population
2. Questions that seek to quantify the nature of relationships between variables or between subjects
3. Questions that seek to investigate causality or the effects of interventions or risk factors

Descriptive Research

Descriptive research is appropriate when very little is known about the question at hand. Often, researchers seek to fix problems without understanding the current problem as it exists. Descriptive research can help the investigator discover a baseline performance level, describe a subject's responses to treatment, or determine the desirability of a new service. Research questions that begin with "what" and "why" generally indicate a descriptive study. **Descriptive studies** set out to describe in detail some process, event, or outcome. They document the characteristics of a "subject" of some sort. Subject is in quotes because it represents a broad range of possibilities other than individuals. For example, a subject may be a child, a patient, a patient care unit, an emergency department, a county's health, or a unit's adverse event rate. Once a subject of interest has been described, an exploratory study sets out to discover as

Descriptive studies: Research designed to describe in detail some process, event, or outcome. The design is used when very little is known about the research question.

much about the subject as possible and to find themes that can help the researcher effectively derive meaning from the study.

Descriptive qualitative studies rarely have detailed procedures identified up front; the design of a qualitative study is "emergent" in that the details of the study emerge as information is gathered and the nature of the information is evaluated. The qualitative researcher will identify a specific approach to data gathering and a philosophical basis for the approach, but it is unusual for a researcher to create a detailed plan prior to initiating a qualitative study. Most quantitative descriptive studies, however, have a clear plan for implementation that outlines the sample, the measurement procedures, and statistical processes that will be used to summarize the data.

Descriptive studies are often exploratory, but they can also be confirmatory, meaning the researcher suspects that a phenomenon or event exists in a population, and he or she sets out to confirm those suspicions. Most often, however, descriptive studies are applied when very little is known about the situation, and baseline knowledge is required to be able to design effective nursing practices. Chapter 12 will cover common designs for descriptive research in detail, and Chapter 13 will explicitly describe the analytic techniques used for summarizing and interpreting descriptive data. **Table 7.2** depicts a summary of the common descriptive designs and characteristics of each.

Table 7.2

Some Common Descriptive Designs

Design	Description	Example of a Research Question	Strengths	Limitations
Survey design	Describes the characteristics of a sample or event at a single point in time through self-report.	What coping strategies do adults use when diagnosed with cancer?	Description of current state provides a basis for planning interventions	Unable to determine causes of change or differences between groups
Cross-sectional study	Describes the characteristics of samples that differ on a key characteristic, measured at a single point in time.	What are the coping strategies that adults use when newly diagnosed with cancer?	▪ Uncomplicated to manage ▪ Economical	Does not capture changes that occur over time
Longitudinal study	Data are collected from a sample at selected points over time to describe changes in characteristics or events.	What coping strategies do adults use when managing their cancer in the 5 years after diagnosis?	Enables exploration of issues affected by human development	▪ Affected by attrition of subjects ▪ Extended time period required for data collection

Table 7.2

Some Common Descriptive Designs *(Continued)*

Design	Description	Example of a Research Question	Strengths	Limitations
Case study	Explores in depth a single individual, program, event, or action through the collection of detailed information using a variety of data collection techniques.	What are the responses of a group of adults to a holistic treatment support group?	■ Enables evaluation of rare events or conditions ■ Allows for the study of the uniqueness of individual people or situations	Time-consuming, requiring extended study
Single subject design	Studies the response of a single individual to an intervention, based on measurement of a baseline and ongoing measurement after introducing a treatment.	What are the responses of a 30-year-old woman diagnosed with breast cancer after introduction to a holistic treatment support group?	■ Allows for the study of the unique responses of individuals to interventions ■ Enables the determination of timing of responses after an intervention	Does not enable generalization to larger populations
Phenomenology	Investigates the meaning of an experience in a group that have all experienced the same phenomenon.	What is the meaning of the experience of receiving a diagnosis of cancer?	■ Produces rich data from the informant's perspective ■ Can be used to study a wide range of phenomena	Requires a high level of analytic skill
Ethnography	Intensive study of the features and interactions of a given culture by immersion in the natural setting over an extended period of time.	How do women in Muslim society respond to a diagnosis of breast cancer?	Produces rich data that enable the development of culturally sensitive interventions	Requires extensive contact over long periods of time

Research That Examines Relationships

The research question often reflects a need to go beyond describing single characteristics to determining if a relationship exists between variables or between subjects. This type of research can fall into two categories: correlation research or predictive research. **Correlation research** involves the quantification of the strength and direction of the relationship between two variables in a single subject or the relationship between a single variable in two samples. For example, a researcher might want to determine if there is an association between anxiety and blood pressure in the preoperative patient, or the researcher may study the nature of anxiety between mothers and daughters.

> **Correlation research:** Research designed to quantify the strength and the direction of the relationship of two variables in a single subject or the relationship between a single variable in two samples.

Predictive research: Research designed to search for variables measured at one point in time that may forecast an outcome that is measured at a different point in time.

The purpose of **predictive research** is to search for variables measured at one point in time that may predict an outcome that is measured at a different point in time. For example, given a patient's total cholesterol, could the occurrence of myocardial infarction be predicted?

Both correlation and predictive research are considered descriptive because the variables are not manipulated and the relationships are not controlled. Correlation and predictive research also may be used legitimately to search for suggested causal relationships that may subsequently be studied through experimental designs. Experimental designs will be discussed in more detail later in this chapter. Table 7.3 depicts a summary of common designs that are used to describe relationships and their associated characteristics.

Research That Examines Causality

Evidence-based nursing practice is commonly focused on determining the effectiveness of nursing interventions. This requires a research design that can establish and quantify causality. Measuring cause and effect is complex, however; several requirements must be met before a researcher can conclude that the cause did, indeed, result in the effect to the exclusion of all other causes. To establish that a causal relationship exists, several criteria must be met. These criteria form the basis for the elements that make up the set of research designs that are known as the experimental and quasi-experimental methods. The criteria include:

- *Temporality:* The time sequence between independent and dependent variables must support causation.
- *Influence:* The effect that the independent variable has on the dependent variable can be detected statistically, and the probability that the relationship was caused by chance is small.
- *Specificity:* Rival explanations for the specific relationship between independent and dependent variables have been eliminated or controlled (Hartung & Touchette, 2009).

The temporal relationship that is required for causality is reflected in the sequence of events in an experiment. In short, the cause must precede the effect. Although this seems self-evident—an effect cannot be exhibited until its cause has occurred—this criterion is the reason that some types of research (for example, correlation, case–control, or causal comparison) cannot be considered experimental. Unless clear evidence exists that the cause preceded the effect, the relationship cannot be truly described as causal.

Influence is established primarily through statistical methods. The researcher cannot directly measure the effect that a cause produced, but he or she can determine the probability that the effect was caused by something else (for example, random events, error, or sampling issues). Inferential statistics has as its goal the measurement of this relative probability. The researcher rules out rival explanations by controlling as many aspects of the research study as can reasonably be controlled. The most common rival explanations are related to bias. **Bias** occurs when true findings are distorted due to a factor other than the one being studied. Many elements related to the

Bias: The distortion of true findings by factors other than those being studied.

| Table 7.3 | | | | |

Some Designs That Describe Relationships

Design	Description	Example of a Research Question	Strengths	Limitations
Correlation	Describes the relationship between two variables in a single population or the relationship between a single variable in two populations	Are coping skills and socioeconomic status related in a sample of adults newly diagnosed with cancer?	▪ Enables scrutiny of a large number of variables in a single study ▪ Provides an evaluation of the strength of relationship between two variables ▪ Provides a basis for subsequent experimental testing	▪ May be affected by extraneous variables ▪ Does not enable a conclusion about causality
Predictive study	Describes the relationship between a predictor variable (or group of predictor variables) and an outcome variable	Can coping skills in adults with newly diagnosed cancer predict their level of compliance with the treatment plan?	Describes the predictive capacity and quantifies the explanatory ability of a variable or group of variables	May be affected by extraneous variables
Grounded theory	Qualitative method in which the researcher attempts to develop a theory of process, action, or interaction based on in-depth analysis of the words of informants	How do social support systems affect the development and use of coping skills in adults newly diagnosed with cancer?	Enables development of theoretical models of action and interaction	▪ Requires sophisticated analytic skill ▪ Involves collection of large amounts of data
Tests of model fit	Test theories of causal relationships between variables based on fitting data to a preconceived model	Does the introduction of a support group affect the type and effectiveness of coping skills used by adults with newly diagnosed cancer?	Enable quantification of the fit of a theoretical model to real life	Complex studies that require large samples, statistical sophistication, and specialized software

research study can be biased; the researcher, measurement tools, subjects, sample, data, or statistical analyses may all introduce bias. This bias is most often unintentional and unconscious, and so researchers cannot assume that bias is controlled simply because they are aware it might happen. To ensure causality, the researcher must build important controls for bias into the design.

Other sources of rival explanations are extraneous variables. Their control is a central part of experimental design. The control of rival explanations is an important concern in establishing that the independent variable—and only the independent variable—produced the effect that was observed.

gray matter

Bias may be introduced in research by the following sources:
- Researcher
- Measurements
- Subjects
- Sampling procedures
- Data
- Statistical analysis
- Extraneous variables

The research question that requires establishing causality forces the researcher to consider how all these elements will be managed in an experiment. The more carefully thought out the details of a study, the stronger the design will be and the more confidently the nurse can apply the findings as evidence for practice. Once the considerations that are inherent in the research question have been made explicit, the researcher can begin focusing even more closely on the structure of the explicit design that will be used to answer the question. Chapter 14 will explore research designs that measure effectiveness in detail. Chapter 15 will review the statistical methods available to analyze and report experimental data. Table 7.4 depicts a summary of the common designs for examining causality and the characteristics of each.

Table 7.4

Some Designs That Examine Causality

Design	Description	Example of a Research Question	Strengths	Limitations
Experimental design	Studies causality by introducing an intervention to one group (the treatment group) and comparing an outcome to another group that has not experienced the intervention (the control group); subjects are randomly assigned to groups.	Does coaching to improve coping strategies result in increased compliance with the treatment program for adults with newly diagnosed cancer?	Provides the most rigorous test of effectiveness of interventions	■ Difficult to implement. ■ It may be impossible or ethically undesirable to withhold treatment from the control group.
Quasi-experimental design	A treatment is introduced to a group, but random assignment and/or a control group are missing.	Does coaching improve coping strategies in adults with newly diagnosed cancer who are participating in a support group?	Enables scrutiny of causality	■ Cannot definitively determine causality. ■ Level of evidence provided is weaker than experimental designs.
Causal-comparative design/case control	Nonexperimental study in which groups are selected because they do or do not have a characteristic of interest and are examined for a dependent variable; groups are carefully matched based on the independent variable.	Do adults with newly diagnosed cancer who have supportive spouses comply with their treatment plan more effectively than those without supportive spouses?	■ Is useful when the independent variable cannot be manipulated ■ Provides evidence that suggests causal relationships that can be tested experimentally	■ Inferences about causality are limited. ■ Extraneous variables may affect the outcome. ■ May be difficult to find matched controls.

Table 7.4

Some Designs That Examine Causality *(Continued)*

Design	Description	Example of a Research Question	Strengths	Limitations
Time series analysis	Studies the effects of an intervention by measuring a baseline, implementing a treatment, and collecting data about an outcome at specified periods over time.	Does coaching to improve coping skills introduced after initial treatment improve compliance with the treatment plan for adults with cancer?	■ The treatment group serves as its own control group, so subjects' effects are minimized. ■ Extended time period for measurement strengthens the capacity to attribute effects to the intervention. ■ More powerful in detecting changes over time.	■ May be affected by attrition of subjects. ■ Historical events or maturation of subjects may affect the outcome. ■ No comparison group is measured to determine the effects of extraneous variables.

Develop Detailed Plans for Implementation of the Study

Many of the decisions that guide the research will be dictated by the type of design chosen. For example, an experimental design requires a random sample or random assignment of subjects to groups, whereas a qualitative study will have purposeful sampling. Even after an explicit design is chosen, however, there are still many decisions to make. These decisions include the procedures selected for recruiting subjects, applying interventions, and measuring outcomes, to name a few. Other decisions are required to ensure that an adequate sample can be accessed and that ethical considerations are addressed.

A research plan guiding implementation of the study describes the following design elements:

- The sampling strategy
- The measurement strategy
- The data collection plan
- The data analysis plan

The research plan is used like a road map to ensure that all the steps of the research process are systematically and rigorously applied. The research plan provides documentation of steps that were taken and the rationale for specific decisions, and this plan is the primary way a researcher can support replicability of the study. A detailed research plan also helps the researcher recall the decisions that were made and procedures that were carried out when the time comes for writing the final report of the research.

Reading Research for Evidence-Based Practice

The research report should provide a clear description of each step that was taken in the design and implementation of the research study. This description is often summarized in the abstract of the article under the heading "methods." The methods section is relatively standard; a good quantitative methods section will review the sampling strategy, design of the study, instruments, procedures, and analysis. A qualitative methods section should describe the sampling criteria, the method for gathering information, and an overview of data coding procedures. Although length limitations imposed by journals may restrict the depth of detail an author can provide, the nurse reader should be able to determine enough key elements to assess the validity or trustworthiness of the study.

Validity is primarily a quantitative concern. A valid study is one in which enough control has been exerted so the effect of the concepts under study can be isolated from other effects. Trustworthiness is the primary concern in qualitative studies. A trustworthy study is one in which the researcher has drawn the correct conclusions about the meaning of an event or phenomenon. Neither is a minor task, but each is essential for the respective application of the evidence to practice. Judging the validity or trustworthiness of the data is primarily based on how well the study design accomplished the purpose of the study and how thoroughly the design allowed for the answer to the research question.

Several steps can guide the nurse when he or she is evaluating the study design.

- The methods section should be complete. It should present an accurate and thorough account of every important step in the design and conduct of the research. This thorough account allows the reader to make decisions about accepting the results of the study. Providing sufficient detail about the methods used in the study enables readers to decide for themselves how much confidence they have that the experimental treatment did indeed lead to the results.
- A strong methods section supports replication, one of the hallmarks of sound research that contributes to an overall professional body of knowledge. In practical terms, the nurse should be able to get enough information from the description of the methods to conduct the study exactly as the author did, using

 Where to Look

Where to look for information about the methods and procedures:

- The design of the study is usually described in the abstract of the study and again in the introduction. It should be identified in a straightforward way and clearly described. If not, it should be described early in the section labeled "methods."
- The design section may be called "research design" or "plan." Other words may appear in the heading, such as "methods and procedures" or "methods and materials."

- The description of the design should be easily identifiable and a major part of the research study write-up. The description may be concise, but it should have enough detail that an informed reader could replicate the study.
- If the intervention or measurement is complex, the write-up may include a separate section for procedures, which may be labeled as such or called "protocols." This section may describe the specific steps for applying the treatment, the specific steps for measuring its effects, or both.

Checklist for Evaluating the Design of a Research Article

✔ The design is clearly identified and described using standard language.
✔ A rationale is provided, or can be easily inferred, for the choice of a design.
✔ The characteristics of the design can be clearly linked to the nature of the research question.
✔ The variables are explicitly identified and definitions are written for each.
✔ Enough detail is provided that an informed reader could replicate the study.
✔ If qualitative, the researcher has documented the basis for decisions as the design emerged.

different subjects, to determine whether the results can be generalized to another population.

■ A thorough methods section allows comparison of findings across studies. This is critical for the systematic review process. A thorough account of the subjects, intervention, measurement, and analysis allows for a comparison across studies to draw conclusions about both the size of the treatment effect and the consistency with which outcomes are achieved (Fain, 2008).

This section of a research study is the basis for conclusions about the validity and trustworthiness of the findings. A critical appraisal of study methods should lead the nurse to the conclusion that inconsistency in procedures is not an explanation for the results. In other words, can all other rival explanations for the outcome be eliminated, except that of the intervention? If the methods section is sound, the answer to this question should be an unequivocal "yes," giving the nurse confidence to apply the findings to practice.

Using Research in Evidence-Based Practice

All types of research designs are useful in application to practice. The hierarchy of evidence puts more weight on the results of experimental designs, but all types of knowledge can contribute to the effective practice of nursing. The task of the nurse is to choose the type of knowledge—and therefore the range of designs—that produces the kind of information needed to solve a clinical problem.

Descriptive research is useful when determining the characteristics of specific populations, identifying the practices that are used at other organizations, or measuring baseline performance. This type of research is helpful when little is known about the existing state of a phenomenon or when exploring perceptions, attitudes, or beliefs. Descriptive research focuses on what is, and so it is not used for quantifying the effectiveness of interventions, but nevertheless can provide valuable information about the status quo. This baseline information is often necessary to establish the overall desirability of a change in practice.

When the focus of the nurse is on improving a clinical intervention, then quantitative research is more valuable. Quantitative research enables the nurse to determine whether an intervention has produced a desired effect and the probability that it will continue to do so, even with different populations. If the nurse needs to change a procedure, standardize practices, measure relationships, or determine cause and effect, then quantitative studies are the most useful.

Often, the nurse also needs to determine the acceptability of a nursing intervention. If the goal is to provide emotional or social support for patients and their families, then qualitative research is more likely to produce the evidence needed for practice. When design of an appropriate intervention requires that the nurse understand the meaning of a life event for a patient, then qualitative studies are more likely to provide the insight that is needed to design acceptable treatments.

The nurse should evaluate the soundness of the design for answering the specific research question to determine whether it can be applied to nursing practice. This includes

---

SKILL Builder | Design a Stronger Study

Although the hierarchy of evidence-based practice identifies randomized controlled trials as the strongest designs, they are not always possible or even desirable. Although experimental designs do make for strong evidence for nursing practice, it is difficult to conduct a pure experimental design. There may not be enough subjects to attain sufficient power, and those who are available may not consent to be in the study. Extraneous variables abound, and it is often unethical to withhold treatment from a control group. Once the study has begun, it is hard to ensure that the experimental group always gets the exact same treatment, particularly in an applied setting. Time constraints and availability of individuals to collect data can hinder the validity of the experiment. Although it may be challenging to conduct a true experiment in a nursing practice environment, there are still measures that can strengthen the validity of a study:

- Use a comparison group of some kind. Although it may be difficult to randomly assign patients to groups, the use of a comparison group does strengthen validity, even if it is a convenience sample.
- If using a nonrandom comparison group, match the groups as closely as possible on potential extraneous variables (for example, age, severity of illness, and number of co-morbid conditions).
- Measure a baseline in a group of subjects, which becomes your comparison group, and then repeat the measures as the treatment is applied. This design, called a repeated measure design, has a great deal of power.
- If the sample is less than desirable, use a strong and valid measurement system. Sampling error can be balanced somewhat by a reduction in measurement error.
- Clearly identify the variables of interest and write formal operational definitions of each. These definitions can help determine criteria for inclusion in the study, treatment protocols, and measurement systems. For a qualitative study, explicitly identify the concepts that are of interest to the researcher.
- Replicate the studies of others whenever possible. Finding a similar study can help jump-start the study by describing procedures and measures that you might be able to use.
- Use standard designs, methods, and procedures whenever possible, even if they do not exactly match your question. Standardized approaches allow for the aggregation of like studies into practical guidelines that make a contribution to the overall body of nursing knowledge.

an appraisal of the match between the purpose of the study and the kind of knowledge generated for it, the links between the nature of the research question and the explicit design chosen to answer it, and the appropriateness of the specific procedures put in place to carry out the study.

Creating Evidence for Practice

Creating an effective research plan involves a systematic process of considering the purpose of the study and the nature of the question and then making decisions about the way the study will be carried out to draw the correct conclusions. These designs are rarely clear cut; almost always the investigator is charged with weighing the relative strengths and weaknesses of various design elements to arrive at the best possible decision given the specific characteristics of the study at hand. That said, the researcher is well served by spending the time to consider and create a careful research plan because it will serve as a blueprint for the study as well as its documentation.

The researcher needs to determine the answers to the following questions:

1. What is the nature of the knowledge that will be required to address this research problem? Quantitative studies are needed to test interventions; qualitative ones to discover the meaning of phenomena.

2. What concepts are involved in answering this question? Describing the variables that will be studied, or the phenomena of interest, guides the measurement strategy.

For More Depth and Detail

For a more in-depth look at the concepts in this chapter, try these references:

Creswell, J. (2008). *Research design: Qualitative, quantitative and mixed methods approaches* (3rd ed.). Thousand Oaks, CA: Sage.

Endacott, R. (2007). Clinical research I: Research questions and design. *Accident and Emergency Nursing, 15*, 106–109.

Fain, E. (2008). *Reading, understanding, and applying nursing research*. Philadelphia: F.A. Davis.

Hartung, D., & Touchette, D. (2009). Overview of clinical research design. *American Journal of Health System Pharmacy, 66*(15), 398–408.

Knight, K. (2010). Study/experimental/research design: Much more than statistics. *Journal of Athletic Training, 45*(1), 98–100.

Leykum, L., Pugh, J., Lanham, H., Harmon, J., & McDaniel, R. (2009). Implementation research design: Integrating participatory action research into randomized controlled trials. *Implementation Science, 4*, 69.

Munhall, P. (2006). *Nursing research: A qualitative perspective* (4th ed.). Sudbury, MA: Jones & Bartlett.

Romeiser, L., Hickman, R., Harris, S., & Heriza, C. (2008). Single-subject research design: Recommendations for levels of evidence and quality rating. *Developmental Medicine and Child Neurology, 50*(2), 99–103.

3. What is the nature of the research question? A descriptive design is required for research questions that ask about what is or that are exploratory. If the question is focused on the nature of relationships, then correlation studies are needed. Questions related to causality or the effectiveness of interventions demand experimental designs. The specifics of the design will be based on the accessibility of the population, the skills and resources of the researcher, and the expectations of the ultimate audience for the research.

4. What specific procedures will be required to answer the question? Once a design is selected, the researcher must determine how the subjects or informants will be recruited, how the concepts will be measured, and how data will be analyzed.

Once these decisions have been made, the research design is translated into a specific plan of study—one that can be used to guide and replicate the study.

Summary of Key Concepts

- A design is a plan that outlines the overall approach to a study, grounded in a set of beliefs about knowledge and inextricably linked to the nature of the research question.
- The research design is focused on answering the research question with the greatest level of credibility.
- Selection of a design is based on the purpose to be achieved by the study, the availability of subjects, ethical limitations, the skills and resources of the researcher, the time frame, the amount of control required, and the expectations of the audience for the research.
- The phases of the research process include identifying assumptions about the knowledge needed, selecting an overall approach that serves the purpose, specifying an explicit design for the study, and developing detailed plans for implementation.
- Assumptions about the knowledge needed to answer the research question will result in the choice of a quantitative, qualitative, or mixed method approach.
- The overall approach of the study is determined by considering whether a study is exploratory (generating new knowledge) or confirmatory (testing theories or hypotheses).
- The concepts reflected in the research question are translated into measurable variables for a quantitative study. These variables may be descriptive, independent, dependent, or extraneous. The concepts in qualitative questions describe characteristics, experiences, or phenomena that are of interest to the researcher.
- The three major classifications of research questions are those that seek to describe a phenomenon or population, those that seek to quantify the nature of relationships, and those that seek to investigate causality.
- Three conditions must be met to establish causality: The cause must precede the effect; the probability that the cause influenced the effect must be established; and rival explanations for the effect must be ruled out.

CRITICAL APPRAISAL **EXERCISE**

Retrieve the following full text article from the Cumulative Index to Nursing and Allied Health Literature or similar search database:

Pauly, B., Varcoe, C., Storch, J., & Newton, L. (2009). Registered nurses' perceptions of moral distress and ethical climate. *Nursing Ethics, 16*(5), 561–573.

Review the article, looking for information about the research design. Consider the following appraisal questions in your critical review of this element of the research article:

1. How would you classify the design of this study? Is the design clearly discernible early in the article? Is it described using accurate and standard language?
2. Do the authors provide a rationale for their choice of this design? If not, can you provide reasons for its selection?
3. Is there a clear link between the research purpose and questions and the choice of this design?
4. Are the primary variables of interest clearly identified? Were the variables manipulated?
5. Identify potential extraneous variables that may have affected the outcome of the study. Are any of these strong enough that they might affect the credibility of the study?
6. What are the strengths of this research design for answering this question? What are the limitations of this research design?
7. Could the study be replicated from the information provided in the description of the design and methods?

- Detailed plans for research implementation form a road map for the research and include specification of procedures for sampling, measurement, and analysis.

For a full suite of assignments and additional learning activities, use the access code located in the front of your book to visit this exclusive website: http://go.jblearning .com/houser. If you do not have an access code, you can obtain one at the site.

References

Creswell, J. (2008). *Research design: Qualitative, quantitative and mixed methods approaches* (3rd ed.). Thousand Oaks, CA: Sage.

DelBoca, F., & Darkes, J. (2007). Enhancing the validity and utility of randomized clinical trials in addictions treatment research: I. Treatment implementation and research design. *Addiction, 102*, 1047–1056.

Endacott, R. (2007). Clinical research 1: Research questions and design. *Accident and Emergency Nursing, 15*, 106–109.

Fain, E. (2008). *Reading, understanding, and applying nursing research.* Philadelphia: F.A. Davis.

Hartung, D., & Touchette, D. (2009). Overview of clinical research design. *American Journal of Health System Pharmacy, 66*(15), 398–408.

Iversen, M., & Petersson, I. (2006). Design issues and priorities in team and nonpharmacological arthritis care research. *Journal of Rheumatology, 33*(9), 1904–1907.

Miller, S., & Fredericks, M. (2006). Mixed-methods and evaluation research: Trends and issues. *Qualitative Health Research, 16*(4), 567–579.

Munhall, P. (2006). *Nursing research: A qualitative perspective* (4th ed.). Sudbury, MA: Jones & Bartlett.

Parfrey, P., & Ravani, P. (2009). On framing the research question and choosing the appropriate research design. *Methods in Molecular Biology, 473,* 1–17.

Speziale, H., & Carpenter, D. (2006). *Qualitative research in nursing: Advancing the humanistic perspective.* Philadelphia: Lippincott Williams & Wilkins.

Weaver, K., & Olson, J. (2006). Understanding paradigms used for nursing research. *Journal of Advanced Nursing, 53*(4), 459–469.

part III

Research Process

chapter 8

The Sampling Strategy

CHAPTER OBJECTIVES

The study of this chapter will help the learner to

- Define a population and discuss the rationale for sampling.
- Contrast probability sampling with nonprobability sampling.
- Describe methods for estimating necessary sample size.
- Discuss methods for avoiding selection bias.

KEY TERMS

Convenience sampling	Population	Sample
Ecological validity	Population validity	Sampling error
Effect size	Power	Sampling frame
Exclusion criteria	Probability or random sam-	Selection bias
External validity	pling	Snowball or referral sampling
Inclusion criteria	Purposive selection	Unit of analysis
Independence	Random selection	

Introduction

No aspect of the research plan is more critical for assuring the usefulness of a study than the sampling strategy. It will determine whether the results of the study can be applied as evidence and contributes to the trustworthiness of the results. Good sampling is critical for the confident application of the study findings to other people, settings, or time periods.

❝ *Voices from the Field* ❞

After having my first baby, I became very interested in studying the kind of care given to mothers during the first stage of labor. I worked in obstetrics (OB) for several years, and I guess I took this stage of care a bit for granted until I had my own experience. When I was on the other side of the bed I remember thinking that the supportive kinds of things the nurses did meant more to me than all the activity and data they were collecting. So I became interested in better understanding what type of care nurses give to patients in their first stage of labor, and how they rate that care in terms of priority and importance.

I raised the topic at a staff meeting during a conversation about evidence-based practice, and there seemed to be quite a few people interested in the topic. Some of the physicians were interested in addition to the nurses on the floor. Many of them believed that the right kind of supportive care in the first stage of labor could have a significant impact on both mother and baby during the delivery process. I even informally asked some of the laboring mothers what they thought about the idea and their positive response is what made me believe I should actually carry out the study.

I started with the exploratory question, "What types of care provided by nurses to mothers in the first stage of labor can be classified as supportive care?" I thought that I would start with an exploratory study to observe and describe what was happening, with the idea that in the future we might design strategies to improve and enhance this care. So I could see there was a lot of potential for studying this topic.

When I started planning, I thought getting a sample would be easy because we have a busy mother/baby unit. What I discovered as I began getting specific about the study was not a problem with access, but really with too much access. I couldn't possibly study all of the nurses in the birthing unit every minute of every day. Yet, I knew if I picked the times and the nurses myself that there was likely to be some bias in the study, particularly because I worked with many of these nurses. So I knew I would have to have some element of random selection, both to reduce the size of the potential sample to a manageable size and to remove any effect I might have on sample selection.

Even though I knew it was the best approach, it was a little overwhelming to think about drawing a random sample from all of those mothers. I consulted with a nurse researcher and found out there were several ways I could go about sampling. I could do a systematic random sample, picking the first mom randomly and then every tenth or so after that. That seemed like an easy process, but I was not sure how I could keep track of the mothers when I was not working the shift. The researcher suggested that I could randomly select blocks of time, or nurses, or even rooms that I would then periodically use for data collection. It seemed more doable, then, when I considered the range of possibilities.

I planned to eventually report my data in terms of "proportion of time spent in supportive care," so I figured that clear time periods of data collection were required. I decided to randomly select blocks of time for observation. Further, to ensure there was not any bias, I decided to randomly select a nurse that was taking care of one patient in the first stage of labor during that time period for observation.

I knew that all shifts needed to be equally represented, to capture variations that were due to time of day. To begin with, I randomly chose 2 months out of the next six. All the shifts for all the days in those months were grouped together and numbered. The nurse researcher helped me find a table of random numbers that I used to select the shifts. Hours of the day on those shifts were assigned sequential numbers and random numbers were again generated, and I selected the time periods. So I knew before the study started the exact days and times I would be involved in data collection, which was very helpful from a personal organization standpoint.

I was afraid it would get complicated in terms of picking the nurses to observe, though. The nurse researcher was available to help with the random sample of dates and times, but would not be there to help me select the exact nurse to observe. Further complicating the process was the fact that each shift has a different number of nurses and a different number of mothers in the first stage of labor, so it was impossible to select the nurses ahead of time. Instead of using a complicated mathematical method, the nurse researcher told me I could use something as simple as rolling dice or tossing coins. I decided to literally pick the subjects out of a hat. When I arrived for an observation period, the charge nurse helped identify all the nurses taking care of mothers in the first stage of labor. Those names were written on strips of paper that were folded and put in a container. The container was shaken and the charge nurse drew a name. The selected nurse was approached and asked for consent. Those who agreed to were observed during the selected time period.

It still sounds complicated, but it actually was not too difficult to do. After the initial random sample of dates and times was drawn, all I needed were slips of paper and a shoebox to find my sample. Previously, I had thought it would be a really complex procedure to get a random sample; instead, I found it wasn't that bad. I am also much more confident now that the sample I have is representative, and that my biases are not affecting the outcome.

Andrea Lee, MS, RN

Samples are drawn to represent populations in a research study. A population, sometimes called the target population, is the entire set of subjects that are of interest to the researcher. It is rarely possible, or even necessary, to study the entire population of interest. It is more likely that the researcher will study a subset of the population called a sample. Samples, if selected carefully, can represent the population. Because samples are more efficient and economical to study, their use enables researchers to study phenomena when reaching the entire population would be impossible.

Sampling has a downside, however. Measures acquired from a sample cannot be as precise and accurate as those drawn from the entire population. The results from a sample will never match the population values perfectly. Researchers use statistics to measure and account for this difference, resulting in a value called sampling error. Sampling error is key in hypothesis testing; sampling error is sometimes

Population: The entire set of subjects that are of interest to the researcher.

Sample: A carefully selected subset of the population that reflects the composition of that population.

Sampling error: A statistical value that indicates differences in results found in the sample when compared to the population from which the sample was drawn.

referred to as "chance" or "standard error," and is the criterion used to determine whether statistical results are a result of real effects. It is critical, then, to use a selection strategy that minimizes sampling error by maximizing the chance that the sample will represent the population well.

The sampling plan is important whether the research is qualitative or quantitative; the plan serves different purposes, however, based on the type of research. In qualitative research, the sampling plan is central to establishing credibility. The individuals who participate are referred to as informants or respondents and are chosen specifically for their capacity to inform the research question. In a quantitative study, the sampling strategy is aimed at maximizing the potential for generalization or the ability to apply the findings to larger groups. The individuals who participate are referred to as subjects and are chosen using methods that ensure the sample adequately represents the overall population. Therefore, the way samples are recruited and selected will determine the overall confidence we have in the results.

The sampling strategy is the primary way that researchers control selection bias. Selection bias occurs when subjects are selected for the study or assigned to groups in a way that is not impartial. When subjects are assigned to treatment groups using a random method, selection bias is reduced. Selection bias poses a threat to the validity of a study and is controlled almost exclusively by a sound sampling strategy.

Selection bias: A condition that occurs when subjects are selected for a study or assigned in groups in a way that is not impartial. This may pose a threat to the validity of the study.

No less critical is the sample's capacity to detect the effects of the intervention. Having an adequate number of subjects provides the study with power, or the ability to detect effects. Power increases confidence in the results of the study and is dependent on an adequate sample size. Power is controlled by the researcher by ensuring that an adequate number of subjects are represented in the sample.

These aspects of research design—the method for selecting subjects and assigning them to groups and the number of subjects studied—are the most important considerations in the sampling strategy. Frequently, however, the sampling strategy gets little attention in a research study and is often the weakest aspect of otherwise well-designed projects. One researcher assessed the sampling adequacy of all the research studies published in a nursing journal over a 7-year period and found that only 32 percent of the studies used samples that were appropriate for the type of statistical analysis used (Williamson, 2003).

This may not be a reflection on the efforts of the researchers. Even when effort is spent to design an effective sampling strategy, conditions beyond the researcher's control may limit the capacity to apply the sampling strategy as planned. In one study of a nursing intervention in a population of HIV-positive persons, 639 clients were eligible for the study. Despite multiple attempts to recruit subjects, only 43 agreed to participate and, of those, only 16 finished the study (Nokes & Nwakeze, 2007). The authors noted the multiple challenges of sampling in this highly marginalized population and concluded that less rigorous sampling strategies may be the only recourse for studying their care.

When reading research, the sampling strategy is assessed to determine the confidence that the results are accurate and potentially valuable to practice. A sampling strategy that is not representative limits the ability to use the research results in nursing practice. Creating an adequate sampling strategy requires that the nurse researcher maximize representativeness and sample size. This frequently requires creativity and persistence, but is critical to ensure that the results can be confidently applied to nursing practice.

Selection Strategy: How Were the Subjects Chosen?

The first step of a sampling strategy is to clearly define the population of interest. Often, this definition begins during development of the research question. The definitions should be clear, unambiguous, and detailed enough to avoid misinterpretation. Populations are frequently defined in terms of age (for example, adults, children, and neonates), diagnosis, setting, or geographic location. The available population is called the sampling frame; these are the potential participants who meet the definition of the population and are accessible to the researcher. This does not necessarily mean physically accessible; for example, the sampling frame for the population of critical care nurses in acute care might be the membership roster for the American Association of Critical Care Nurses.

> **Sampling frame:** The potential participants who meet the definition of the population and are accessible to the researcher.

Once the population is clearly defined, a selection strategy is designed to choose the actual subjects from the sampling frame. The selection strategy involves making decisions about how subjects will be recruited, selected, and, if appropriate, assigned to groups. These decisions are based on the type of study design and the goals of the research. The goal of the selection strategy is to prevent bias, support the validity of the study, and enhance the credibility of the results.

All samples may be threatened by selection bias, meaning the sample is not an accurate representation of the population. This may occur for many reasons—some related to design of the study and some related to execution of the study procedures. Selection bias can occur when a researcher can affect the selection of the subjects for the study and/or the assignment of subjects to groups. This may result in a sample that is biased toward success of the experiment. For example, a researcher may select an intervention group consisting of individuals who are healthy and therefore more likely to improve, and select a control group of sicker patients who are unlikely to experience unaided improvement. This bias may be conscious, but it is more commonly unconscious. It is of particular concern when the researcher has preconceived ideas about how the study will turn out.

Inadequate sampling can also lead to sampling bias. A biased sample under- or over-represents some characteristic in the sample. Unfortunately, samples that are the easiest to recruit may introduce sampling bias into a study. Convenience samples run the risk of overrepresenting characteristics that are local to the study. For example, subjects that are recruited primarily from a tertiary care center may inherently include more seriously ill patients. Conversely, recruiting from outpatient settings may under-represent the severity of a condition. Sampling bias increases sampling error as well as the chance the researcher will draw misleading conclusions.

Even with a rigorous sampling plan, certain segments of the population may refuse to participate or be unable to participate. Sampling bias may be present when a group is too

Selection bias may occur under the following conditions:
- The sample is not an accurate representation of the population.
- The researcher is able to influence selection or assignment of subjects.
- The numbers in the sample are inadequate.
- The ease of recruitment skews subject characteristics.
- The subjects elect not to participate or drop out of the study.

homogeneous, so that it does not reflect the diversity in a population. A homogeneous sample is one in which the subjects are very similar in characteristics, and it makes generalizing to other populations difficult. Historically, samples for medical research have been heavily weighted with white males. In the past decade, researchers have become more sensitive to the need for a broad representation of ethnic and gender groups in research, but gaps in representation still exist.

Another kind of selection bias occurs when subjects elect not to participate. Systematic sampling error can occur when response rates are low or attrition is high. There are many reasons that subjects may decline to participate in a study or drop out once it has started. A certain amount of refusal and/or nonresponse is to be expected in any study. However, the researcher should describe the reasons for refusal or attrition to ensure that systematic sampling error is not exhibited. For example, if all the individuals who refuse to participate are from a particular ethnic group, socioeconomic status, or educational level, then the final sample is not representing the entire population.

The Sample Selection Strategy

A sound selection strategy is one of the best ways to control bias in an experiment. Several aspects of the strategy enhance validity and control bias. The use of objective selection criteria and sound recruitment methods are appropriate for all types of research. These should be some of the earliest decisions made about the study because objective selection criteria help minimize bias in both qualitative and quantitative studies.

The sampling strategy for a qualitative study has a different goal than quantitative research, so the sampling procedures for these two types of studies can be quite different. In the case of qualitative research, the goal is credibility rather than generalizability, so selection methods are purposive (Gerrish & Lacey, 2006). This makes the sampling strategy less complicated for qualitative studies, but no less thoughtful. Careful attention to selection criteria can help minimize the effects of both researcher bias and selection bias in a qualitative study (Creswell, 2008).

For quantitative studies, the use of probability in sample selection or group assignment reduces bias and enhances the representativeness of the results (Lohr, 2009). In addition, subjects are recruited and selected for the study based on criteria that are carefully considered to represent the population under study while minimizing the effects of extraneous variables. The criteria are applied objectively, and all subjects who meet the criteria are generally invited to participate.

Inclusion criteria: Guidelines for choosing subjects with a predetermined set of characteristics that include major factors important to the research question.

Exclusion criteria: Characteristics that eliminate a potential subject from the study.

Objective selection criteria may involve inclusion criteria, exclusion criteria, or both. The use of inclusion criteria provides guidelines for choosing subjects with a predetermined set of characteristics. These criteria define the major factors that are important to the research question and may include clinical, demographic, geographic, and temporal criteria as appropriate. The primary function of inclusion criteria is to limit the potential for selection bias by objectively identifying who can be considered a subject.

Many authors also include exclusion criteria, or characteristics that exclude a potential subject from the study. Some individuals are not suitable for the study, even though they meet the inclusion criteria. These subjects might have clinical exclusion criteria (for example, co-morbid conditions that might affect the study) or behavioral exclusion criteria (for example, high likelihood of being lost to follow-up). Exclusion criteria fulfill the same function as inclusion criteria and help to control extraneous variables.

Sampling in Qualitative Studies

Although objective criteria for recruitment and selection strengthen the credibility of a qualitative study, informants are selected from the potential pool of subjects in a way that is controlled and executed by the researcher. This is described as **purposive selection** and has as its aim the selection of subjects most likely to inform the research question. Criteria for selection of informants often look quite different for a qualitative study than for a quantitative one. Qualitative selection criteria may include requirements that an individual has experienced a phenomenon, possesses a particular attribute, or even expresses a willingness to talk openly about sensitive issues. Qualitative selection criteria are formulated through a thoughtful reflection on the type of individual who is most likely to inform the research question. The researcher then seeks out these individuals and invites them to participate in the study. FIGURE 8.1 depicts the general progress of a sampling strategy.

> **Purposive selection:** A technique used in qualitative research in which the subjects are selected because they possess certain characteristics that enhance the credibility of the study.

The following primary aspects must be considered in the qualitative sampling strategy:

- The characteristics or experiences of the individuals who will be asked to participate
- The setting within which the researcher will expect to find the participants
- The process of approaching, inviting, and securing consent of the participants (Creswell, 2008)

A purposive sample is in some ways easier to procure than a probabilistic one, but that does not imply the process is not systematic. The researcher has an obligation to design a sound sampling strategy that will meet the goals of the research regardless of the nature of the research.

Sampling in Quantitative Studies

Quantitative samples are best when they are selected and assigned to groups randomly. These are often referred to as probability samples. In quantitative studies, the development and use of inclusion and exclusion criteria are only the first steps in a highly controlled, objective selection strategy. The goal

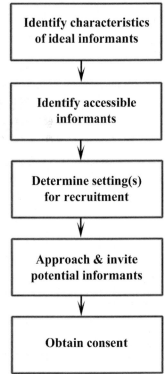

FIGURE 8.1 Stages of the Qualitative Sampling Strategy

Probability or random sampling: A sampling process used in quantitative research in which every member of the available population has an equal probability of being selected for the sample.
Random selection: A method of choosing a random sample using mathematical probability to ensure the selection of subjects is completely objective.

of quantitative studies is representation of the population, and the use of probability in sample selection or group assignment helps the researcher achieve this goal (Levy, 2009).

Probability sampling (also called random sampling) refers to a sampling process in which every member of the available population has an equal probability of being selected for the sample. A sample that is drawn randomly will represent the characteristics of the population and can be used to draw conclusions about the larger group, even when the entire population cannot be included (Lohr, 2009). FIGURE 8.2 depicts the general steps of the quantitative sampling strategy.

The only way to be sure a sample represents a population is if it incorporates two essential criteria: Each member of the population has an equal probability of

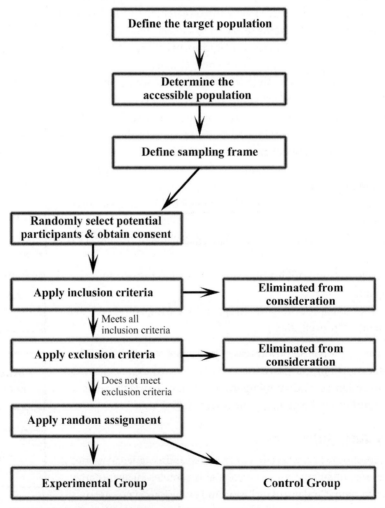

FIGURE 8.2 Stages of the Quantitative Sampling Strategy

selection for the sample, and each subject selection is an independent event. A random sample is one in which mathematical probability is used to ensure that selection of subjects is completely objective. Independence is ensured when the selection of one subject has no effect on the selection of other subjects. In other words, each member of the population has exactly the same chance of being in the sample, and the selection of one subject has no influence on the selection of another. For example, if a subject were asked to recruit his or her friends and family members for the study, the assumption of independence has been violated. Both randomness and independence are central to ensuring that a sample is representative of the population and are also underlying assumptions of most inferential statistical tests.

> **Independence:** A condition that occurs when the selection of one subject has no influence on selection of other subjects; each member of the population has exactly the same chance of being in the sample.

The best quantitative studies have samples that are either randomly selected or randomly assigned to experimental groups. A researcher might have no choice but to ask accessible subjects to join the study—and so potentially introduce bias. But if the researcher randomly assigns the subjects to experimental groups, then any differences between the sample and the population are evenly spread out over all groups in the experiment.

Random sampling and/or assignment do not have to be complicated processes. Several types of random samples meet the essential criteria of both equal probability and independence.

Simple Random Sampling

Simple random sampling is used when a table of random numbers (either from a textbook or generated by a computer program) is used to select subjects from the sampling frame. The sampling frame includes the entire population that is eligible for the study. The researcher must have access to a listing of all eligible individuals that are both part of the population and meet the selection criteria. The subjects are then numbered. Random numbers are drawn, and the subjects with the drawn numbers are asked to participate in the study. For example, the drawn set of random numbers "21, 11, 143, 86 …" means that the 21st, 11th, 143rd, and 86th subjects on the list would be asked to participate in the study. Common statistical texts generally include a table of random numbers as an appendix that can be used for a manual process. Most spreadsheet programs can generate a list of random numbers, and statistical software can automatically select a simple random sample from an imported list of potential subjects.

To draw a simple random sample from a population, the researcher must have access to a list of the individuals who are in the population; however, access to a listing of the entire sampling frame is rarely available to the researcher. For example, how would a researcher get a list of all people with hypertension? All nurse managers that work in critical care units? All adolescents who are sexually active? In addition to these logistical problems, most researchers do not have unlimited access to the population. If nothing else, most studies are limited by geography or availability of resources. In these cases, other varieties of random samples that do not require access to a list of the sampling frame may be more efficient and feasible. Table 8.1 depicts the major types of random sampling methods and examples that demonstrate the characteristics of each.

Table 8.1

Types of Random Samples and Examples

Type of Random Sample	Example
Simple random sample	The researcher wants to survey 40 percent of the nurses regarding their perceptions of the work environment. A list of all the nurses who work on the patient care units is generated by the human resources department. The list is numbered. Random numbers are generated by computer, and the nurses with those numbers by their names on the list are invited to participate in the study.
Systematic random sample	The researcher is studying the relationship between time spent in an examining room and patient satisfaction, and wants a 10 percent random sample of patients who will present in the next 6 months. The nurse selects the number 5 from a table of random numbers. The 5th patient to present to the clinic is invited to participate. Every 10th patient who presents is invited to participate until the 6 months have passed.
Stratified random sample	The researcher is studying the relationship between educational level and the identification of early symptoms of myocardial infarction. The researcher wants to ensure that neither gender is overrepresented. A list of individuals who have presented to the emergency department with symptoms of myocardial infarction is generated by the health information management department. The list is divided by gender. A 20 percent random sample is selected from each list so that gender is represented in the sample.
Cluster random sample	The researcher is studying the baseline knowledge of school nurses relative to managing childhood diabetes. A list of all school districts in the state is generated, and the districts are numbered. Random numbers are generated and the associated school districts are identified. All school nurses in the selected school districts are invited to participate.

Systematic Random Sampling

Systematic random sampling is useful when the researcher is unsure how many individuals will eventually be in the population or if there is an indefinite sampling frame. It is also a practical way to draw a sample from a prospective group (that is, a group that will be created in the future). In systematic random sampling, the first subject is drawn randomly, and remaining subjects are selected at predetermined intervals. For example, if a researcher needed a 10 percent random sample from the visitors to the emergency department over 12 months, the researcher might select the random number of 6 from a table of random numbers. In this case, once the study began, the researcher would invite the 6th visitor to the emergency department and every 10th visitor after that. Systematic random sampling is not considered a strict probability sample, but for all practical purposes it is usually just as good. It has the advantage that it is a relatively uncomplicated way to draw a representative sample.

Stratified Random Sampling

Stratified random samples are structured so that important characteristics are evenly distributed across all groups. It is a good way to reduce the probability that a subgroup will be under- or overrepresented in some way. Stratification based on some important characteristic helps ensure that all subgroups are represented in proportion to their prevalence in the defined population. Stratified random samples are more difficult to accomplish than simple or systematic random samples, and involve two steps. The researcher first divides the population into groups based on some characteristic (for example, gender, ethnicity, and diagnosis), and then picks a representative sample from each group. Often, a proportion from each subgroup is predetermined and is used to control a potential extraneous variable. For example, in a study of community-acquired pneumonia, the researcher might want to ensure that nonsmokers and smokers are represented in the sample in the same proportion as they appear in the general population. If the population had a 17 percent smoking rate, then the researcher would first identify the smokers and nonsmokers in the sampling frame and randomly select subjects from each group so that the sample had 83 percent nonsmokers and 17 percent smokers.

Cluster Random Sampling

Sometimes it is impossible to draw single subjects from groups, because of either geographic limitations or accessibility issues. In cluster sampling, the researcher randomly selects entire groups and then randomly selects subjects from only those groups. For example, an organizational researcher might want to study the effect of care delivery models on patient satisfaction among Magnet facilities. Instead of randomly selecting from all patient care units in all Magnet facilities, the researcher would first randomly select Magnet facilities and then solicit participation from all the units in those facilities. Cluster random sampling is useful when subjects naturally fall into groups (for example, schools, hospitals, and counties) because it is both relatively uncomplicated and efficient (Rose & Bowen, 2009).

Ensuring Independence

Independence, the second criterion for a probability sample, is a statistical concern rather than one of representation. Independence is violated if subjects are related in some way or if more than one score is collected from the same subject. It would be expected that subjects that are not independent share some characteristic. When data are not independent, then the score on one measure shares some characteristic with the score on another measure. This means their results might be correlated in a way that is unrelated to the study. The most common nonindependent sample is a pretest/posttest design. Time-series data, or data collected on the same sample over time, are also nonindependent. A researcher can compensate for nonindependence with specific statistical tests, but the nonindependent nature of the data has to be recognized and dealt with.

The Most Common Sample: Convenience Sampling

When random sampling is not realistic, the researcher often relies on convenience sampling. **Convenience sampling** is based on subjects that are accessible to the researcher. Sometimes called accidental sampling, convenience samples have

Convenience sampling: A nonprobability method of selecting a sample that includes subjects who are available conveniently to the researcher.

obvious advantages over probability samples, primarily with respect to logistics and cost. However, selection using convenience methods can introduce bias into the sample. Even greater potential for selection bias exists if the researcher is involved personally in selecting the subjects. Consciously or unconsciously, the researcher's predetermined ideas about the research might affect subject inclusion.

A specific kind of convenience sample that violates both randomness and independence is snowball sampling (also called referral sampling). In snowball sampling, each subject is asked to recruit other subjects. Although this may be the only way to reach some groups that possess sensitive characteristics (for example, alcoholics, drug addicts, or sexually active teens), the subjects are not independent and randomly selected, and so generalizing the results may be limited.

Snowball or referral sampling: A nonprobability sampling method that relies on referrals from the initial subjects to recruit additional subjects.

Convenience sampling is often used in pilot studies when the specifics of a research study have yet to be completely determined. A small study conducted with a convenience sample can help guide the specifics for a larger study. In this situation, convenience sampling is acceptable and expected. However, even in pilot studies when convenience sampling is necessary, the researchers should do as much as possible to limit the bias that is inherent in this sampling method.

The best way to reduce bias in a convenience sample is to assign subjects to groups randomly once they have been recruited. A simple flip of a coin is considered a random event and can be used to assign subjects to groups. Using random assignment minimizes the bias of a convenience sample because extraneous variables are randomly spread over both groups.

Other Sample Selection Considerations

Although it is most likely that the subjects in an experiment are people, this is not necessarily the case. Populations and samples are not restricted to human beings. Subjects might refer to documents (such as medical records), counties, or whole hospitals. In a particular kind of evidence-based research called meta-analysis, the subjects are actually research studies. When the subject is something other than an individual human being, it is referred to as the unit of analysis. If a researcher wants to study the relationship between socioeconomic status and teen pregnancy rates in counties, then the researcher needs a sample made up of whole counties; in this case, the unit of analysis is a county. The unit of analysis may be groups of people, whole organizations, or cities. When the unit of analysis is quite large, then it becomes more difficult to recruit an adequate sample. For example, if the unit of analysis is a hospital, and the researcher needs a sample size of 60, then 60 hospitals will have to be recruited for the study. Careful consideration of the unit of analysis involves thought about the difficulty of recruitment as well as the characteristics that are needed in the sample.

Unit of analysis: The definition of the major entity or subject that will be analyzed in the study.

Regardless of the unit of analysis, the sample should be selected based on preset criteria. The selection process may be purposive in qualitative studies. For quantitative studies, the best samples are selected with some element of randomness. However, the sampling strategy is not of much use, no matter how well it is constructed, if an inadequate number of subjects agree to be in the study.

Sample Size and Power: How Many Subjects Are in the Sample?

Although subject selection determines whether the results can be generalized to a larger population, the number of subjects in the sample affects whether the results can be trusted. Sample size affects whether significant findings can be detected and the level of confidence with which we can incorporate results into practice and expect the same outcome.

Sample Size in Qualitative Studies

In qualitative studies, sample size is rarely predetermined. Although a researcher may have a general number of informants in mind—and although some standards have been set for particular kinds of qualitative studies such as phenomenology—criteria are generally not strict. The standard for sample size in a qualitative study is the achievement of saturation. Saturation has been achieved when the researcher concludes that responses are repetitive, and no new information is being generated. Determining when an adequate sample has been achieved is the responsibility of the researcher. Documenting saturation is one of the ways that qualitative researchers can improve the trustworthiness of a study, and it may be achieved with as few as six or eight subjects or may require much larger numbers. As the complexity of a phenomenon under study increases, it will be more likely that a larger number of subjects will be required to achieve saturation.

Sample Size in Quantitative Studies

In quantitative studies, the standard for determining sample size adequacy is power. Adequate power means there are enough subjects to detect a difference in the outcome variable. The calculation of power is a mathematical process and may be calculated prospectively (to determine how many subjects are needed) or retrospectively (to determine how much power a sample possessed).

> **Power:** An analysis that indicates how large a sample is needed to adequately detect a difference in the outcome variable.
> **Effect size:** The measurement of the magnitude of the impact of an intervention.

The calculation of power involves making several decisions about accuracy and tolerable error, as well as consideration of some characteristics of the population. In general:

- Adequate power is harder to achieve when results must be very accurate. When the significance level is set very low—for example, at 0.01 or 0.001—then larger samples are needed to meet the more stringent standard.
- The number of variables to be examined simultaneously and the number of subgroups to be compared increase demands for power. When a large number of characteristics will be compared among several subgroups, then samples have to be larger. This means that focusing a research question carefully is important and can reduce the size of the sample needed to answer the question.
- A highly heterogeneous population—one that has a lot of diversity—is not represented well by a small sample, and so will have less power. The chances are greater in a diverse population that some group will be under- or overrepresented, and larger samples can help ensure this does not happen.
- Very strong effects are easier to detect with small samples, but more subtle effects are hard to detect without large ones. Called effect size, big effects are easier to see

in the data, just as a large object is easier to see than a small one. When small effects are expected, then larger samples are needed to find them (Connelly, 2008).

- Research designs that involve dependent data (for example, repeated measures or pretest/posttest design) are associated with greater statistical power than those involving independent groups.

Low power reduces the likelihood that the researcher will find significant results and also affects the confidence the reader can have in the findings (Holm & Sorenson, 2007). The best samples are based on a power analysis that estimates the size of sample needed, taking into consideration the characteristics of the study and the population.

Researchers can use other methods to estimate sample size needs by applying some rules of thumb. It is generally considered sufficient to have 15 subjects per variable, although some researchers estimate this number to be as high as 50 (Hulley, Cummings, Browner, & Grady, 2006). In general, samples with fewer than 30 subjects are not considered powerful enough to detect changes in an outcome variable. On the other hand, samples that exceed 200 subjects generate only marginal improvements in power.

If power is insufficient, then Type II error is more common. A Type II error occurs when there is a difference between groups but the researcher does not detect it. In other words, the intervention works, but the researchers do not conclude that it does. Power is primarily a function of sample size, and so inadequate samples are most suspicious when results are *not* significant. The potential for a Type II error should be considered any time a researcher is working with a small sample of subjects and cannot find any significant differences or relationships. This issue can be addressed by increasing the sample size until sufficient power is ensured. Of course, if findings were significant, then the sample obviously had enough power to detect them, and calculation of power retrospectively is not required.

In general, larger samples are more desirable from many perspectives. Larger samples have more power and less sampling error. Larger samples are more likely to be normally distributed (to fall in a bell curve), which is an assumption of many statistical tests. Larger samples generally represent the population better, especially if it is a highly diverse population.

However, when samples are very large, then standard error (the basis for statistical significance) becomes very small. When standard error is very small, even inconsequential differences between groups may be statistically significant. Statistical significance only ensures that a difference is real, not that it is clinically important. This is a particularly important consideration in very large samples.

Reading the Sampling Section of a Research Study

The way a sample is selected allows for generalization of the results; the size of a sample allows trust in the results. Both are considerations when reading and evaluating the sampling section of a research study. A representative sample may not be trustworthy if it is too small, but even a large sample may not be applicable if it does not represent the population well.

That is not to say that every member of a target population needs to be included in every study. It is rarely practical (or even possible) to include every potential subject in a study. Most research studies use a subgroup—a sample—to draw conclusions about a larger group—a population. The key consideration in appraising the sampling strategy is whether the researchers have managed to represent the target population well.

The most important considerations in evaluating a research sample are whether the sample is biased and whether the results can be trusted. Bias is minimized by the use of objective inclusion and exclusion criteria. Confidence in the results is based on an adequate sample size. When reading the sampling section of a research article, the nurse researcher should evaluate both sample selection methods and sample size.

When critically reading a quantitative research study, ask the following questions to guide the evaluation of the sampling strategy:

- Were the subjects selected in an objective way?
- Was the sampling strategy applied consistently?

 ### Where to Look

Where to look for information about the sample:

- A description of the sampling strategy should appear in the methods section. It may be labeled "sample," "subjects," or "participants." The researcher should describe inclusion and exclusion criteria in this description.
- The descriptive characteristics of the actual sample will likely appear in the results section. If the researcher has conducted statistical tests of group equivalency, the results of those tests will appear with the overall results. This is to demonstrate that the experimental and control groups have roughly the same characteristics. It is a good thing when these tests of group equivalency show no differences between groups; that indicates the groups were alike in every way except group assignment. In other words, tests for group equivalency should *not* be statistically significant.
- The sampling strategy may not be described at all. This is particularly true if a convenience sample was used. If a description is not clear, then it is safe to assume the sample was not selected randomly and is a convenience sample. Random samples can be complex and difficult to accomplish, and so the researcher will almost certainly report it if a random sample was accomplished.

- The words *probability sample* and *random sample* mean the same thing. Conversely, the words *nonprobability sample* indicate the sample was one of convenience. This is the most common kind of sample in a qualitative study and is not a weakness in that context. Instead, the sample will appear to be one that best informs the research question.
- It is common that specific calculation of power is not reported. This is not a problem if the results are statistically significant; if results are significant, then the sample had adequate power (even if the sample was small). If results are not statistically significant, then reporting of power calculation is essential to avoid a Type II error. It cannot be assumed that negative results are conclusive without calculated power of at least 80 percent or 0.80. Because power can be calculated retrospectively, there is no reason not to report it.
- The sampling plan is critical for generalization to other patients and settings. If the sampling plan is seriously flawed, then it is wise to be cautious in generalizing results unless they have been replicated in other, more representative samples.

- Were the subjects assigned to treatment groups in an impartial manner?
- Were enough subjects included to be comfortable with the conclusions?

When critically reading a qualitative research study, ask the following questions to guide the evaluation of the sampling strategy:

- Were criteria established for the characteristics that were desirable in informants?
- Did the researchers apply effort to find respondents who could best inform the question?
- Was saturation achieved and documented as a standard for sample size?

The ideal sample for qualitative research is purposively selected based on selection criteria, and saturation is documented. The ideal sample for a quantitative study has objective selection criteria, is randomly selected and/or assigned to groups, and has at least 80 percent power. The authors should report these elements of the sampling strategy in clear, straightforward terms in the methods section of the research article.

Using Research as Evidence for Practice

The sampling strategy is a key determinant of whether the research findings can be used in a specific patient care environment. Using research as evidence for practice is based on studies that are well designed and that consider populations similar to the user's population. The appropriate use of research as evidence requires that the study possess external validity. External validity is the link between finding knowledge through research and using knowledge in practice. Whether a research project can be used in a specific situation with a specific group of patients is a function of external validity. External validity refers to the ability to generalize the findings from a research study to other populations, places, and situations.

External validity: The ability to generalize the findings from a research study to other populations, places, and situations.

It is obvious that research studies done in limited settings or with small, convenience samples may not generalize well to other populations. However, external validity may

---

Checklist for Evaluating the Sampling Strategy

✔ The target population is clearly and objectively identified.

✔ Inclusion criteria are specific and relevant.

✔ Exclusion criteria are specified to control extraneous variables.

✔ Procedures for selecting the sample are specified. (If not, assume a convenience sample.)

✔ Sampling procedures are likely to produce a representative sample for a quantitative study.

✔ Sampling procedures are likely to produce the best informants to answer the qualitative research question.

✔ Potential for sampling bias has been identified and controlled by the researcher.

✔ The sample is unaffected by common sources of bias such as homogeneity, nonresponse, and systematic attrition.

✔ The sample is of adequate size, as documented by power for a quantitative study or saturation for a qualitative study.

✔ Power analysis is conducted and reported and is at least 80 percent (unnecessary if results were statistically significant).

Table 8.2		

Threats to External Validity Addressed with Sampling Strategies

Threat	What It Is	How It Is Controlled
Selection effects	The way subjects are recruited and selected may limit generalization to all populations (for example, volunteers and compensated subjects may have motives that are different from the population in general).	▪ Select samples randomly. ▪ Choose samples from real-world settings. ▪ Report descriptive data for subjects so external validity can be evaluated objectively.
Refusal and attrition	Subjects may refuse to participate or drop out of a study in a way that introduces systematic bias; those that refuse may share some characteristic that would inform the study. As the proportion who do not participate increases, external validity decreases.	▪ Limit the investment demands (time, effort, and discomfort) on subjects to improve participation. ▪ Report descriptive data for those who refuse to participate and those who do not complete the study to judge the impact on the generalization. ▪ Report overall refusal and attrition rates.
Setting bias	Settings that encourage research subjects to agree to participate may introduce bias via shared characteristics; research-resistant organizations may not be represented at all.	▪ Consider the characteristics of the setting when discussing generalization of the study to other organizations. ▪ Use random selection when possible.

be limited even in large, multisite studies. Table 8.2 reviews common threats to external validity that are dealt with via the sampling strategy.

The two types of external validity are ecological and population. Ecological validity refers to findings that can be generalized to other settings. For example, a study has strong ecological validity if it is conducted in an acute care setting in a tertiary care center, and the findings will be applied in a similar setting. That same study may have weak ecological validity for a small, rural skilled nursing facility. Ecological validity is evident if a study done in one geographic area can be generalized to other geographic areas. For example, studies conducted in the Rocky Mountains of Colorado might reasonably be generalized to other western states at similar altitudes but may not apply as well to patients at sea level.

Population validity means that a study done in one group of subjects can be applied to other subjects. A study has strong population validity if it was conducted on a population that has characteristics similar to the nurse's patients. Age, gender, ethnicity, or diagnoses are examples of characteristics that might limit external generalization. Samples that are more diverse generally have more external population validity; highly homogeneous subjects, on the other hand, limit generalization.

Although many considerations affect external validity, the strongest element is the sampling strategy. The sampling process determines whether subjects are representative of the larger population and whether they can reasonably be expected to represent all patients.

Ecological validity: A type of external validity where the findings can be generalized and applied to other settings.
Population validity: A type of external validity where the findings can be generalized and applied to other subjects.

Unfortunately, many of the measures used to control internal validity (for example, very tightly drawn inclusion and exclusion criteria, sample matching, and stratified random sampling) make it difficult to maximize external validity. When samples become so homogeneous that most extraneous variables are controlled, they no longer represent the real world very well. Generating research that is generalizable, then, requires a balance between control of internal validity and real-world sampling.

To determine if a research study can be used in a specific setting, the nurse should consider these elements:

1. *How is the population defined?* It is easiest to determine if a study can be generalized to a specific group of patients if the researchers have clearly and thoroughly defined the population under study.

2. *Are there extraneous variables in the research situation that could affect the outcome?* For example, a specific region may have a high proportion of non-English-speaking patients or a large proportion of older patients. If so, are these patients well represented in the sample? On the other hand, an extraneous variable may exert no effect. Deciding whether a variable exerts an effect requires clinical judgment.

3. *Is the setting one that is reasonably similar?* If there are differences, they may not have any impact at all, or they may render the study virtually inapplicable. For example, findings from a critical care unit will generally not be useful in a long-term care setting.

4. *Have the findings been replicated with a range of subjects in different settings?* Continued testing of findings in multiple studies or in multiple sites increases the ability to transfer results to more diverse situations. Replication is both a hallmark of scholarly work and a source of increased confidence in the findings. Multisite studies provide some of the strongest evidence for both generalizability and support for practice change because they represent such a diversity of subjects.

To determine if the study results can be used, evaluate whether the sample and environment of the study are similar enough that the results could reasonably be expected to apply. If the defined population and environment are considerably different, then results that were achieved in the study may not be replicated.

How similar do the study specifics have to be for successful generalization? Those who develop guidelines based on research rarely find studies that have exactly the same patient mix in an identical situation. Critical judgment is used to evaluate whether the results of a study can be used in practice. Although the authors might suggest extensions of the study or potential sites for application, final responsibility lies with the reader to decide if a study can be translated from research into reality.

Creating an Adequate Sampling Strategy

Although the sampling strategy is critical to ensure that the findings will be applicable, it does not have to be complicated. The researcher can take many steps to ensure that the sample is as unbiased as possible, achieves maximum representation of the population, and is adequate to find statistical significance or achieve saturation. Most of these decisions are made during design of the study; careful consideration of the sampling strategy is well worth the effort.

Define the Population

A clear definition of the population of interest drives the sampling strategy. Often called the target population, the definition may include clinical, demographic, or behavioral characteristics. The target population is the whole set of people to whom the results will be generalized, although it may be defined broadly (for example, all people with type 2 diabetes) or more narrowly (for example, all people with type 2 diabetes who present to the emergency department with hyperglycemia).

Create Inclusion Criteria

The inclusion criteria define the main characteristics of the desired population. The development of inclusion criteria often requires clinical judgment about which factors are most closely related to the research question. Inclusion criteria involve a tradeoff between generalizability and efficiency. Very specifically designed inclusion criteria will limit those available for the study; very broad ones will increase the chance that extraneous variables are introduced.

To develop inclusion criteria, consider the factors that are most relevant to the research question. These may include

- *Demographic characteristics:* Ethnicity, gender, socioeconomic status, and educational level are all examples of demographic characteristics that might define a desirable subject set.
- *Clinical characteristics:* The specific clinical conditions under study should be specified.
- *Temporal characteristics:* The specific time frame for the study is identified.
- *Behavioral characteristics:* Certain health behaviors (for example, smoking or alcoholism) may be essential considerations for a study. In qualitative studies, a

---

SKILL Builder | Strengthen a Convenience Sample

When selecting a random sample is not possible, the following methods enhance the validity and representativeness of a convenience sample:
- Develop inclusion and exclusion criteria and apply them consistently. This will lower the risk of selection bias.
- Use an element of randomness. Although the subjects may not be selected randomly, they can be assigned to groups randomly. The process does not have to be complicated; flipping a coin or rolling dice are both acceptable methods of randomization.
- Conduct a power calculation to determine adequate sample size. If it is not possible to prospectively identify sample size, use power calculation to determine how much power the sample did have, particularly if no significant findings were produced.

legitimate behavioral characteristic is the informant's willingness to talk with the researcher about the phenomenon under study.

- *Geographic characteristics:* Practical considerations generally form geographic criteria for a study.

Develop Exclusion Criteria

Exclusion criteria indicate subjects that are not suitable for the research question, and so these criteria eliminate individuals from consideration in the study rather than identify them for recruitment. These criteria may improve efficiency, feasibility, and internal validity of a study at the expense of its generalizability, so they should be used sparingly. Exclusion criteria are generally clinical (for example, certain co-morbid conditions) or behavioral (for example, a high risk of loss to follow-up).

Design a Recruitment Plan

Once the eligible population has been identified, a specific plan is needed to recruit subjects for the study. The goals of recruitment are twofold:

1. Represent the population.
2. Recruit enough subjects to attain adequate power or saturation.

From a practical standpoint, recruitment of a sufficient sample depends on finding the individuals who are eligible and making contact with them. Often, this may involve educating staff members to identify potential subjects and inform them of the study and following up with frequent contact to ensure ongoing efforts.

Clinical nurses are in a unique position to understand and influence the attitudes of patients toward participation in research, and nurses bring a broad range of skills that can be applied to recruitment for clinical research. Recruiting a sample from a population that has sensitive characteristics (for example, drug users) or from minority or immigrant populations may present a particular challenge. These populations are sometimes called "hidden" because it is rare that the sampling frame is available for random selection. However, these patients make up a substantial part of the healthcare population, and such populations may be disproportionately affected by some important health problems. Designing culturally sensitive approaches to recruitment can enhance the potential for ensuring these populations are represented appropriately in healthcare research (Calamaro, 2009). Other factors such as cultural appropriateness, safety of the investigators, time, and expense also may pose barriers to random sampling. Furthermore, some members of these populations are purposefully hidden for personal, legal, or social reasons. In these cases, a purposive sample may be the only possible approach to gain access to an adequate sample.

Spring et al. (2003) studied sampling strategies in hard-to-recruit populations. They found that establishing rapport and trust between the investigator and participant was the key element in recruiting an adequate sample. Furthermore, building a trusting relationship between the researcher and subject supported a high participation rate and a lower attrition rate. Although this approach required additional time and effort on the part of the researcher, the authors found few statistical differences in outcomes between samples recruited through a carefully planned purposive sampling method and a cluster random method. Although true randomized sampling remains more likely to result in a representative sample, when dealing with hidden populations or difficult-to-recruit samples, a thoughtful, carefully executed purposive sample may generate results that are transferable.

Subjects also may be recruited through advertisements and flyers or by mailing surveys directly to them. Recruitment may include compensation if the study is burdensome or involves effort on the subject's part. Recruiting through compensation, however, adds bias because those most financially needy will be overrepresented in the sample.

Determine the Number of Subjects Needed

The number of subjects needed for a qualitative study will be an emergent characteristic. As the study proceeds, an analytic method is generally used that involves continuously comparing results to those that have already been recorded. This method, called constant comparison, allows the researcher to evaluate when saturation has been achieved (that is, when no new information is being gathered). Generally, it is wise to continue collecting data for one or two additional subjects to confirm that saturation has been achieved. The number may be quite small, or a study may require a large number of informants. The researcher, using his or her knowledge of the population characteristics and the phenomenon under study, determines whether saturation is achieved.

Determining the number of subjects needed for a quantitative study is part mathematics, part judgment. If power analysis is not available, an estimate can be achieved by applying the broad rule of thumb of using 15 subjects for every variable that will be studied. Include at least 30, but using more than 200 subjects is rarely necessary. Although this rule of thumb produces a very general estimate, it can be useful as an initial projection of necessary sample size.

An actual calculation of statistical power is superior to general rules of thumb. Calculating the sample size needed to carry out a strong study helps avoid wasting resources on studies that are unlikely to detect significant outcomes (particularly if the intervention is inconvenient or ineffective for the patient). Decisions and some "educated" guesses about the sample must be made by the researcher to complete a power analysis. Prior to calculating power, the researcher must know the planned analytic method, the level of acceptable error, the amount of power desired, and the effect size expected (Holm & Sorenson, 2007). Estimates of the amount of variability in the outcome variables must also be determined by finding similar or concurrent studies of the same phenomena.

Sample size tables may also be used and can be found in many advanced texts on clinical research design. These have the advantage of being less complicated (but somewhat less accurate at predicting power) than power calculations.

Power calculation is more accurately called an "estimation," and it is mathematically complex. As a result, some researchers use a rule of thumb to guide the number of subjects recruited and then calculate a retrospective power analysis based on the actual findings (Connelly, 2008). This is only necessary if no statistically significant findings

For More Depth and Detail

For a more in-depth look at the concepts in this chapter, try these references:

Connelly, L. (2008). Research considerations: Power analysis and effect size. *MED-SURG Nursing, 17*(1), 41–42.

Heiney, S., Adams, S., & Cunningham, J., et al. (2006). Subject recruitment for cancer control studies in an adverse environment. *Cancer Nursing, 29*(4), 291–299.

Hulley, S., Cummings, S., Browner, W., & Grady, D. (2006). *Designing clinical research: An epidemiological approach.* Philadelphia: Lippincott Williams & Wilkins.

Levy, P. (2009). *Sampling of populations: Methods and applications.* Hoboken, NJ: Wiley.

Lohr, S. (2009). *Sampling: Design and analysis.* Pacific Grove, CA: Duxbury Press.

Shah, K., & Batzer, F. (2009). Improving subject recruitment by maintaining truly informed consent: A practical benefit of disclosing adverse clinical trial results. *American Journal of Bioethics, 9*(8), 36–37.

were achieved; when significant differences are detected, the sample is considered to have possessed adequate power.

Apply the Selection Methodology

Once a potential sample has been recruited, then the specific selection methodology is used to identify the final participants. If a purposive sampling method is used for a qualitative study, the researcher invites participants directly from the eligible pool, based on a judgment as to the credibility of the informant. For quantitative studies, some element of randomness either in selection or group assignment will strengthen the representativeness of the sample. A table of random numbers can be used, either from a textbook or generated by computer. Simpler methods are also acceptable. A systematic random sample can be determined using a roll of dice. Considered a random event, the roll of dice can be used each time a potential subject is recruited; it is a simple and straightforward way to determine if he or she should be part of the sample. Likewise, a flip of a coin is acceptable for assigning subjects to treatment groups randomly. One researcher, studying the validity of a pain instrument in long-term care, stood in the doorway of each eligible patient's room and flipped a coin. If the coin landed on heads, the researcher entered the room and informed the patient about his or her eligibility for the study. If the coin landed on tails, the researcher moved on.

Implement Strategies to Maximize Retention

When an adequate number of acceptable subjects have been identified, recruited, and enrolled in a study, the researcher maintains an adequate sample through strategies that maximize retention. Subjects may move away, withdraw for personal reasons, or die during the course of the study. Attrition is particularly problematic in intervention studies and time-series studies.

Subjects who have a personal interest in the study are more likely to complete it. A combination of personal enthusiasm and nurturing by the researcher is often necessary to keep subjects in a study. Keeping procedures for data collection simple and hassle-free, designing clear collection methods, and minimizing any inconvenience to the subjects may all reduce subject attrition. Efforts to follow up with subjects using multiple methods and reminders may also prevent loss of subjects. Regardless, it is generally agreed that maintaining an adequate sample of subjects throughout the life of an experiment is challenging and requires effort and attention on the part of the researcher.

> **gray matter**
>
> The following methods reduce subject attrition in research samples:
> - Keeping procedures for data collection simple and hassle-free
> - Designing clear data collection methods
> - Minimizing any inconvenience to the subject
> - Following up with subjects using multiple methods and reminders

Summary of Key Concepts

- Sampling strategy is critical for application of research findings to larger or different populations.
- The way a sample is selected is the major control for selection bias and is the primary determinant of whether results from a sample can be generalized to a population.
- The goal of the sampling strategy for a qualitative study is credibility and requires that the researcher use judgment in the purposeful selection of individuals who can best inform the research question.
- Objective inclusion and exclusion criteria can reduce the potential for selection bias in any type of study.
- An element of randomness in sample selection for a quantitative study strengthens the potential for generalizability.
- If random selection is impossible, random assignment may evenly distribute population characteristics across all treatment groups.
- Random selection is possible through several methods, including simple random, systematic random, stratified random, and cluster random sampling methods.
- Sample size is an important consideration in power, or the ability to detect differences using a sample. Samples with at least 80 percent power are desirable.
- Power is only a concern if no statistically significant results were reported; if statistical significance was achieved, the sample had sufficient power.
- Several characteristics of the design and the population affect how much power a study has, including effect size, variability in primary outcome measures, and the level of certainty required.
- The criterion for sample size in a qualitative study is saturation, which is the point at which no new information is being generated.
- The sampling strategy should be clearly described in a research study, along with a rationale for each sampling decision. It is the basis for trusting the results and applying them to specific patients.

CRITICAL APPRAISAL **EXERCISE**

Retrieve the following full text article from the Cumulative Index to Nursing and Allied Health Literature or similar search database:

Hess, R., Weinland, J., & Saalinger, N. (2010). Knowledge of female genital cutting and experience with women who are circumcised: A survey of nurse-midwives in the United States. *Journal of Midwifery and Women's Health, 55*(1), 46–54.

Review the article, focusing on information about the sampling strategy. Consider the following appraisal questions in your critical review of this element of the research article:

1. What is the population for this study?
2. What is the sampling frame for this study?
3. What method was used to select subjects from the sampling frame? What are the strengths and weaknesses of this sampling strategy?
4. Discuss any characteristics of the sample that may have affected response rates. How might the different response rates affect the outcome of the study?
5. What are indications that the sample size is adequate for the quantitative portion of this mixed method study?
6. What are indications that the sample size is adequate for the qualitative portion of this mixed method study?
7. What type of external validity does this sampling strategy support?

For a full suite of assignments and additional learning activities, use the access code located in the front of your book to visit this exclusive website: http://go.jblearning.com/houser. If you do not have an access code, you can obtain one at the site.

References

Calamaro, C. (2009). Cultural competence in research: Research design and subject recruitment. *Journal of Pediatric Healthcare, 22*(5), 329–332.

Connelly, L. (2008). Research considerations: Power analysis and effect size. *MEDSURG Nursing, 17*(1), 41–42.

Creswell, J. (2008). *Research design: Qualitative, quantitative and mixed method approaches* (3rd ed.). Thousand Oaks, CA: Sage.

Gerrish, K., & Lacey, A. (2006). *The research process in nursing.* Malden, MA: Oxford Press.

Holm, K., & Sorenson, M. (2007). Research corner: Toward understanding and using statistical power analysis. *SCI Nursing, 24*(3), 2–4.

Hulley, S., Cummings, S., Browner, W., & Grady, D. (2006). *Designing clinical research: An epidemiological approach* (3rd ed.). Philadelphia: Lippincott Williams & Wilkins.

Levy, P. (2009). *Sampling of populations: Methods and applications.* Hoboken, NJ: Wiley.

Lohr, S. (2009). *Sampling: Design and analysis*. Pacific Grove, CA: Duxbury Press.

Nokes, K., & Nwakeze, P. (2007). Exploring research issues: In using a random sampling plan with highly marginalized populations. *Journal of Multicultural Nursing and Health, 13*(1), 6–9.

Rose, R., & Bowen, F. (2009). Power analysis in social work intervention research: Designing cluster-randomized trials. *Social Work Research, 33*(1), 43–52.

Spring, M., Westermeyer, J., Halcon, L., et al. (2003). Sampling in difficult to access refugee and immigrant communities. *Journal of Nervous and Mental Disease, 181*(12), 813–818.

Williamson, G. (2003). Misrepresenting random sampling? A systematic review of research papers in the *Journal of Advanced Nursing*. *Journal of Advanced Nursing, 44*(3), 278–288.

chapter 9

Measurement Strategies

 CHAPTER OBJECTIVES

The study of this chapter will help the learner to

- Determine the major elements of a measurement strategy.
- Discuss the link between the research question and the measurement strategy.
- Identify the level of measurement of research variables and implications for analysis.
- Describe the types of reliability and validity and how they are assessed.
- Evaluate sources of measurement error and plan strategies to minimize its effect.
- Review methods to establish trustworthiness of qualitative data collection processes.

 KEY TERMS

Calibration	Internal reliability	Primary data
Classification measures	Interrater reliability	Random error
Conceptual definition	Interval data	Ratio data
Concurrent validity	Measurement	Responsiveness
Construct validity	Measurement error	Secondary data
Content validity	Nominal data	Sensitivity
Credibility	Operational definition	Specificity
Criterion-related validity	Ordinal data	Systematic error
Dependability	Precision	Test blueprint
Discriminate validity	Predictive validity	Validity

Introduction

Measurement: Determination of the quantity of a characteristic that is present; involves assigning of numbers or some other classification.
Classification measures: Measures that involve sorting of subjects into categories based on their characteristics.

There is an old saying among performance managers: You get what you measure. This is never truer than with the measurement strategy in nursing research. The credibility of a study is almost completely dependent on identifying, measuring, and collecting the right things. A strong measurement strategy is critical for good research. The process of measurement allows the researcher to determine if and in what quantity a characteristic is present, and to provide evidence of the characteristic, usually represented by a number. If that measurement is not correct, or if it is inconsistent, then the researcher may draw the wrong conclusions.

Measurement is based on rules. Often, measurement is about assigning numbers or some other classification to subjects in a way that represents the quantity of the attribute numerically. When we think of measurement, it often brings to mind equipment or tools applied to some concrete physical manifestation. Indeed, measures used for the sciences involve very strict rules about assigning numbers to characteristics in a completely unbiased way. Not all measurement, though, is quite so straightforward.

There are many forms of measurement, and not all of them involve quantifying a trait; a considerable number of measures involve sorting subjects into categories based on their characteristics. For example, using a thermometer measures the amount of heat in the body, whereas asking about religious affiliation seeks to classify the subject based on his or her belief system. **Classification measures** are frequently used in nursing. Subjects may be classified by some neutral observer, or they may classify themselves via an instrument that asks for a self-rating of perception of attributes.

gray matter

The following standards should be specified to guide measurement:
- The way a measure is administered
- The timing of the procedure
- The exact protocol for collecting the results
- The specific wording of questions
- Directions for how the interviewer should read a question

Rules are used to guide the determination of measures, whether they are collected by instrumentation or classification. Detailed rules exist for all aspects of a measurement. These may include the way a measure is administered, the timing of the procedure, the exact protocol for collecting the result, and even such details as how questions are worded and how the interviewer should read a question.

Whether data are collected by calculation of a value or classification into groups, they will likely be represented by a number. Numbers are key elements of measurement in nursing for several reasons. Numbers are objective, often standardized, and therefore consistent. Numbers can serve as a universal language and as a means of communication. Statistical tests can be applied to numbers, resulting in quantification of how much error a measure represents. Numbers are precise and can accurately represent attributes.

gray matter

Numbers are a key element of measurement in nursing because they are:
- Objective
- Standard
- Consistent
- Precise
- Statistically testable
- An accurate representation of attributes

Regardless of the type of measure, numbers are useful only to the extent that they represent the underlying characteristic they are intended to represent. This means they must be clearly linked to the research question, appropriate to represent the variable of interest, and consistently accurate.

❝ Voices from the Field ❞

I became interested in the topic of teamwork very early in my career. Even when I was a novice nurse, I vividly remember that there were times when the people I worked with seemed to "click," and we were able to get an enormous amount of work done without any unit strife. Other times, when there were particular groups of nurses working together, we couldn't even get an average amount of work done without conflict of some sort. So I began wondering about the effects of teamwork on productivity, and whether improving teamwork would result in a more efficient unit. When I later became a department manager myself, it was important to me to build and maintain good team relations, and I believe that is why I had a unit that had a reputation for getting a lot of work done.

I did one study in particular that was focused on how teams function at night versus on days. I have worked both shifts and I know the environment, the way people relate, the work to be done—it is radically different on the two shifts. It is literally like night and day. So I wanted to see if I could differentiate team behaviors that happen at night from those during the day.

I could not find exactly the instrument I wanted; I did not find any, in fact, that broke teamwork down by the behaviors I was interested in. There were some that came close but none that I thought asked the particular questions I had. I was a bit cocky, I guess, when I decided I would just write my own. I had looked at quite a few, and I thought, how hard can it be? So I set out to develop my own instrument for measuring team behaviors.

I did it quite logically. I consulted a friend of mine who was nursing faculty and she helped me develop a test outline and gave me advice on the wording of questions. Still, it took me almost a month to get a first draft done. I knew I had to test it for reliability, and my faculty friend helped me find a statistician. I was really excited up to this point. I thought I might try to copyright my instrument, use it as a teambuilding basis, that kind of thing. We gave the instrument to about a dozen nurses and the statistician ran reliability statistics for me. What a nightmare! The number came back at 46 percent, which is woefully inadequate for any kind of research. I was really crestfallen; I thought I had done a pretty good job.

The statistician was really nice about it. He showed me how some of the questions were written in a confusing way. I had some double negatives in the questions; they were confusing even to me when I reread them. Some of the words could be interpreted several different ways, and there were some typos that I just flat overlooked. It was a humbling experience. I persisted, but it took a couple of revisions and about 6 months before I could get my little instrument where I was comfortable using it.

After I had the results, it was a bit more of a disappointment, because I didn't have anything to compare the numbers to. Since it was a totally unique instrument, the numbers I produced were isolated; I had no way to put them into context. In retrospect, it would have been much easier and stronger if I had just used an existing instrument, even if it wasn't exactly what I needed. "Close enough" actually would have been better than what I wound up with. In hindsight, I should have balanced the weaknesses of a unique tool with the little bit I would have lost from using a standard one.

Since then, I've done quite a bit of work measuring teamwork. I found a standard tool that enables me to measure teamwork reliably while having a large, national database to compare scores to. It also means that studies I have done can be replicated, and that some of my studies have been used in meta-analyses and integrative reviews.

Overall, developing my own tool was a good experience. Painful but good; I learned a lot. I would say my strongest lesson was this: If you need to write your own instrument—and you may—then be sure it is for a really good reason, and that you have the time, energy, and know-how to put into it. Measurement is not as easy as it looks.

Janet Houser, PhD, RN

The Measurement Strategy

The actual measure of an attribute is only one part of a measurement strategy. The complete measurement strategy is critical to the design of a valid research study, and so considerable time and energy should be applied to its planning and execution. The measurement strategy involves the following steps:

1. Thoughtful determination of the most relevant attributes that demonstrate the answer to the research question
2. Definition of the attributes in terms of the operations used to demonstrate them
3. Selection of an instrument that will reliably capture an accurate representation of the attribute
4. Documentation that the instrument and measurement procedure are reliable and valid
5. Development of protocols to guide the process of gathering data
6. Quality checks to ensure the data collection process results in an accurate and complete data set

Define the Research Variables

gray matter

To represent the underlying characteristics, numbers used in research measurements must be:

- Clearly linked to the research question
- Appropriate to represent the variable of interest
- Consistently accurate

The first step of the measurement strategy is to give careful thought to the concepts represented in the research question. The research question will describe the phenomena or characteristics of interest in a study. For a successful measurement strategy, these phenomena or characteristics must be translated into observational attributes before they can be measured (Mlinar, Schmelzer, & Daniels, 2007). Eventually, these concepts may be represented as a physical attribute (for example, blood sugar), a perception (for example, pain), a behavior (for example, a gait), or a response (for example, recall). These are called, logically enough, attribute variables. To ensure that everyone is interpreting the attribute in the same way, the researcher must write definitions that represent the characteristic in such a way that it cannot be misinterpreted.

There are two kinds of definitions for attribute variables. The first is a **conceptual definition**, which describes the concept that is the foundation of the variable by using other concepts. For example, a conceptual definition of depression might include the presence of sadness, lack of pleasure, and changes in eating or sleep habits. An **operational definition**, on the other hand, defines the operations that must be performed to accurately represent the concepts. An operational definition of depression might include using a scale to record weight loss or gain in kilograms or using a log to record hours of sleep per night. It is useful to begin the process by describing conceptual definitions because these can help ensure the researcher is measuring the right things. Operational definitions ensure that the researcher is measuring attributes reliably.

> **Conceptual definition:** Clearly stated meaning of an abstract idea or concept used by a researcher in a study.
> **Operational definition:** An explanation of the procedures that must be performed to accurately represent the concepts.

Determine a Measurement

After writing an operational definition, the researcher defines the procedure for collecting and recording the data. Measurements may be primary or secondary. Primary data are recorded directly from a subject. The researcher uses specific rules to collect the data and makes and maintains a record of the responses. Measures for primary data can involve the following tools:

- Calibrated instruments, such as a thermometer
- Equipment, such as a digital camera
- Paper-and-pencil or online tests, questionnaires, surveys, or rating scales, such as a pain scale
- Observation, rating, and reporting characteristics or behaviors, such as a skin assessment
- Counting the frequency of an attribute or exhibited action, such as the number of falls on a unit

Primary data are considered most reliable because the data are collected by the researcher for a single, specific purpose, but primary data do have limitations. Primary data are time consuming to collect, and the quality of the data depends on many factors. Some of these factors are related to subjects, and some are due to those conducting the measure. The subject's recall of a physical reaction or an event may be quite different from reality. Some subjects may not be able to communicate clearly, or language barriers may be present that distort reporting. A subject may have a mental condition that prohibits accurate and clear reporting of data. Subjects may misrepresent sensitive data, respond dishonestly, or simply give an answer they think the researcher wants to hear. However, although self-reports of behavior, beliefs, and attitudes are prone to biases, there are no acceptable alternative means of measurement for many constructs of interest to nurse researchers, such as satisfaction, pain, depression, or quality of life (Kimberlin & Winterstein, 2008).

> **Primary data:** Data collected directly from the subject for the purpose of the research study. Examples include surveys, questionnaires, observations, or physiologic studies.

The data collectors can also affect the accuracy of primary data. The individual making the recording may not use consistent language or a consistent approach. Inflection or wording may inadvertently lead a patient to an inaccurate answer. For example, the question, "Do you abuse alcohol?" will elicit a far different response than "How many alcoholic drinks do you have in a week?" The response to either can be affected by the tone of voice of the questioner. Those doing the data recording must be carefully trained in data collection techniques. The consistency of data captured by multiple raters must be checked by measures of interrater reliability; this is important in any measure where different individuals will be asked to score observations (Salmond, 2008).

Secondary data: Data collected for other purposes and used in the research study. Examples include patient medical records, employee or patient satisfaction surveys, organizational business reports, or governmental databases.

Secondary data are often easier and quicker to collect. **Secondary data** are retrieved from data sets that have already been collected, usually for another reason. The following list gives examples of secondary data sources:

- Information documented in the patient record (for example, laboratory values or operative reports)
- Public or commercial databases of health data (for example, the renal dialysis data set or the behavioral risk factor data set)
- Registries or other outcomes measurement systems (for example, the National Database of Nursing Quality Indicators or tumor registries)
- Government sources of health data (for example, the Census Bureau or the Healthy People 2010 database)

Many times, secondary data are recorded for specific research purposes and then made available to the research community after the primary research is complete. Secondary data can reveal important relationships and offer a good way to retrieve data efficiently and effectively.

The key consideration when deciding whether secondary data can be used is to verify that the data set includes measures of the specific variables needed to answer the research question (Kimberlin & Winterstein, 2008). Although secondary data are attractive because of their convenience, they hold several limitations. Secondary data may be incomplete or inaccurate, and the researcher cannot control the conditions and rules under which they were collected. The data are necessarily retrospective because they have been collected in the past. Eder et al. (2005) identified five assumptions that must be met before it can be assumed that secondary data are valid:

1. The data that are needed are present in the record.
2. The data in the record are in a form that can meet the variable definitions.
3. The data are accurately recorded.
4. If data are recorded in more than one place in the record, the multiple entries will be consistent.
5. The data are recorded in a manner that is interpreted in a common way by the reader.

When data do not meet all the assumptions, then error is introduced into the data collection process. As with primary data collection, interrater reliability is also a concern. This potential for error is increased if a large number of practitioners have recorded data; if there are multiple locations, forms, or formats for the record; or if the data are collected over a long period of time.

There are ways to promote the validity of secondary data collection. Those who are retrieving the data should be thoroughly trained in the data collection process. Processes such as quality checks and periodic reassessment of interrater reliability should be in place to sustain a high level of reliability when gathering data. Development of a glossary or data dictionary can help the data collector identify equivalent forms of a single variable, and a glossary or dictionary is also helpful in maintaining data integrity. For example, the glossary might note that dyspnea, SOB, and shortness of breath are all acceptable representations of the concept *difficulty breathing*.

In general, the patient record is the best and most sensitive source of objective data regarding patient conditions. Laboratory values, procedures, vital signs, and other documentation of physiological processes are accurately retrieved from the record. Processes that are more subjective may be unavailable or unrecorded in the patient record and are more accurately retrieved via primary data collection. For example, patient education, discharge planning, and counseling may not be recorded consistently in the patient record, but such information can be retrieved directly from patients.

Regardless of the type of data collected, the information must be recorded in a way that lends itself to analysis using acceptable statistical techniques. This requires that thought be given to the nature of the measurement so that subsequent analysis is accurate and precise.

Identify the Level of Measurement

Defined variables must be turned into numbers or classifications to be analyzed statistically. Not all numbers are created the same, and not all numbers in a research study can be treated the same way mathematically. The level of measurement should be determined when the variable is defined so the appropriate statistical test can be applied to answer the research question (Mlinar et al., 2007).

Nominal data are those that can be placed into categories but cannot be ranked. Nominal data include, for example, gender, marital status, ethnicity, diagnosis, and other variables that can be named but not measured on a scale. Each subject can be classified into one category, and the categories are mutually exclusive, meaning a subject cannot be in more than one category. These numbers are sometimes called categorical or classification variables. When nominal data can fall into only two categories (for example, gender or mortality) then they are referred to as binomial or dichotomous. Nominal data are attractive because they are easy to collect and summarize. However, they are the least sophisticated type of measure and only a limited range of analytic methods can be used to analyze them.

Ordinal data are categorical data that can be put in rank order. A pain scale is an example of ordinal data. Patients are asked to place themselves in one of the categories represented by the scale, denoting a relative value from a great deal of pain to very little pain. There is a high and low end of the scale—or good and bad, big and little—so the categories can be ranked. These data are also referred to as categorical because each subject response can be placed at only one place on the scale.

Nominal data: Data that can be named and placed into categories but cannot be ranked or measured on a scale.
Ordinal data: Categorical data that can be put in rank order. The scales contain intervals between entries that vary, limiting statistical analyses and comparisons across the scales or between subjects.

The primary distinction of ordinal data is that the entries on the scale cannot be directly compared across the scale or between subjects because intervals between entries may not be the same. For example, is the difference between "strongly agree" and "agree" exactly the same amount of agreement as the difference between "disagree" and "neutral"? Is the difference between 7 and 8 on the Beck Depression Scale the exact same amount of depression in an elderly patient and a postpartum mother? Is an independent chair-to-bed transfer Functional Independence Measure (FIM) score the same for a patient with a head injury and a stroke victim? The researcher cannot determine that each score or interval is comparable. Although there is a larger range of analytic methods for ordinal data than nominal data, this mathematical limitation restricts the operations that are available for statistical analysis.

Nominal and ordinal data are attractive because they are simple to collect. Subjects are placed in categories or some response is placed in rank order. The attractiveness of their simplicity is balanced by the relative insensitivity of the measures and the limitations on the statistics that can be used.

Interval data: Data measured on a scale. The scale theoretically has an infinite number of entries, limited only by the sensitivity of the measurement instrument. A subject can fall anywhere on the scale (not just in categories). The size of intervals between measurement units is identical, no matter where an individual response falls on the scale. For example, a centimeter will always be a centimeter, no matter whether it falls between 10 and 11 centimeters or between 150 and 151. The intervals between entries are also proportional, meaning that 20 units are twice as big as 10, which are twice as big as 5. The equality of intervals gives the researcher a broad selection of mathematical operations and, therefore, analytic options. The continuous nature of the scale increases the sensitivity of the instrument to changes in the underlying trait.

Ratio data are measured on interval scales that have a true zero. Interval and ratio data together are often referred to as continuous data. They are considered discrete if the units can only be measured in whole numbers, such as number of children or treatment rooms in a trauma center. FIGURE 9.1 summarizes levels of measurement and gives examples of each.

Interval data: Data measured on a scale that has consistent intervals between measurement units and allows for broad selection of mathematical operations and analytic options.

Ratio data: Data measured on interval scales that have a true zero.

Measurement error: The difference between the actual attribute (true score) and the amount of attribute that was represented by the measure (observed score).

Random error: A nonreproducible error that arises from a variety of factors in measurement. These errors do not affect average scores in a data set but do affect the variation that exists around the average.

Strategies to Minimize Measurement Error

Measurement error is the amount of difference between the true score (or the actual amount of the attribute) and the observed score (or the amount of the attribute that was represented by the measure). This difference between the true score and the observed score is called measurement error. Measurement error is a threat to the internal validity of a research study, so minimizing measurement error means that the overall study results are more credible (Alwin, 2007).

Error is present in every instrument to some degree or another. Measurement error may be random or systematic. Random error is expected and is affected by a host of influences that may be present in an experiment. Random error may be due to the following factors:

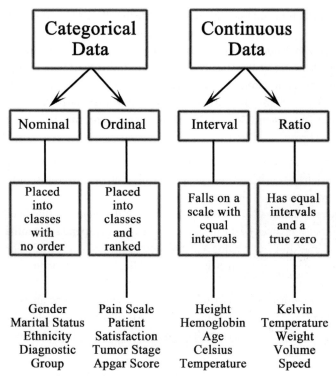

FIGURE 9.1 Levels of Measurement

- Human factors that are personal and transient, such as mood, fatigue, and workload
- Confusion as to how to respond to the instrument, such as complex wording or questions written in a foreign language
- Bias in the way the individual responds to measures, such as the desire to be socially accepted
- Variations in the environmental conditions under which the instrument is applied
- Bias because the respondent is consistently harsh or lenient in rating some characteristic
- Variation in the procedure used for the measure, such as the conditions under which the measure is taken or inconsistencies in directions given to the subject
- Errors in data processing, including data entry errors and missing data

Random error by and large does not affect the average scores in a data set, but it does affect the amount of variation that exists around the average (Viswanathan, 2005). The researcher should minimize random measurement error as much as possible so the responses of subjects are consistent and credible.

Systematic error has a more serious effect on the results of a research study because measures with systematic error may appear to be accurate. **Systematic error** is any error that is consistently biased. In other words, the measure is consistent

Systematic error: A bias in measurement that is consistent but not accurate and that underestimates, overestimates, or misses data in a way that is not random.

but not accurate. The measure may cons   it,
or miss data in a way that is not random   lls
may elect not to participate in a study t   s-
ing data are not random; they are syste   ot
read well. In the case of systematic error   ld
provide information but does not. This is   s
or when investigating sensitive issues (C   lt
of the following factors:

- *Measures that are consistent but in   s
  been used so often it has stretched.   ,
  it will routinely overestimate the l

- *Measures that have complicated or*   .ividuals
  who are greatly inconvenienced by   .... who have to expend substantial
  energy to respond may drop out, leaving only the most motivated in the study. For
  example, asking a subject to maintain a daily diary will likely result in incomplete
  or hastily collected data.

- *Measures that reflect sensitive or socially taboo topics:* The subject may be able but
  unwilling to respond, and missing data may affect the results. For example, self-
  report of tobacco and/or alcohol abuse will often underrepresent the prevalence
  of the behavior in the population.

Instruments are used to measure variables directly from subjects. The primary way
to minimize measurement error with physical instruments (for example, a blood glucose
monitor) is through proper calibration. Keeping instruments in top working condition
and well calibrated minimizes measurement error. Using instruments may lead the reader
to believe that the measures are automatically more reliable because they record objective
biological data. Yet one researcher found less than half of all nursing research studies
using calibrated instruments reported the methods for assuring accuracy and precision
of the data that were collected (Liu & Chen, 2009). When biological measures are collected, the researcher must still assure that instruments are working properly, calibrated
frequently, and tested for reliability.

Measurement error is minimized by creating measures that are closely linked to
the concepts in the research question. Ensuring that measures are simple and clear and
that procedures are convenient can reduce systematic error. Using multiple instruments
reduces measurement error because reliability increases when agreement is observed
across multiple ways of measuring the same concept.

Measurement error is the quantification of unexplained variability. Variability that
is due to anything other than a change in the underlying attribute represents error. It is
important, then, to find instruments that measure characteristics consistently and with
minimal unexplained variability. An instrument is not reliable when there is a discrepancy
between the real attribute and its representation by the results.

A second way to minimize measurement error is to maximize reliability. Reliability
affects the precision of a measure. When measures are highly reliable and precise, then

measurement error is reduced, and it becomes easier to detect the true effects of an intervention. Validity, on the other hand, enhances the accuracy of the measure. When an instrument is highly valid, then it is known to represent the underlying attribute well. Validity increases the credibility of the conclusions and supports application of the results to practice.

Use Properly Calibrated Equipment and Instruments

Calibration of an instrument reduces the discrepancy between the true score and the observed score. Calibration, or the use of objective procedures to verify that an instrument is measuring a characteristic accurately, is highly structured. Laboratory instruments may be calibrated using samples with known quantities; blood glucose monitors often come with calibration samples for quality assurance. These procedures ensure that the instrument is consistent (reliable) and accurate (valid).

However, not all instruments are easily calibrated. For example, how do you calibrate an instrument to measure depression? In the case of instruments that measure characteristics or traits, the calibration concern is replaced with an emphasis on reliability and validity. These are the most important issues to consider when selecting an instrument to measure nonphysiologic characteristics.

Ensure Reliability: A Focus on Consistency

Instruments are considered reliable if they consistently measure a given trait with precision. When a measure is reproducible, that is, when it generates a consistently accurate value every time it is used appropriately, it is considered precise. When a measure is precise, then the reader has a level of confidence that differences between groups are not explained by differences in the way the trait was measured. Reliability analysis and the resulting statistics ensure that an instrument is stable. Reliability statistics document the degree to which an instrument is stable internally, among individuals, between raters, and over time.

Stability Within an Instrument

Stability within an instrument is called internal reliability, and it is measured with the alpha coefficient statistic. This coefficient may be called Cronbach's alpha, coefficient alpha, or internal reliability, and it should have a value of 0.7 or greater. Cronbach's alpha represents the extent to which the variability on individual items represents the variability in the overall instrument (Cronbach, 1951). In other words, the way that responses vary on one item should demonstrate the same pattern as the way that responses vary on the entire instrument. This indicates that changes from item to item represent real changes in the subject and not changes in the way the questions are interpreted (Ponterotto & Ruckdeschel, 2007).

The coefficient alpha has an additional use: It allows the researcher to calculate the amount of measurement error inherent in the instrument (Alwin, 2007). One minus the coefficient alpha quantifies error for this sample using this instrument. For example, if the coefficient alpha were 0.92, then measurement error is equal to 1 minus 0.92, or 8 percent. The smaller the amount of measurement error, the stronger the internal validity of a research study. The reverse is also true. When measurement error is high—in general, more than 20 to 25 percent—then the conclusions of the study may be suspect.

Calibration: The use of procedures to minimize measurement error with physical instruments by objectively verifying that the instrument is measuring a characteristic accurately.

Precision: The degree of reproducibility or the generation of consistent values every time an instrument is used.

Internal reliability: The extent to which an instrument is consistent within itself as measured with the alpha coefficient statistic.

If differences are found, are they due to the intervention or to inconsistencies in the measurement procedure? It is desirable, then, to use an instrument that has as large a coefficient alpha as possible.

Stability Among Individuals

Stability among individuals is measured by an item–total correlation, which should have a positive sign and an absolute value close to 0.5. An item–total correlation represents whether performance on a single item is consistent with the individual's performance on all items.

Stability Between Raters

> **Interrater reliability:** The extent to which an instrument is consistent across raters, as measured with a percentage agreement or a kappa statistic.

Stability between raters is documented as interrater reliability or scorer agreement (Salmond, 2008). This specific type of reliability assessment is indicated when multiple raters observe and record a variable. Interrater reliability quantifies the stability of a measure across raters. For example, the degree of agreement between two or more nurses who are staging a pressure ulcer should be documented. A simple percentage agreement can be used to document interrater reliability, but a kappa statistic is even better. Specifically called Cohen's kappa, this statistic focuses on the degree of agreement between raters and generates a p value, reflecting the statistical significance of the agreement (Cohen, 1968). A kappa can be interpreted like a percentage, and in either case (percentage agreement or kappa) a value of 0.85 or greater is considered acceptable. An associated small p value indicates the agreement was not due to chance. A high kappa (greater than 0.85) with a low p value (less than 0.05) reflects good reliability between multiple raters in an experiment. Ongoing training and monitoring of raters can improve agreement and reliability between raters over time.

Stability over Time

Stability over time is quantified by a test-retest correlation coefficient. Although the usual standard for any reliability coefficient is 0.7, some measurement experts argue that a lower standard—as low as 0.5—can be applied to test-retest correlations because of the attenuation that naturally occurs over time (Schultz & Whitney, 2005). Test-retest correlation is accomplished by administering an instrument, waiting a reasonable period of time, and then readministering the instrument. A correlation coefficient is then calculated between the two sets of item scores.

At least one test of reliability should be performed and reported for the instruments used in an experiment. **Table 9.1** summarizes the primary reliability tests and their interpretation. The gold standard is to assess consistency within the instrument and among individuals over time. Efficiency, resources, and time often limit the capacity to run multiple tests of reliability.

If the instrument has been developed by the researcher, it should be pilot tested on a small group of subjects for assessment of reliability. These pilot tests should be performed and reported as part of the methods section. If a subject participates in the pilot, he or she should be excluded from the primary study to avoid a potential pretesting effect.

An instrument will only be as strong as its reliability. If an instrument does not measure a characteristic reliably, then it cannot be expected to represent the true score for

Table 9.1		

Reliability and Validity Statistics

Test	What It Means	Interpretation
Cronbach's alpha/ coefficient alpha	Internal reliability: Are the individual items consistent with the overall test results?	▪ Coefficient alpha should exceed 0.7 as a minimum ▪ < 0.4 is unacceptable ▪ 0.4 to 0.7 is weak reliability ▪ 0.7 to 0.9 is moderate reliability ▪ > 0.9 is strong reliability
Guttman split half/split half alpha	Internal reliability: Is the first half of the test as reliable as the second half or are odd-numbered items as reliable as even-numbered items?	Split half will be lower than coefficient alpha, but should exceed 0.6 as a minimum.
Test-retest reliability	Is the instrument stable over time? If used repeatedly, are the results due to actual changes in the subject, not the instrument?	Yields a correlation coefficient, which should equal or exceed 0.5.
Criterion-related	Does the instrument measure actual performance or presence of the characteristic it is intended to measure?	Yields a correlation coefficient, which should exceed 0.5.
Interrater reliability	Do two or more raters agree on the ratings?	Percentage agreement of 0.85 or greater; Cohen's kappa ≥ 0.80 with a p value < 0.05.

an individual subject (Salmond, 2008). Measuring the characteristic accurately requires validity, or assurance that the instrument measures the concept it is supposed to measure.

Ensure Validity: A Focus on Accuracy and Truth

An instrument has to be consistent to be precise, but a measure can consistently measure the wrong thing. For example, it is difficult to measure the length of a neonate. A squirming baby is measured from the tip of the heel to the crown of the head, which is not exactly a precise description. Measuring over the head to the tip of the nose would be more reliable—it is easy to find the end of the nose—but it would not be an accurate representation of the baby's length. Reliability tells us an instrument will be consistent; validity tells us the instrument will consistently measure the right thing.

Reliability constrains, but does not ensure, validity. An instrument cannot be more valid than it is reliable. For example, a scale may weigh kilograms and accurately represent the concept of weight. But if the scale consistently weighs

Validity: The ability of an instrument to consistently measure what it is supposed to measure.

light or heavy, then the observed score is not matching the true score, no matter how relevant the measure itself. Simply possessing reliability does not ensure validity; separate tests of each are required to draw a comprehensive conclusion about the usefulness of an instrument. Even so, it is not uncommon for reliability to be reported without comment on validity. Both are required to trust the outcome of a study.

The search for a valid measure begins by determining all of the most important aspects of the phenomenon under study. For example, a study of quality of life in hospice patients might include instruments to measure physical symptoms, social support, spirituality, and mental state. The study may require multiple instruments to confidently measure all the concepts related to the research question, and each instrument must be reliable and valid.

Validity is harder to test than reliability. Complicating the process is the need to test validity on multiple populations to determine who it is valid for and under what conditions. Consider the pain scale in **FIGURE 9.2**; the scale shows six faces, with the lowest end a smile and the upper end a face with a frown and tears. The instrument is intended to represent the quantity and nature of pain reported by pediatric patients. Is the instrument interpreted the same way by children and by adults? Might some groups of patients interpret the crying face as sadness instead of pain? Does the instrument represent pain for someone with dementia or in rehabilitation or from another culture? The validity of the instrument must be tested and retested to ensure it is effective across settings and situations.

A researcher can use several methods to document validity. One or all types may be used in the same study.

Content Validity

Content validity: A subjective judgment about whether a measurement makes sense by assessing that items of the instrument are the attributes being measured (face validity) or by verifying items with a panel of experts.

Content validity involves a subjective judgment about whether a measurement makes sense. Content validity can mean that face validity has been assessed ("This instrument looks like it should measure pain") or that a panel of experts has verified that the correct concepts are included in the measure.

Content validity may be developed from a thorough review of the literature on the concept or from qualitative research findings where representatives of the

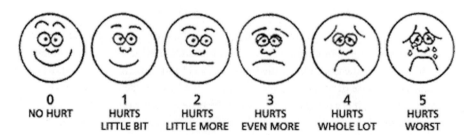

| 0 | 1 | 2 | 3 | 4 | 5 |
| NO HURT | HURTS LITTLE BIT | HURTS LITTLE MORE | HURTS EVEN MORE | HURTS WHOLE LOT | HURTS WORST |

FIGURE 9.2 Wong-Baker Faces Pain Rating Scale
Source: From Hockberry, M.J., Wilson, D., & Winkelsstein, M.L. (2005). *Wong's Essentials of Pediatric Nursing* (7th ed.). St. Louis, MO: 1259.

relevant population provide data on the experience (Salmond, 2008). In this way, basic content validity is established. But it is necessary to go beyond a review of the basic concepts; an external panel of reviewers should evaluate the fit of the tool with the underlying concepts.

A helpful tool in determining content validity is the test blueprint. A test blueprint can help the researcher determine if items in the instrument represent all the basic content that must be represented. Often, the test blueprint and the instrument are reviewed by an impartial reviewer, who evaluates whether all the items in the blueprint are reflected in the content of the instrument. **Table 9.2** shows a test blueprint for the measurement of fatigue in oncology patients.

Construct Validity

Construct validity indicates that a measurement captures the hypothetical basis for the variable. This is, as it sounds, abstract and very difficult, but extremely valuable. Construct validity may be the most important type of validity test to ensure that results will represent reality. Researchers can take years to validate the constructs represented by an instrument. A common method of construct validation is factor analysis, which groups items within the instrument according to their shared variability (Salkind, 2007). The researcher can then review the factor groups and determine whether they represent the conceptual basis of the instrument.

Criterion-Related Validity

Criterion-related validity is the correlation of the instrument to some external manifestation of the characteristic. For example, a newer instrument may be compared with an older, more established instrument. There are several ways to measure criterion-related validity:

- Concurrent validity is present when an instrument reflects actual performance. An example might be when the reading from a temporal thermometer is correlated with the reading from a rectal thermometer.

> **Test blueprint:** An outline for determining content validity that includes the analysis of basic content and the assessment objectives.
>
> **Construct validity:** An indication that a measurement captures the abstract concept that is the basis of the study. A common method of construct validation is factor analysis.
>
> **Criterion-related validity:** A correlation of the research instrument to some external manifestation of the characteristic.
>
> **Concurrent validity:** A measurement of criterion-related validity that is present when an instrument reflects actual performance.

Table 9.2

A Test Blueprint for Measurement of Fatigue

	Critical Concepts	Critical Concepts	Critical Concepts	Critical Concepts
Physical manifestations	Feeling tired	Drowsiness	Naps in daytime	Nauseated
Emotional reactions	Anxiety	Depression	Shortness of breath	Irritability
Mental state	Difficulty concentrating	Lack of interest	Lack of pleasure	Withdrawn
Vigor and energy	Lack of appetite	Sedentary behavior	Boredom	Lack of well-being

Predictive validity: A measurement of criterion-related validity that is indicated when an instrument can predict future performance.

Discriminate validity: A measurement of criterion-related validity that is demonstrated by the instrument's capacity to differentiate those who have a characteristic from those who do not.

- Predictive validity indicates that a measure can predict future performance. For example, predictive validity for an instrument measuring professional competency for a new graduate would be a valid measure if it correlated with the actual competency of the nurse as measured by appraisal at the end of orientation.

- Discriminate validity demonstrates the capacity to differentiate those who have a characteristic from those who do not. An instrument has good discriminate validity if it can successfully sort subjects into classifications. For example, an instrument to measure the presence of a disease would have discriminate validity if it could accurately diagnose the disease when present and also definitively confirm when the disease is absent.

Most validity tests use the correlation coefficient to represent the degree of relationship between the instrument and the reference. Unlike reliability, when a 0.7 is considered the cutoff for acceptability, it is uncommon for a validity coefficient to be greater than 0.5 (Schultz & Whitney, 2005). The seminal works of Cohen (1988) established the standard for interpretation of a validity coefficient: Greater than 0.5 is strong, 0.3 to 0.5 is moderate, 0.1 to 0.3 is small, and less than 0.1 is trivial. **Table 9.3** depicts the types of validity tests, a description of each, and implications for use.

The correlation coefficient has the added advantage of being the basis for the coefficient of determination, or the amount of variance in the criterion that is explained by this instrument. This is calculated by squaring the correlation coefficient, represented as r^2. For example, if the correlation coefficient between a score on a thermometer and a reading of core body temperature were 0.9, then 0.9^2 or 81 percent of the variance in core body temperature will be explained by this instrument.

Taken together, reliability and validity tests ensure that results are consistent and accurate. Both are key to supporting the internal validity of a research study.

Sensitivity and Specificity

Sensitivity and specificity are measures of validity used in the biomedical sciences because they measure characteristics of diagnostic tools used to detect disease. Sensitivity and specificity are types of discriminate validity. Sensitivity is the capacity of an instrument to detect a disease if it is present. A diagnostic tool such as a mammogram must be sensitive enough to detect breast cancer if it is present. Specificity is the capacity of an instrument to differentiate when the disease is not present. A diagnostic tool is specific if it can definitively conclude that the disease is not present when it is not. In other words, sensitivity helps the researcher avoid false negatives, and specificity helps the researcher avoid false positives. Both sensitivity and specificity are needed to be confident that results accurately represent the distribution of the disease in the sample (Forthofer, 2007). In general, the larger the sensitivity and specificity statistics, the better the test. However, there are tradeoffs; when sensitivity becomes very high, then specificity often suffers, and vice versa. An ideal test will balance sensitivity and specificity, with high scores on each.

Sensitivity: A measure of discriminate validity in the biomedical sciences that indicates an instrument has the capacity to detect disease if it is present.

Specificity: A measure of discriminate validity in the biomedical sciences that indicates an instrument has the capacity to differentiate when the disease is not present.

Table 9.3

Tests of Measurement Validity

Test	How It Is Done	Implications
Face validity	Subject-matter experts review the instrument and conclude that it appears valid.	■ Accurate conclusions are heavily reliant on the competence of the subject-matter expert. ■ Is considered an essential element of validity testing.
Content validity	■ Subject-matter experts review the instrument and conclude that the content of the instrument represents the concepts of interest. ■ Often, raters are asked to rate each item as "essential," "useful," or "not necessary" and to give feedback about the usefulness of the overall instrument.	■ Accurate conclusions are heavily reliant on the competence of the subject-matter expert. ■ Helps determine which items should be included in the final instrument and which may be deleted. ■ Results in feedback on both content and form of the instrument.
Criterion-related: Predictive validity	Correlation or regression statistical analysis is applied to determine if the instrument is correlated to or can predict an objective measure of performance.	Is important for tests that will be used to predict who is successful (e.g., pre-employment tests or college admission tests) or who will exhibit a condition in the future (e.g., cardiac risk assessment).
Criterion-related: Concurrent validity	■ Collect test and criterion scores at the same time. ■ Correlation analysis is applied to determine if the instrument reflects current performance.	Is important for tests of conditions that are difficult, expensive, or painful to detect (e.g., heart disease) or when tests are not available in an appropriate form (e.g., patients for whom English is a second language).
Criterion-related: Discriminate validity	■ Collect test and criterion scores. ■ Discriminate analysis is applied to determine if the instrument can accurately sort subjects into groups that do and do not have the criterion condition.	■ Is important for tests of sensitivity and specificity of diagnostic tests. ■ Is useful when differences between groups are subtle or difficult to detect (e.g., between a B+ and an A– score).
Construct validity	Difficult to evaluate, but may be based on studies of group differences, studies of internal structure, factor analysis for subscale structure, or studies of the stability of test scores.	■ Is best suited to the instances when test scores assess an attribute or a quality that is not easily or objectively measured. ■ Is often used for psychological or social conditions.

Responsiveness

A final assessment of validity for clinical measurements is responsiveness. **Responsiveness** is the ability of a measure to detect change over time in the construct of interest (Kimberlin & Winterstein, 2008). When an outcome measure is intended to capture the effect of an intervention, the capability to detect changes in the subject over time is critical. There are multiple ways to measure responsiveness, including the standardized response mean, Cohen's d, and responsiveness indices (Husted, 2000). Responsiveness is a highly desirable characteristic in a measure, particularly when it will be used to determine the effect of interventions over time.

Responsiveness: A measure that indicates change in the subject's condition when an intervention is effective.

Reading the Measurement Section of a Research Report

The measurement section is generally identified in a straightforward way and labeled "measures." Other words may appear in the heading, such as "methods and measures" or "measures and materials." The measures may be called "instrumentation" or "tests." It should be an easily identifiable part of the write-up. If the measurement is complex, the write-up may have a separate section for measurement procedures, which may be labeled as such or called "protocols." This section may describe the specific steps for measuring variables and may include photographs or figures to support an objective process.

The researcher should describe his or her rationale for the selection of the instruments and provide a summary of the concepts that were the focus of the measurement. The instruments and their content should be clearly linked to the research question and to the conceptual and operational definitions of the variables.

At a minimum, calibration and/or internal reliability should be reported for any instruments used in the experiment. The study becomes stronger as more documentation of the reliability and validity of the instrument are provided. The tests and their actual results should be reported; jointly they are called the *psychometric properties* of the instrument.

If a survey is used, a separate section should describe the development of the instrument as well as its pilot testing. Unless the properties of the instrument have been determined, the results are suspect, and so author-developed instruments should be subjected to the same scrutiny as publicly available tests. If the instrument has been used before, then information about reliability and validity should be provided with the description of the instrument. The actual statistics should be reported with the names of the tests that were

Where to Look for Information About the Measurement Strategy

- A thorough description of the measurement procedures should appear in the methods section.
- The measures may be called "instrumentation," "tools," or "tests." If the measurement procedure is complex, it may have its own section called "protocols" or "procedures."
- Physiologic measures that are not standard may have accompanying photographs or figures to depict the measurement procedure.
- If a survey is used, a separate section may describe the development of the instrument, any pilot tests that were conducted, as well as procedures for its completion by subjects.
- Information about reliability and validity should be provided with the description of the instrument.

- Description of the psychometric properties of the instruments should appear regardless of whether the instrument was developed specifically for the study or was already developed.
- It is not unusual to find that the author describes the instrument rather than providing a copy; this is not a weakness. The survey may be copyrighted or proprietary, or limitations on the length of the article may preclude its inclusion.
- The measurement strategy should be explained in sufficient depth that the reader could re-create the measure with accuracy. If the instrument is a survey, an explanation of content and scales should enable the reader to grasp the concepts measured by the survey.

run. Even if prior statistics are available, reliability and validity should be retested on the specific population used in the study. For example, an instrument designed to measure satisfaction for an acute-care patient may not be as reliable or valid if used in long-term care.

It is not uncommon to see instruments that, from a statistical standpoint, are considered borderline acceptable. This does not mean the researcher has designed the measurement strategy poorly, but rather that strengths and weaknesses of the measures have, by necessity, been balanced. Many factors in instrument use should be considered in addition to the reliability and validity properties. Feasibility of administration, costs of instruments, and the type of measures considered professionally acceptable also drive the selection of an instrument. If stronger tests were available but not used, the author should describe the rationale for his or her choice of a specific instrument. Determining which instrument to use generally involves trade-offs between conceptual purity and research reality.

gray matter

The following considerations drive selection of instruments used in research studies:

- Reliability properties
- Validity properties
- Feasibility of administration
- Acceptability for the subjects
- Instrument costs
- Professional acceptance of types of measures

Although reliability and validity are critical aspects of a measurement, the practicality of the tool may be a major consideration in its selection. The instrument should be as efficient and easy to use as possible. Schmelzer (2007) identified five aspects of practicality that should be considered when selecting a measurement instrument:

- The time required of the subject to complete the tool
- Ease of use in completing the tool
- Interference of the data collection process with usual clinical activities
- Items that cause confusion
- Problems created for statistical analysis

Acceptability for the subject is a strong consideration. It might be more accurate to use urine collected before dawn because it is more concentrated, but it is not acceptable to wake a patient at 4 a.m. to solicit a urine sample. The acceptability of a measure can affect patient responses and attrition of study subjects.

The author may describe the instrument rather than provide a copy, but this is not a weakness. The instrument may be copyrighted or proprietary, or limitations on the length of publication may preclude its inclusion. The author should give enough information that the reader could determine how to obtain a copy of the instrument. The source of instrument or a citation for its publication should be included.

Using Measurements from a Research Study

Research procedures may be applied to practice just as research findings are. Instruments for measuring patient responses to interventions may be used by the clinician to monitor the effectiveness of nursing interventions, diagnose patient problems, and measure outcomes. Appropriate application of a measurement instrument in practice requires that the nurse evaluate conceptual congruence of the instrument as well as the populations for which the instrument is effective.

Checklist for Evaluating the Measurement Strategy

✔ The instruments are clearly linked to concepts in the research question.
✔ Instruments and measures are described objectively.
✔ Reliability of the instrumentation is described and supporting statistics are provided.
✔ Validity of the instrumentation is described and supporting statistics are provided.
✔ A detailed protocol for the use of each instrument in the measurement is described.

Bolton et al. (2009) conducted a literature search and reviewed the use of measurement instruments as evidence in nursing practice. The strongest evidence was for the use of patient risk-assessment tools and interventions implemented by nurses to detect complications and prevent patient harm. For example, prediction rules for risk of falls or for early signs of oversedation can be extremely helpful in clinical nursing practice.

Instruments can be used for purposes other than the original research. For example, the SF-36 measure of functionality can be used to determine general quality of life across a variety of conditions. To determine if an instrument is applicable to a specific practice setting, evaluate its conceptual and operational definitions for fit with the clinical situation. If the phenomenon being evaluated is based on similar concepts, then instruments may be useful to monitor effectiveness in the clinical setting.

Instruments should be reevaluated if applied to radically different problems, populations, or practice settings. For example, an instrument intended for the measurement of anxiety may not be useful in a test of panic disorder. On the other hand, the instrument may measure preoperative anxiety as well as anxiety disorder. Repeated use and testing of the instrument strengthens its ability to apply to different problems.

An instrument should be reevaluated before using it in a different setting than the original use. For example, an instrument intended for use in acute care may not be applicable in a skilled setting; measures used in inpatient settings may not be relevant to outpatient settings. Testing the instrument properties in a new setting prior to its use can verify its applicability in diverse settings.

Finally, an instrument should be rechecked before using it on a different population. Instruments written in English may not be reliable when translated into another language, or tests used with one age group may not be effective with younger or older groups. Reliability and validity are sample-specific and so should be checked with a pilot test before application to practice.

Of course, the instrument itself should be acceptably reliable and valid before its use is considered in any setting—research or practice. Finding suitable measures is also critical to creating valid nursing research projects.

Creating Nursing Research Measures

A strong measurement strategy involves a systematic approach to linking the concepts in the research question to a specific manifestation as a measure. This process begins by breaking down the research question into underlying concepts. For each concept, an

Table 9.4

Translation of a Research Question into Operational Variables

Research Question	Concepts	Operational Variables
Do patients in palliative care who report fatigue have more physical symptoms than similar patients who do not report fatigue?	Palliative care	**Palliative care:** Patients who have been admitted to a home-based palliative care service based on a physician's assessment that their condition is terminal and they are within 6 months of death
	Fatigue	**Fatigue:** Reports of feeling tired and/or drowsy that disrupt the subject's life, as measured by the Fatigue Disruption Score of the Fatigue Symptom Inventory
	Physical symptoms	**Physical symptoms:** The number of symptoms reported, as manifested by physical, emotional, mental, or vigor scales of the Edmonton Symptom Assessment Scale

operational definition is written. An operational definition gives a clear, unambiguous description of the steps needed to quantify the characteristics of a population. Table 9.4 depicts the process of translating a research question into operational definitions.

Once the concepts in a question are defined, a search for an existing instrument is carried out. Instruments may be found in many locations, but it is always best to start with a literature review. The literature can help identify potential instruments and their psychometric characteristics, but it can also point to experts in the field for further contact. Direct contact with instrument developers is a helpful step in the process, and test developers are generally willing to discuss their research and give advice. This initial contact is also helpful to begin the process of seeking permission to use the instrument.

A comprehensive source of both measurement instruments and their evaluation is the *Mental Measurements Yearbook*, which has been published for decades and serves as a source of instruments and critical reviews. Information can be found online for a small fee or in hard copy in most academic libraries. The online version has a search engine to help find instruments based on key concepts. The review includes psychometric statistics about the instrument and recommended applications of the tool. General advice regarding where to find instruments and their cost is also included.

The ideal situation is to find a suitable instrument that has already been validated and determined reliable. When actual test statistics are reported, the researcher can be comfortable using the instrument for measurement of similar concepts in similar settings and patients. Finding an existing instrument is highly efficient and reduces the complexity of a study. Using an existing instrument makes the study consistent with previous studies and therefore easier to compare in the systematic review process. Using standard measures helps the study make a strong contribution to evidence-based practice. In addition, grants and publications are often based on having credible procedures, represented by strong, established measures.

SKILL Builder | Develop a Strong Measurement Strategy

Every measurement system has some inherent error—particularly when the measure is applied to unique human beings in applied settings. The following list includes ways to minimize measurement error through instrument selection and research design:

- Select measurement instruments that have been developed and tested over time. Look for measures that have been administered to large, diverse samples and in multiple studies. Continued testing and refinement decrease measurement error, increase reliability, and ensure validity. Standard measurement instruments also allow aggregation of results into evidence-based practice.
- Develop a custom instrument only as a last resort. Attempt to find an existing instrument, even if it does not match the study goals exactly. An existing instrument may be modified, a subset of items or scales may be used, or questions may be added to customize the instrument to the study. Be sure to contact the author for permission before altering an instrument. These actions require that the revised instrument be pilot tested again for reliability and validity.
- Standardize the measurement methods. Develop guidelines for using the measurement instruments, including verbatim instructions to be given to subjects who complete surveys individually. Use photographs and drawings if necessary; media such as video demonstrations also help train data collectors. The less variability there is within measures, the stronger the reliability of the measure.
- Train and certify observers and data collectors. Minimize the error from multiple raters by ensuring they have a consistent and complete approach to data collection. Measure interrater reliability and do not allow data collectors to conduct measures independently until they have achieved a preset competency level.
- Automate data collection. Use data from existing sources for efficiency and quality. Develop data definitions to ensure the data retrieved from different databases are identical in content.
- Repeat measures. Efficiency can be increased even more if the data collector has the capacity to measure several times and take a mean value. This must be balanced with the pretesting effect, which affects repeated administrations of a test.
- Blind the data collectors. The Hawthorne and/or testing effect can contribute to rater bias just as it can affect subject responses. Data collectors who are unaware of group assignment will yield more objective results with less interrater error.

It is rare, however, to find an instrument that meets the exact purposes of the researcher. The efficiencies of existing instruments then must be balanced with the fact that they may be outdated or may not measure the concepts of interest exactly. The selection of an instrument is always a balance between efficiency and accuracy.

Test Measurement Psychometric Properties

If an existing instrument is used, then the reliability of the instrument for a specific population should be documented. If the author develops the instrument, the reliability of the instrument must be documented with a pilot study. The instrument is administered to a pilot group and its psychometric properties tested. At least one test of internal reliability, and ideally one measure of validity, should be conducted in the pilot phase. Changes are made to the instrument before the selection is finalized. Internal reliability coefficients from the pilot quantify the amount of error in the measurement and document the acceptability of the instrument for use in the research. The extent to which the researcher is able to vigorously reduce error must be balanced with available resources, the importance of the variable, and the magnitude of impact of an error.

A Note About Qualitative Data

Qualitative research is generally not concerned with a measurement strategy. In qualitative research processes, the researcher is the measurement instrument, and so reliability is directly related to his or her skill at eliciting and describing information. Qualitative data involve a naturalistic inquiry that bases results on the analysis of meaning, generally in words, so there is little reliance on numbers. However, qualitative researchers are interested in the pursuit of truth, and to the extent that data collection represents truth, qualitative research is also concerned with sound data collection.

For More Depth and Detail

For a more in-depth look at the concepts in this chapter, try these references:

Alwin, D. (2007). *Margins of error: A study of reliability in survey measurement.* Hoboken, NJ: Jossey-Bass.

Brown, D., Hofer, T., Thomson, R. et al. (2008). An epistemology of patient safety research: A framework for study design and interpretation. Part 3. End points and measurement. *Quality and Safety in Health Care, 17*(3), 170–177.

DiIorio, C. (2005). *Measurement in health behavior: Methods for research evaluation.* Hoboken, NJ: Jossey-Bass.

Houser, J., & Kotzer, A. (2008). Precision, reliability, and validity: Essential elements of measurement in nursing research. *Journal for Specialists in Pediatric Nursing, 13*(4), 297–299.

Lake, E. (2006). Multilevel models in health outcomes research. Part I: Theory, design and measurement. *Applied Nursing Research, 19*, 51–53.

Mittleman, M. (2008). Psychosocial intervention research: Challenges, strategies, and measurement issues. *Aging and Mental Health, 12*(1), 1–4.

Salkind, N. (2007). *Encyclopedia of measurement and statistics.* Newbury Park, CA: Sage.

Strickland, O., DiIorio, C., Coverson, D., & Nelson, M. (2007). Advancing nursing science in vulnerable populations: Measurement issues. In Fitzpatrick, J., Nyamathi, A., & Koniak-Griffin, D. (Eds.). *Annual Review of Nursing Research: Vulnerable Populations* (p. 27). New York: Springer.

Wilson, M., Allen, D., & Li, J. (2006). Improving measurement in health education and health behavior research using item response modeling: Comparison with the classical test theory approach. *Health Education Research, 21*(Suppl 1), i19–i43.

Qualitative research is not focused on reliability and validity so much as trustworthiness of the data. Lincoln and Guba (1985), in their seminal work on naturalistic inquiry, identified criteria that are used to evaluate data collection in qualitative studies that are analogous to the methods used in quantitative studies.

Dependability: A qualitative data measure focused on the stability of the information across individuals or over time.
Credibility: A qualitative data measure focused on ensuring that the results represent the underlying meaning of the data.

- *Dependability:* Like reliability, dependability of qualitative data is focused on the stability of the information across individuals or over time. Methods to demonstrate dependability include achieving saturation, member checking, and using an audit trail.
- *Credibility:* Like validity, credibility of qualitative data is focused on ensuring that the results accurately represent the underlying meaning of the data. Credibility is improved by prolonged engagement in the data collection process, triangulation, and negative case analysis.

Summary of Key Concepts

- Measurement is the process of quantifying characteristics that can answer the research question. The measurement strategy involves defining the research question in conceptual and operational terms and finding instruments to express these characteristics as variables.
- Data collected as primary data are solicited directly from the subject for the specific purpose of the research study. Secondary data collection involves retrieving information from data sets that were originally collected for purposes other than the research.
- The level of measurement may be nominal, ordinal, interval, or ratio. The level of measurement drives the type of statistical analysis that can be conducted to answer the research question.
- Measurement error can be random or systematic. It may be due to human factors, problems with the instrument, variation in procedures, or data processing error. Random error is expected in a research study, but systematic error will bias the results.
- Reliability is a reflection of the consistency with which the instrument records the measure. It may take the form of calibration with technology or tests of reliability for other kinds of instruments. Instruments may have internal reliability, reliability across subjects, reliability among raters, or reliability over time.
- Instruments must be reliable to be valid. Validity indicates the extent to which a measure accurately measures what it is supposed to measure. Types of validity testing include content validity, construct validity, and criterion-related validity.
- The reliability and validity of an instrument are the most important characteristics, and they should be documented in the research report. Using an existing instrument is desirable for its efficiency and the capacity to provide a comparison with existing studies.

CRITICAL APPRAISAL **EXERCISE**

Retrieve the following full text article from the Cumulative Index to Nursing and Allied Health Literature or similar search database:

Voepel-Lewis, T., Zanotti, J., Dammeyer, J., & Merkel, S. (2010). Reliability and validity of the face, legs, activity, cry, consolability behavioral tool in assessing acute pain in critically ill patients. *American Journal of Critical Care, 19*(1), 55–61.

Review the article, focusing on the section that describes the testing of the instrument. Consider the following appraisal questions in your critical review of this research article:

1. The FLACC instrument had already been validated. Why did these authors choose to undertake this examination of the instrument's psychometric characteristics?
2. What controls did the researchers put in place to control the effect of the nurse's biases in using the FLACC instrument?
3. The authors note that the FLACC and CNPI are ordinal data. What are the implications of these kind of data for analysis? What is the distinguishing characteristic of ordinal data?
4. What measure of interrater reliability was used to determine reliability of the FLACC? Was this an appropriate test to use for the purposes of the study? Why or why not?
5. Explain how the authors tested criterion validity. Was this an appropriate way to measure validity for this instrument? Would another method have been more appropriate in this situation?
6. Explain the other tests of reliability and validity that were applied in this study. Were these appropriate for this instrument?

- Qualitative research is concerned with discovering truth and so focuses on the trustworthiness of the data. Methods for ensuring trustworthiness include establishing dependability and credibility of the data.

For a full suite of assignments and additional learning activities, use the access code located in the front of your book to visit this exclusive website: http://go.jblearning .com/houser. If you do not have an access code, you can obtain one at the site.

References

Alwin, D. (2007). *Margins of error: A study of reliability in survey measurement.* Hoboken, NJ: Jossey-Bass.

Bolton, L., Donaldson, N., Rutledge, D., Bennett, C., & Brown, D. (2009) The impact of nursing interventions: Overview of effective interventions, outcomes, measures, and priorities for future research. *Medical Care Research and Review, 64*(2 Suppl), 123S–124S.

Cohen, J. (1968). Weighted kappa: Nominal scale agreement with provision for scaled disagreement or partial credit. *Psychological Bulletin, 70*(4), 213–220.

Cohen, J. (1988). *Statistical power analysis for the behavioral sciences* (2nd ed.). Hillsdale, NJ: Lawrence Erlbaum.

Colbert, A. (2009). Measurement challenges in forensic nursing research. *Journal of Forensic Nursing, 5*, 51–52.

Cronbach, L. (1951). Coefficient alpha and the internal structure of tests. *Psychometrika, 16*, 297–334.

Eder, C., Fullerton, J., Benroth, R., & Lindsay, S. (2005). Pragmatic strategies that enhance the reliability of data abstracted from medical records. *Applied Nursing Research, 18*, 50–54.

Forthofer, R., Lee, E., & Hernandex, M. (2007). *Biostatistics: A guide to design, analysis and discovery*. Boston: Elsevier Academic Press.

Husted, J., Cook, R., Farewell, V., & Gladman, D. (2000). Methods for assessing responsiveness: A critical review and recommendation. *Journal of Clinical Epidemiology, 53*, 459–468.

Kimberlin, C., & Winterstein, S. (2008). Validity and reliability of measurement instruments used in research. *American Journal of Health System Pharmacies, 65*, 2276–2284.

Lincoln, T., & Guba, E. (1985). *Naturalistic inquiry*. Thousand Oaks, CA: Sage.

Liu, Y., & Chen, M. (2009). Biological measures in nursing research: A discussion of accuracy and precision. *Journal of Nursing, 56*(5), 60–68.

Mlinar, S., Schmelzer, M., & Daniels, G. (2007). Are your measurements reliable? *Gastroenterology Nursing, 30*(5), 382–384.

Ponterotto, J., & Ruckdeschel, D. (2007). An overview of coefficient alpha and a reliability matrix for estimating adequacy of internal consistency coefficients with psychological research measures. *Perceptual and Motor Skills, 105*, 997–1014.

Salkind, N. (2007). *Encyclopedia of measurement and statistics*. Newbury Park, CA: Sage.

Salmond, S. (2008). Evaluating the reliability and validity of measurement instruments. *Orthopaedic Nursing, 27*(1), 28–30.

Schmelzer, M. (2007). Measurement tool requirements. *Gastroenterology Nursing, 20*(2), 136–138.

Schultz, K., & Whitney, D. (2005). *Measurement theory in action*. Thousand Oaks, CA: Sage.

Sim, J., & Wright, C. (2005). The kappa statistic in reliability studies: Use, interpretation and sample size requirements. *Physical Therapy, 85*(3), 257–268.

Viswanathan, M. (2005). *Measurement error and research design*. Thousand Oaks, CA: Sage.

Weir, J. (2005). Quantifying test-retest reliability using the intraclass correlation coefficient and the SEM. *Journal of Strength and Conditioning Research, 19*(1), 231–240.

chapter 10

Data Collection Methods

Introduction

The conclusions from a research study will only be as good as the data that were used to draw them. A research study can be beautifully designed, well-controlled, and impeccably executed, but if the data that are collected are not consistent and accurate, then the results will be suspect. The data collection plan, then, is integral to producing reliable evidence for nursing practice.

❝❝ *Voices from the Field* ❞❞

The first study I had exposure to was several years back, and my role was purely data collection. It was a good way to break into the idea of doing research because I really just had to follow directions. I was able to sit in on research design meetings and measurement selection, and I had a chance to absorb it all without being responsible for making decisions.

This particular study was looking at the role of nutritional support in the length of time critical patients spend on a ventilator. The advanced practice nurses, nutritionists, and physicians had care conferences, and one particular physician kept encouraging them to consider more aggressive nutritional supplementation for patients. So they decided to look at it, mostly to appease him, I think. The group identified several indicators they thought might be related to length of time on a vent—age, diagnoses, type of admission, and so on—and we retrieved the data from the patient's chart.

The procedure for selecting charts and collecting data was very precise. I carried the directions with me so I was sure I did not skip a step; even if I did 12 charts in a row I still went through the whole checklist. The team really impressed upon me the need to be consistent in the way the data were collected, and I took them seriously. There were definitions for each of the events and characteristics, and they had to be rated numerically. That was sometimes a challenge, because documentation was not always standard, so finding the right data could be hard. I also was concerned that some events may not have been recorded, because there appeared to be a consistent picture of events happening, and then a gap, so you wondered if it did not happen or was just not written down. If it was not written down, no matter how much you might infer it happened, you could not include it.

At first, I tried to find the time to do data collection during work, but that just did not work out. I made a personal decision to come in and help on my time off. If you told me I would be willing to do this when I first volunteered for the team, I'm not sure I would have believed you, but participating in the discussions really got me curious, and I wanted to see it through.

One of the nurses on the team was working on her doctorate, and so she ran the statistics for us. She used a technique to see if she could predict length of stay with any of these indicators. Days to nutrition support came out on top of the list—they did find the doctor was right. The sooner these patients got adequate nutritional support, the more quickly they got off the vent. He gloated (deservedly) and presented the findings at a couple of professional conferences. I was proud to be part of the team; I really enjoyed the experience.

I was surprised at how engaged I got in this idea, even though most of my work is in neonatal ICU. I began to think of ways I could transfer this information to my unit, so it got me motivated to think of my own studies, too.

Irene Burch, RN, MSN

After design and measurement strategies are chosen, the next step is to identify an appropriate, effective method for data collection. The specific method chosen to collect data will be guided by the design and enhanced by the literature review. Ultimately, however, the researcher must design a data collection procedure that is clear, unbiased, reliable, and valid—and it must produce evidence that answers the research question. This chapter describes common data collection methods, procedures, and management issues. The most common data collection methods will be reviewed here, including physiologic measurement, psychometric instrumentation, surveys, questionnaires, interviews, focus groups, observation, and secondary data reviews.

Data collection methods are used to gather information in a systematic way. Regardless of its design, all research has a specific goal for the data collection process: high-quality data. There are many ways to collect data, and the choice of a data collection strategy depends on the nature of the research question, the specific information being gathered, and the resources available to the researcher. Whether the researcher is conducting a quantitative or a qualitative design, it is necessary to identify the best type of data collection method. Data methods used in quantitative studies will be of a numeric nature and subject to statistical analysis. Data methods used in qualitative studies will be of a text-based nature and subject to coding.

> **gray matter**
>
> Effective data collection must be designed to
> - Be clear
> - Be unbiased
> - Be reliable
> - Be valid
> - Answer the research question

The research question guides the data collection method. To specify a particular data collection method, the researcher needs to answer some key questions:

- Are the data primarily objective or subjective?
- Will the data collection process be highly structured or minimally structured?
- Will the data be retrieved by trained data collectors or via self-report?
- Is the analysis statistical or narrative?

To answer these questions, the researcher must be clear about the purpose of the research and the information that is needed to answer the research question. Once clarity of purpose and question is achieved, then the researcher must select the type of data that are required.

The following are the most common data collection methods:

- Physiologic measurements
- Psychometric instrumentation
- Questionnaires
- Interviews
- Focus groups
- Observation

Physiologic Measurement

Evidence-based practice focuses attention on the use of physiologic measurements from patients for clinical research efforts. Physiologic measurement involves the assignment of a number or value to an individual's biological functioning. The measure can be self-reported, observed, directly measured, indirectly measured, electronically monitored, or obtained through diagnostic tests.

Nurses commonly rely on physiologic measurements to make patient care decisions. They take vital signs, read lab results, and measure blood glucose. The measurement of a patient's biological functioning involves the use of specialized equipment and often requires specific training in the use of that equipment. The specialized equipment used to measure a patient's biological functioning is likely to be accurate, precise, and sensitive. It can provide valid measures for variables related to physical functions. Physiologic measurements are readily available for the clinician researcher and provide objective data. To use the data for research purposes, the data are collected from each participant in exactly the same way. Consistency in the data collection process is very important.

Limitations on using physiologic measurements include the need for calibration of the equipment, the use of different equipment on different study participants, and the variability of multiple data. For example, if the research involves measuring the temperature of all study participants, the researcher should ensure that all temperatures were taken with the same type of instrument and taken in exactly the same way. An example of an undesirable situation is one in which one data collector obtains temperature using an oral thermometer while another data collector obtains the temperature using a tympanic thermometer. The researcher's goal is to have minimal variability in the data collection procedure by ensuring all data collectors use the same steps.

Psychometric instruments: Instruments used to collect subjective information directly from subjects; they are tested for reliability and validity.

Physiologic measurement can also be self-reported for variables such as pain, nausea, and dizziness. These variables are often a critical part of research but are subjective in nature and depend on the participant understanding what is being asked of him or her. These types of measures are usually collected using instruments, but these are of a different nature. Instruments used to collect subjective information directly from subjects are referred to as **psychometric instruments**.

Psychometric Instrumentation

In the case of instruments that measure characteristics or traits, the calibration concern is replaced with an emphasis on reliability and validity. Many instruments exist whose reliability and validity have been verified. Before a researcher begins to develop his or her own data collection tool, a literature review and query of research instrument databases is justified to see if an instrument exists that will answer the research question. If an instrument is located, its properties may be found using reports from various instrument evaluation companies or from the original author. Permission must be obtained from the original author before the instrument can be used in a publishable research study. The psychometric properties of the instrument are documented in the research write-up to assure the reader that measurement error is not responsible for the findings. At a minimum, internal reliability should be reported for any instrument used in the research study.

The advantages of using an existing instrument are many. It saves the researcher time in the development and validation of a new instrument, which may be substantial. Development of a new instrument for a research study involves developing a test blueprint, creating questions, soliciting feedback about the fidelity of the instrument to the blueprint, pilot testing the instrument, and making revisions. This process can be burdensome, can delay the research, and should be undertaken only when a thorough review of the literature reveals no acceptable instruments.

In addition, the use of existing measurement tools allows for the replication of a study and a contribution to aggregate studies. Results of the research can be compared to the work of others if the procedure uses the same instrument. Limitations of using a previously developed instrument include cost of the instrument, measures that may not address all the research interests, feasibility of administering the instrument, and an inability to locate psychometric information or the original author.

Psychometric instruments encompass a variety of methods and may vary widely in complexity. Surveys, questionnaires, and scales are all examples of instruments that must possess adequate psychometric properties to be useful in research.

Survey

The most common data collection method is the survey. The survey method is an approach in which a systematic tool is used to gather information directly from respondents about their experiences, behaviors, attitudes, or perceptions (Lavrakas, 2008).

Depending on the types of questions used, survey research can be a quantitative design, a qualitative design, or a mix of both. Surveys may be personally distributed, distributed through the mail, or delivered online. They can be administered during a face-to-face interview or in a telephone survey, or the respondents may complete the surveys on their own. Responses of participants are described in numeric terms and/or in words. Important characteristics of numeric research surveys are that they use a systematic approach and allow for a quantitative analysis of reliability, validity, and statistical conclusions (Fowler, 2008). A systematic approach to developing survey questions appears in Table 10.1. FIGURE 10.1 depicts a decision-tree approach to determining the survey method and outlines the qualities of a good question.

Table 10.1

Guidelines for Creating a Survey

Step 1
- Identify the objectives of the survey.
- Identify demographic characteristics.
- Identify the dependent variable (if applicable).
- Identify variables of interest or the independent variables (if applicable).

Step 2
- Envision how the data will be analyzed.
- Create data definitions.
- Design a data tabulation form.

Table 10.1

Guidelines for Creating a Survey *(Continued)*

Step 3

- Draft a set of questions.
- Check to make sure all the variables are addressed.
- Modify wording on questions.

Step 4

- Group the questions to reflect each major topic of the survey.
- Organize questions from general to specific.
- Format the survey so it is easy to follow.
- Write clear instructions for completion of the survey.

Step 5

- Distribute a preliminary draft of the survey to a group of colleagues.
- Solicit their review of the document and identify problems with questions, including the way the questions and the directions are worded.
- Provide the group a copy of the objectives so they can determine if the questions will address each of the objectives.

Step 6

- Revise the survey.
- Test the survey on a pilot group of subjects.
- Measure the reliability of the survey and make any changes based on the statistical analysis and the feedback of the pilot group.
- Analyze the results of the pilot group, looking for patterns of missing the answers or inconsistency in responses, and make final revisions.
- Record the amount of time the subjects take to complete the survey.
- Revise the data tabulation form.

Step 7

- Write instructions for the participants.
- Write an introductory letter.
- Write a consent form, if applicable.
- Distribute the survey.
- Give the participants clear instructions for returning the completed instrument.

Questionnaires

Questionnaires are common survey data collection tools. They are structured surveys that are self-administered by subjects. The questions are identical for all subjects and thus result in consistent responses.

Questions used in surveys can be open-ended or closed questions. **Open-ended questions** are used when the researcher does not know all the possible alternative responses, or if the researcher wants participants to respond in their own words. Typically, open-ended questions are characteristic of qualitative research, but they may be included as part of an otherwise quantitative data collection tool. Responses are analyzed using content analysis to find themes in the words of respondents. Examples of open-ended questions appear in **Table 10.2**.

Open-ended questions:
Questions with no predetermined set of responses.

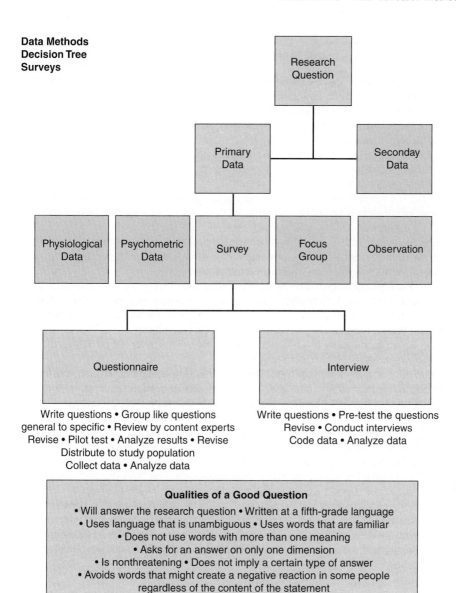

**Data Methods
Decision Tree
Surveys**

Research Question

Primary Data

Seconday Data

Physiological Data

Psychometric Data

Survey

Focus Group

Observation

Questionnaire

Write questions • Group like questions
general to specific • Review by content experts
Revise • Pilot test • Analyze results • Revise
Distribute to study population
Collect data • Analyze data

Interview

Write questions • Pre-test the questions
Revise • Conduct interviews
Code data • Analyze data

Qualities of a Good Question
• Will answer the research question • Written at a fifth-grade language
• Uses language that is unambiguous • Uses words that are familiar
• Does not use words with more than one meaning
• Asks for an answer on only one dimension
• Is nonthreatening • Does not imply a certain type of answer
• Avoids words that might create a negative reaction in some people
regardless of the content of the statement

FIGURE 10.1 Steps in Survey Design

Open-ended questions ask for unprompted opinions. There are no predetermined answers for the respondent to choose from. The advantage is that the researcher gets a wide range of responses. Disadvantages of the open-ended question are that it takes the respondent longer to complete, the respondent may misinterpret the question, and analysis of the data takes longer.

Closed questions are used when there are a fixed number of alternative responses and the respondent has to select from the responses provided by the researcher.

Closed questions: Questions that use a fixed number of alternative responses. Respondents are forced to select answers or ratings on a scale provided by the researcher.

SKILL Builder | Design Better Questionnaires

Questionnaires are not easy to construct; they take a thoughtful, systematic approach. Yet they can be invaluable as a data collection tool for both quantitative and qualitative research. Here are some simple suggestions for designing strong questionnaires that are more likely to be answered accurately and completely, making for stronger research conclusions:

- Keep the questions simple, clear, and easy to answer. Consider the value of each question before including it in the final survey. Write the questions in an unbiased way that does not imply a "correct" answer.
- Assess the reading level of the questionnaire. Unless the reading capacity of the potential subjects is known (for example, all the respondents are college-educated), write the items at a fifth-grade reading level.
- Keep the overall survey short, and ask the pilot test subjects to estimate the time it took them to complete it. Include this time estimate in the introductory letter so subjects will know when they have time to respond.
- Know how each question will be analyzed, and be sure the way the data are collected can be subjected to the specific analytic test. For example, yes/no questions have a very limited range of statistical tests that can be used for analysis; questions on a scale have a broader range of potential analytic procedures.
- Have a plan for handling missing data consistently. Determine ahead of time if you will allow analysis of incomplete responses.
- Group similar questions together. Start with nonthreatening questions, such as demographic information, and work up to more sensitive information at the end of the questionnaire. Avoid emotionally laden words that may imply a judgment.
- Avoid questions that ask about more than one characteristic or dimension. Limit each question to a single concept. Likewise, avoid complex designs for answers that involve multiple categories.
- Write scales so that they have no "neutral" or midpoint response. Often, respondents use the "neutral" category for many meanings—including "this doesn't apply," "I don't know," or "I don't want to tell you." If you need a neutral category, include a separate category that has no numerical value for "not applicable/no answer."
- Provide a well-written cover letter with explicit instructions for both completing and sending back or submitting the questionnaire. The instructions should be clear and concise. Make it a convenient process to respond and get the answers back to the researcher.

Table 10.2

Examples of Open-Ended Questions

- What were your emotional reactions to the initial ultrasound that indicated there was a problem with your baby?
- How did you deal with those emotional reactions?
- In what ways did the nurse practitioner help you deal with the birth of your baby?
- What strategies have you used to deal with the stress of caring for a baby with a significant health problem?

This may involve selecting from a limited number of answers or rating something on a scale. Structured, fixed-response questions are best used when the researcher is investigating a finite number of potential responses. Closed questions are easier than open-ended questions for the respondent to answer and for the researcher to analyze. There are many kinds of closed questions.

- Forced-choice questions require the respondents to select a single response from a list of possible answers.
- Dichotomous questions require the respondents to select from only two choices.
- Scales ask the respondents to rank order their responses on a continuum.

Forced-Choice Questions

Forced-choice questions provide choices that are mutually exclusive and encompass the total range of answers. Respondents should not be confused about whether two or more alternatives appear to mean the same thing. Nor should respondents be looking for an answer that is not among the alternative choices of an answer to the question. Forced-choice questions are used when the researcher wants respondents to choose the best possible answer among all options presented. Forced-choice questions often have right and wrong answers. For example, measuring the amount of knowledge a diabetic retained after a teaching session might be via a forced-choice question.

Dichotomous Questions

Dichotomous questions are those that can be answered by selecting from only one of two choices. These typically are used to determine if a characteristic is present or not or if a respondent belongs to a particular group. Dichotomous questions yield limited information about the respondent and are hard to analyze. Because these questions can be analyzed with a limited range of tests, the use of dichotomous questions should be limited to those situations in which no other type of question is appropriate.

Scales

Scales ask respondents to rank some trait or ability on a continuum of possible responses. The individual entries on the scale correspond to variations in the strength of the response. The most common types of scales are Likert scales, Guttman scales, and visual analog scales.

The Likert scale presents a set of attitude statements, and respondents are asked to express agreement or disagreement on a five-point or seven point-scale (Likert & Hayes, 1957). Each degree of agreement is given a numerical value. Thus, a total numerical value can be calculated from all the responses.

The Guttman scale presents a set of items on a continuum, or it may use statements ranging from one extreme to the other (Guttman, 1947). When a person agrees with one statement, it can be assumed that he or she agrees with all previous questions in the scale. In other words, the responses are progressive. Each item on the scale is worth a point, and the total score is cumulative. So if a respondent's score is five, it means that the respondent agreed with all of the item statements from 1 through 5. Examples of closed questions and scales appear in Table 10.3.

Scales: Type of closed-question format in which respondents put responses in rank order on a continuum.
Likert scale: A scale that uses attitude statements ranked on a five- or seven-point scale. The degree of agreement or disagreement is given a numerical value, and a total can be calculated.
Guttman scale: A scale with a set of items on a continuum or statements ranging from one extreme to another. Responses are progressive and cumulative.

Table 10.3

Examples of Closed Questions

Example of a Forced-Choice Question

What is your current marital status? (Select one.)
- ☐ Single
- ☐ Married
- ☐ Divorced
- ☐ Separated
- ☐ Widowed

Examples of Dichotomous Choice Questions

What is your gender?
- ☐ Male
- ☐ Female

Were you born in the United States?
- ☐ Yes
- ☐ No

Example of Likert Scale

The physical layout of my patient care unit is efficient.

1	2	3	4	5
Strongly Disagree	Disagree	Neither Agree nor Disagree	Agree	Strongly Agree

---

Example of Guttman Scale

Please mark whether you agree with the following statements.

	Yes	No
1. Anyone needing health care should pay out of pocket for the services rendered. (Least extreme)		
2. There should be health insurance for anyone who can afford to pay for it.	___	___
3. Employers should be required to offer healthcare coverage for any employee.	___	___
4. Employers should be required to pay for the healthcare premium of any employee.	___	___
5. Employers should be required to pay for the healthcare premium of any employee and his or her family.	___	___
6. Individuals below the poverty level should have their health care subsidized by the government.	___	___
7. There should be universal healthcare coverage for all, subsidized by the government. (Most extreme)	___	___

Visual analog scale (VAS): A rating-type scale in which respondents mark a location on the scale corresponding to their perception of a phenomenon on a continuum.

The visual analog scale (VAS) is one of the most commonly used scales in health care for measuring perceptual measures such as pain or nausea. The VAS is designed to present the respondent with a rating scale that has few constraints and is easy to use. Respondents mark the location on the continuum corresponding to their perceptions of the phenomenon. The Wong Faces Pain Scale in Chapter 9 is an example of a visual analog scale.

Writing Survey Questions

Whether the questions are closed or open-ended, some issues should be considered when writing questionnaires. Primary among these issues is clarity. Questions must be clear, succinct, and unambiguous (Fowler, 2008). The goal is for all respondents who answer the question to interpret its meaning the same way.

The second issue concerns the use of leading questions or emotionally laden words. A leading question is phrased in such a way that it suggests to the respondent that the researcher expects a certain answer. The adjectives, verbs, and nouns used in a question can have positive or negative meanings and may influence the responder unintentionally. An emotionally laden question is one that contains words that can create a negative reaction in some people regardless of the content of the statement. Some words also have more than one meaning and should be avoided.

Questionnaires are a familiar way to collect information. They are cost effective, minimally intrusive, relatively easy to analyze, and provide objective data. Some of the disadvantages of using a questionnaire include an inability to clarify questions, low response rates, lack of personal contact, and unknown level of literacy skills of the respondent.

Delivery Methods for Psychometric Instruments

Multiple delivery methods are available for the delivery of psychometric instruments. Traditional methods include paper-and-pencil surveys that are subsequently manually entered into analytic software packages. Although paper-and-pencil surveys are still widely used, the contemporary researcher has a wide variety of options for collecting data efficiently and conveniently from subjects.

Online Surveys

The use of web-based surveys is increasing as more individuals use the Internet as a means of communication (Greenlaw & Brown-Welty, 2009). Technology enables the researcher to access millions of potential research subjects in geographically diverse sites. The online environment creates opportunities to collect data globally, especially among difficult to access populations (Cantrell & Lupinacci, 2007). Web-based data entry is efficient and effective, and delivered in a way that is convenient for subjects. Data processing and analysis are expedited when web-based surveys are used because data can be directly downloaded into analytic software. The need for data tracking and transfer are eliminated with online data submission processes (Cooper et al., 2006).

Reynolds and Stiles (2007) found that online survey distribution resulted in statistically equivalent responses to paper-and-pencil surveys, with reliability, validity, and completeness similar to standardized methods. Online methods may help the researcher achieve quicker returns (Lefever, 2007). Hsiao and Moore (2009) found that data collected from web-based studies had many advantages, including:

- Increasing sample size
- Obtaining sample diversity
- Accessing specialty samples

- Encouraging voluntary participation
- Reducing the cost of data collection
- Avoiding experimenter bias

Online data collection is not without drawbacks, however. When data are submitted remotely via the Internet, the researcher is unavailable to answer questions, deal with concerns, or troubleshoot problems. Participants may be confused by online data submission systems, resulting in inaccurate or unusable submissions. The researcher may be unable to prevent multiple submissions, or surveys may be abandoned before they are complete. Online systems may ultimately result in systematic sampling error because only those subjects with some level of computer literacy will be able to participate effectively in the study (Hsiao & Moore, 2009). Some critical problems in using online data submission systems are the difficulty in accessing electronic mail addresses for a sampling frame and the challenges of determining response rates when the actual number of recipients is unknown (Lefever, 2007; Reynolds & Stiles, 2007).

The design and collection of online survey data have been made easier through user-friendly survey applications such as Survey Monkey and Zoomerang. The survey tool itself is created by using web-based tools and the data are then downloaded directly into an Excel spreadsheet or a statistical software package for analysis, thus minimizing data entry error.

Technology-Based Delivery

Other technology-based data collection systems are available for the nurse researcher. Laptop computers can allow subjects to respond to surveys or questionnaires efficiently and accurately. Laptop computers have been demonstrated to be effective means for data collection. Haller and colleagues (2009) found that laptop data entry was fast, accurate, resulted in fewer errors, and had less missing data than handheld devices or paper-and-pencil surveys. In addition, computer-based methods have been shown to elicit higher response rates than other methods in reporting risky or sensitive items (Wu & Newfield, 2007).

Handheld digital devices hold some promise but have distinct drawbacks. Researchers found that data collection via handheld devices lengthened the duration of data entry while increasing typing errors and the quantity of missing data. Most of the problems with handheld devices were caused by technical difficulties, typing errors, and loss or theft of the device. If these problems can be mediated, handheld devices may become a legitimate means of primary data collection (Galliher et al., 2008).

Other technologies available for data collection include audio computer-assisted self-interview (ACASI) and electronic portable information collection audio devices (EPIC-Vox). ACASI has been found to be only modestly better than face-to-face interview in eliciting accurate information, but, in general, it yielded the highest rates for sensitive problems such as social isolation, anxiety, and stress (Kim, Dubowitz, Hudson-Martin, & Lane, 2008). EPIC-Vox also showed similar promise for collecting reliable data from subjects (Pallett, Rentowl, & Hanning, 2009). The advantage of both of these technological systems is that they do not require the respondent to possess basic literacy skills or visual acuity. These systems achieve the advantages of an interview without the time or invest-ment required for real-time face-to-face data collection.

Data collection may often be maximized by using technology-based data collection, but these methods are limited to predetermined surveys, questionnaires, or scales. When exploratory or qualitative data are required to answer the research question, the researcher must use more traditional methods of data collection. Asking questions directly of infor-mants, followed by probing questions (i.e., delving more deeply into the meaning of experiences) requires a face-to-face means of data collection.

Interviews

Interviews are a data collection technique in which the researcher interacts directly with the participant one-on-one via the telephone or in person. The format of the interview can be highly structured or loosely structured depending on the information needed. Types of questions may be closed, open-ended, or probing.

Each question that is asked should relate back to the research question. Types of questions that might be asked in an interview are:

- Information or knowledge questions (for example, How much do you know about mandatory staffing ratios?)
- Opinion questions (for example, What do you think about states mandating nurse staffing ratios?)
- Application questions (for example, How do you develop a schedule that allows for equitable staffing to meet the mandatory levels?)
- Analysis questions (for example, What do you see as the relationship between staffing levels and patient safety?)
- Synthesis questions (for example, What changes would you make to provide an equitable solution to the staffing problem?)

Wording of questions is as important in an unstructured interview as it is in a struc-tured interview or in a questionnaire (Fowler, 2008). In a highly structured interview, questions are developed in the same way as for a questionnaire. For interviews that are less structured, the use of open-ended questions allows the respondent to provide more detailed information. Wording of the questions should be clear and words with double meaning should be avoided. To provide an environment that allows the respondent to answer in a truthful manner, the questions should be as neutral as possible.

The sequence of questions is also important and can set the tone for the interview. After the introductions, it is important to put the respondent at ease so he or she is comfortable when responding to the questions. This may be accomplished by asking informational or factual questions that the participant can easily answer. Ask questions about the present before asking questions about either the past or the future. It is often easier to talk about what is current than to recall the past or predict the future.

As the interview progresses, the interviewer should remain as neutral as possible. Once a question is asked, the interviewer should be sure that the respondent has com-pletely answered the question before asking a new question. Any note taking should be as inconspicuous as possible. Interviews are more personal than questionnaires. Unlike

---

SKILL Builder | Conduct Better Interviews
_____

Word the questions carefully.
- Use open-ended words such as "how," "why," or "what."
- Avoid questions that can be answered with a "yes" or "no."
- Word the questions in a clear, straightforward way.
- Avoid words with double meanings.
- Pose questions using neutral words.

Plan the sequence of the questions.
- Start with questions that will put the respondent at ease.
- Use initial questions that involve informational or factual questions.
- Intersperse opinion, analysis, application, or synthesis questions with factual questions.
- Ask questions about the present before asking questions about either the past or the future.

Carry out the interview.
- Remain as neutral as possible in both verbal and nonverbal communication.
- Ask only one question at a time.
- Allow the respondent plenty of time, but keep the interview on track.
- Take notes inconspicuously or use a recorder.

Wrap up the interview.
- Retrieve the tape recorder.
- Review notes and make additions or revisions immediately.
- Make notes of observations made during the interview.

---

the questionnaire that the respondent completes, interviews give the interviewer the opportunity to ask follow-up questions.

Interviews can be very time consuming, and they are resource intensive. The individual conducting the interview needs to be trained to ask the questions properly, to ask the questions in the proper sequence, and to handle any unanticipated possibilities that might arise during the interview process. Interviews are often used in qualitative studies and provide rich information about the respondents' perceptions and beliefs.

Focus Groups

A focus group is an in-depth, qualitative interview with a small group of people (generally between 6 and 12) that have been specifically selected to represent a target audience. The aim of a focus group is to understand the social dynamic and interaction between the participants through the collection of both verbal and observational data (Redmond & Curtis, 2009). These interactions often result in richer qualitative data because members of the focus groups can consider their own views in the context of the views of others. The interplay of participants in a focus group may reveal ideas, experiences, and meaning that are not apparent when individuals are interviewed in isolation (Ayers, 2007). Focus groups are a way to learn about opinions and attitudes. Participants discuss their own opinions, and they have an opportunity to react to the ideas of others. Other advantages of a focus group:

- The discussion can be recorded with audio, video, or both for later review and transcription.
- The facilitator can observe and note nonverbal behavior, reactions, and interactions of group members.
- Misunderstandings can be clarified immediately.
- Unanticipated but related topics can be explored, and results of the interview are immediate.

Although the data gathered through focus group interviews are rich in meaning, focus groups are time consuming and expensive to conduct. They require a skillful facilitator and often require the presence of two individuals—one to facilitate the discussion and one to record observations and nonverbal behaviors. The quality of the data is influenced by the skills and motivation of the facilitator. Focus groups may not elicit accurate information if the facilitator is inexperienced or introduces his or her bias into the discussion. Recording of the group session may feel intrusive to participants and inhibit them from sharing their opinions, and respondents may hesitate to share sensitive information in a group setting. As with qualitative data in general, the results cannot be generalized to larger groups without careful sample selection and reliable content analysis procedures.

Observation

Observational research is used for studying observable behaviors and is generally a noninvasive method for gathering information (Creswell, 2008). There are two types of observation: direct and indirect. Indirect observation is sometimes called unobtrusive. With direct observation, participants agree to be part of the research and know that the researcher will be watching them. Indirect observation involves recording data unobtrusively so that the subjects either are unaware of or become accustomed to the observation.

Observations can be made continuously or in specific time periods. Both observational methods generally involve extended contact with the subjects of the study. Continuous monitoring involves observing a participant or participants and recording in minute detail (either manually, electronically, or both) as much of their behavior as possible. One of the drawbacks to this method of data collection is that individuals who know their behavior is being watched will not behave as they normally would until there has been a great deal of exposure; this generates a large amount of data to manage. Time periods may be randomly selected for observation so that fewer resources are needed for data collection. Unlike continuous monitoring, participants do not know the time or the place that the researcher will be collecting the data, and so are more likely to behave normally. In either case, ethical conduct dictates that the participants be informed that they will be observed, even if they do not know the particulars of where or when.

Secondary Data Collection Methods

Secondary data are data that were collected for purposes other than the current research. Data are routinely collected by governments, hospitals, schools, and other organizations. Much of this information is stored in electronic databases that can be accessed and

---

A Primary Data Collection Plan

1. How will the data be collected?
   - Describe the source of the data.
   - Write a clear, detailed protocol for the data collection.
   - Train data collectors in use of the protocol.
   - Identify who is responsible for obtaining the data.
   - Determine how the researcher will ensure that all relevant data have been collected.
   - Determine how to handle missing data or inaccurate responses.
2. When will the data be collected?
   - Indicate at exactly what point each piece of data is to be collected.
   - Describe whether data will be collected relative to time or to an event.
3. Who is responsible for collecting and recording the data?
   - Identify who will actually collect the data.
   - Identify who will be responsible for transcribing the data or completing data entry.
   - Describe how anonymity of subjects will be protected.
   - Describe how confidentiality of data will be protected.
4. Where are the collected data stored?
   - Describe any transitional means of data storage such as forms, documents, or e-mail.
   - Give the name and location of the final database.
5. How do we ensure the data are correct?
   - Describe any accuracy checks to be performed.
   - Describe the procedure for dealing with errors and missing data.

---

analyzed. In addition, many research projects store their raw data in electronic form in computer archives so that others may also analyze the data. Data available for secondary analysis might include Census Bureau data, public health data, economic data, consumer data, medical records, or Medicare data.

Secondary data are often easier and quicker to collect than primary data. Particularly in organizations that have made great progress maintaining an electronic patient record, patient-level data may be retrievable. Access is limited by the organization's procedure for research approval and assurance that HIPAA standards are met. Using secondary data to answer specific research questions generally requires a moderate level of skill at writing computer requests and using search engines.

Secondary data collection has its limitations as well. The accuracy and completeness of the data are dependent on individuals capturing and recording the data accurately, completely, and reliably. Physicians' notes, nurses' notes, collaborative plans, and teaching plans are only as thorough as their authors. Gaps in information may mean the event did not happen, or it could mean the clinician simply did not record it. Data retrieval from secondary sources that are on paper provide two sources of potential data error: The data may not be recorded correctly from the primary source, and the individual retrieving the data from the chart may miss it or record it inaccurately.

gray matter

Secondary data collection advantages:
- Data routinely collected for purposes other than the research
- Electronic databases available
- Easier and quicker for one rater to collect

Secondary data collection disadvantages:
- Accuracy, completeness, and reliability depend on the original individual collecting the data.
- Access to information requires skill at writing computer requests using search engines.
- Data inaccuracy introduced during retrieval is a possibility.

Table 10.4

Comparison of Data Collection Methods

Method	Advantage	Limitation(s)
Primary Data		
Physiologic	Objective data	Calibration of equipment
Psychometric	Quantifiable data	Access to instrument acceptable for study
		Objective
Questionnaire	Cost effective	Impersonal
	Anonymous	Biased wording
	Easy to administer	Low return rate
	Works with large groups	Literacy barriers
	Familiar	Time consuming
	Allows generalization	
Interview	Flexible	Costly
	Personal	Small numbers
	Nonverbal behaviors	Results cannot be generalized
	Immediate follow-up	
Focus group	In-depth information	Time consuming
	Nonverbal behaviors	Costly
	Trained facilitators	Training time
	Rich data	Results cannot be generalized
		Not useful for sensitive subjects
Observation	Detailed information	Time consuming
	Trained observers	Labor intensive
	Less biased	Training time
Secondary data	Efficient	Costly
	Increases breadth of the study	Unknown issues with primary data collection
	Multiple uses of data	Concern for accuracy and completeness

In general, automated information retrieval systems offer a better probability that the data will be complete and accurate. **Table 10.4** depicts the major data collection methods with each of their strengths and limitations.

Data Management Procedures

During the development of the data collection tool, the researcher makes decisions about the way data will be recorded, including forms that will be used and procedures for the data collector (Harwood & Hutchinson, 2009a). Adequate time should be planned for data collection. Data collection inevitably takes longer and is more difficult than anticipated. Problems should be expected by the researcher and procedures put in place to

Codebook: Codes established prior to data collection that include definitions, abbreviations, and a range of possible numerical values for the variables.

handle common issues that will arise. For example, the data collectors need a procedure to handle incomplete or incorrectly completed forms and questionnaires.

The researcher develops a **codebook** for data definitions before initiating data collection. Coding is the process of transforming data into numerical symbols that can be easily entered into the computer. For example, a researcher might code "gender male" as 1 and "gender female" as 2. Included in the codebook are definitions of variables, abbreviations for variables, and the range of possible values for the variables. In addition to the codebook, a file is established that contains copies of all scales, questionnaires, and forms used in the study.

After data collection is completed, forms are checked for demographic data, legibility, completeness, unanswered questions, or incorrectly answered questions. A subject may have selected two answers, for example, when he or she should have selected only one. Files are inspected for obvious data entry errors; for example, if age is recorded as "360," then it is clear a data entry error occurred. If more than one data collector was used, interrater reliability is analyzed to ensure consistency in the data.

The original data forms as well as a copy of the database should be stored for 5 years. Storage of data serves several purposes. The data are available to document the validity of the analysis and the published results of the study. The data also may be used as secondary data for subsequent studies or aggregate analyses.

Reading the Data Collection Section of a Research Study

Finding the data collection section of a research report is relatively easy. It is usually labeled "methods," "procedures," or "protocols." The description of the data collection procedure should be clear and complete enough that a relatively well-informed reader should be able to replicate it.

Each protocol—whether it is for the measurement process or the documentation of the results—should be outlined. It is here where the researcher should identify the data as primary or secondary. The protocol should outline what was collected, who collected it, what instrument or questionnaire was used, and how the data were recorded. If the researcher was not the individual doing the actual data collection, the methods for training the data collectors should be described. In addition, any protocols for auditing data accuracy, checking for interrater reliability, and doing quality checks should be clearly described. If these descriptions are not included, it cannot be assumed they were done, and this is a weakness of the data collection plan.

Early in the methods section, the author should provide the reader with a rationale for the decisions made about the data collection procedures. A clear link to the research question should be apparent. It is difficult to judge the quality of a data collection procedure without a careful consideration of the measures that were used. It is helpful to review these two sections together to ensure that reliable, valid measures have been collected in the best way.

The key procedures to evaluate when reading the data collection section of a research study are the measures taken to ensure accuracy, reliability, and freedom from bias.

Where to Look for Information About the Data Collection Procedures

- The methods section is generally identified in a straightforward way and labeled "methods." Other words may appear in the heading, such as "methods and procedures" or "methods and materials."
- This should be easily identifiable and a major part of the research study write-up. The data collection plan should appear early in the description of the methods section. The description may be concise, but it should have enough detail that an informed reader could replicate the data collection procedure.
- If the data collection is complex, there may be a separate section for procedures, which may be labeled as such, or they may be called "protocols." This section should describe the specific steps for collecting and recording the data. On occasion, photographs may be used if procedures are not easily described with words.
- The measures may be called "instrumentation" or "tests." If a survey is used, a separate section may describe the development of the instrument, as well as procedures for its completion by subjects. Information about reliability and validity should be provided with the description of the instrument.

Whether the data collection plan is for words or numbers, these procedures are critical considerations.

Using Research in Evidence-Based Practice

The clinical practice environment has many sources of data. The patient can be observed, interviewed, administered a questionnaire, or monitored for physiologic measures. The medical record contains physiologic measures, objective and subjective results of examinations, evaluation of actions taken, and demographic information. The environment of nursing care can be directly observed.

Nurses are often asked to collect data for the studies of others. This is an excellent way to engage in the research process without having the responsibility for design decisions. Reading the data sections of research reports helps the nurse learn to be a better data collector and improve his or her practice. An awareness of the characteristics of a well-done measurement and data collection system can help the nurse's own assessment practices become more thorough, unbiased, and accurate.

Creating Research as Evidence

The choice of the data collection method depends on the specific information needed to answer the research question and the resources available to the researcher. With the wide variety of data collection methods available, the nurse researcher must use a systematic approach to navigate the choices that must be made in developing a strong data collection system. Harwood and Hutchinson (2009b) recommended steps that can help the researcher develop a sound data collection approach:

1. Define the purpose for collecting the data.
2. Select a feasible data collection approach.
3. Select a delivery method that is appropriate for the design and the subjects.
4. Write realistic, reliable, and thorough protocols for collecting the data.
5. Design forms and instruments for collecting valid and reliable data.
6. Train staff in data collection methods and/or write clear instructions for subjects to guide data submission.
7. Develop a plan to manage data and transfer it to analytic software.

The purpose for collecting the data should be driven by the purpose statement and the research question. A clearly defined problem statement and carefully considered research question are critical factors in shaping the data collection strategy. A study that is focused on measuring the effects of an intervention requires data that can be statistically analyzed using hypothesis testing. An exploratory study, on the other hand, may require narratives that explain the meaning of a phenomenon, or descriptive data that can be used as a baseline measure.

Feasibility of a data collection approach is a practical, yet critical aspect to be considered. The complexity of the study, resources available to the nurse researcher, characteristics of the target population, and skills of the research team are all considerations in determining if a particular data collection system will be a realistic option.

The delivery method for data collection should be consistent with the goals of the study and the research question. Qualitative studies typically involve focus groups, interviews, or participant observation. Quantitative studies may use biological measurements, surveys, questionnaires, or observation. Responses to surveys and questionnaires may be collected via laptop computer, handheld data device, paper-and-pencil tools, or online data submissions.

Once a feasible approach and delivery method have been selected, the researcher must write thorough protocols for the data collectors. Protocols should be clear and unambiguous; all steps of the data collection process should be spelled out in detail. Asking an individual unfamiliar with the research plan to try carrying out the data collection procedure can be a useful exercise to determine where directions are confusing or unclear. The plan should be tested until the researcher is assured it cannot be misinterpreted.

If the data are to be self-reported or an instrument will be self-administered, then clear directions should be developed for the subjects. Writing the directions in simple, straightforward language will support the completeness and accuracy of the responses.

Checklist for Critically Reading the Data Collection Methods of a Research Article

✔ Procedures for data collection are specific enough for replication.
✔ Data collection and documentation protocols are described.
✔ A rationale for selection of the specific data collection method is provided.
✔ Psychometric properties are identified for the instruments used.
✔ If psychometric properties are not identified, the process of instrument development and testing is described.

Forms for collecting the data need to be developed. These may vary from questionnaires to surveys to entry logs. The forms should be self-explanatory and efficient to complete. Training data collectors in the procedures and use of the forms is essential to ensure the accuracy and completeness of the data that are collected. Periodic monitoring for quality control is necessary even when data collectors have been trained; measures to ensure ongoing accuracy and completeness are particularly necessary in lengthy studies (Harwood & Hutchinson, 2009b).

The final step of the data collection plan is the transfer of raw data for analysis. Web-based or computer-based data entry systems are often directly transferrable to analytic software programs. Paper-and-pencil surveys and questionnaires must be entered manually to be prepared for analysis. Quality monitoring for data entry errors should be a part of the data management plan.

Summary of Key Concepts

- Data collection methods are used to gather information in a systematic way. Data used in quantitative studies will be of a numeric nature and subject to statistical analysis. Data used in qualitative studies will be of a text-based nature and subject to coding.

For More Depth and Detail

For a more in-depth look at the concepts in this chapter, try these references:

Barriera-Viruet, H. (2006). Questionnaires vs observational and direct measurements: A systematic review. *Issues in Ergonomics Science, 7*(3), 261–284.

Botti, M., & Endacott, R. (2008). Clinical research 5: Quantitative data collection and analysis. *International Emergency Nursing, 16*(2), 132–137.

Casey, D. (2006). Choosing an appropriate method of data collection. *Nurse Researcher, 13*(3), 75–92.

DeLaRosa, M., Rahill, G., Rojas, P., & Pinto, E. (2007). Cultural adaptations in data collection: Field experiences. *Journal of Ethnicity in Substance Abuse, 6*(2), 163–180.

Endacott, R. (2008). Clinical research 4: Qualitative data collection and analysis. *International Emergency Nursing, 16*(1), 48–52.

Fowler, J. (2008). *Survey research methods* (4th ed.). Thousand Oaks, CA: Sage.

Lavrakas, P. (2008). *Encyclopedia of survey research methods.* Thousand Oaks, CA: Sage.

Musselwhite, K., Cuff, L., McGregor, L., & King, K. (2007). The telephone interview is an effective method of data collection in clinical nursing research: A discussion paper. *International Journal of Nursing Studies, 44*(6), 1064–1070.

Oliver, D., & Mahon, S. (2006). Evidence-based practice. Reading a research article part III: The data collection instrument. *Clinical Journal of Oncology Nursing, 10*(3), 423–426.

Sapsford, R., & Jupp, V. (2006). *Data collection and analysis.* Thousand Oaks, CA: Sage.

CRITICAL APPRAISAL EXERCISE

Retrieve the following full text article from the Cumulative Index to Nursing and Allied Health Literature or similar search database:

Holzhauer, J., Reith, V., Sawin, K., & Yen, K. (2009). Evaluation of temporal artery thermometry in children 3–36 months old. *Journal for Specialists in Pediatric Nursing, 14*(4), 239–244.

1. The authors identify in the literature review a relatively low sensitivity for temporal artery thermometers. What are the implications of low sensitivity for detection of fever in children?
2. How did the authors ensure that the thermometers used in the study were accurate physiologic measures of temperature?
3. How did the authors establish the reliability and validity of the thermometer readings?
4. How were data collectors trained for the study? What are the strengths and drawbacks of this training approach?
5. Describe the data collection procedure. Is the protocol thorough enough to support replication of the study? Why or why not?
6. What was the sensitivity of the temporal artery thermometer in this study? Is this level of sensitivity acceptable for clinical practice?
7. What were potential sources of measurement bias in this study? What elements of measurement error may have been present in this study?

- The most common types of data collection are physiologic measurement, psychometric instrumentation, questionnaires, interviews, focus groups, and observation.
- The advantage of using an existing valid and reliable instrument is that it saves the researcher time in the development and validation of a new instrument and allows the study to contribute to a larger body of knowledge.
- The most common data collection method is the survey. The survey method is an approach in which a systematic measurement instrument is used to gather information directly from respondents about their experiences, behaviors, attitudes, or perceptions.
- A variety of data collection methods are available, including paper-and-pencil, online, computer-based, handheld devices, and audio-delivery devices. Each has specific advantages and disadvantages that should be aligned with the goals of the research study.
- Interviews and focus groups can help the researcher gather rich data directly from the respondent and allow the researcher to explore topics as they arise. The drawbacks of these methods are their time-consuming nature and the demands they place on the facilitator's skill level.

For a full suite of assignments and additional learning activities, use the access code located in the front of your book to visit this exclusive website: http://go.jblearning .com/houser. If you do not have an access code, you can obtain one at the site.

References

Ayres, L. (2007). Qualitative research proposals: Part III: Sampling and data collection. *Journal of Wound, Ostomy and Continence Nursing, 34*(3), 242–244.

Cantrell, M., & Lupinacci, P. (2007). Methodological issues in online data collection. *Journal of Advanced Nursing, 60*(5), 544–549.

Cooper, C., Cooper, S., delJunco, D., Shipp, E., Whitworth, R., & Cooper, S. (2006). Web-based data collection: Detailed methods of a questionnaire and data gathering tool. *Epidemiologic Perspectives and Innovations, 3,* 1.

Creswell, J.W. (2008). *Research design: Quantitative, qualitative, and mixed methods.* Thousand Oaks, CA: Sage.

Fowler, F.J. (2008). *Survey research methods* (4th ed.). Thousand Oaks, CA: Sage.

Galliher, J., Stewart, T., Pathak, P., Werner, J., Dickinson, L., & Hickner, J. (2008). Data collection outcomes comparing paper forms with PDA forms in an office-based patient survey. *Annals of Family Medicine, 6*(2), 154–160.

Greenlaw, C., & Brown-Welty, S. (2009). Comparison of web-based and paper-based survey methods: Testing assumptions of survey mode and response cost. *Evaluation Review, 33*(5), 464–480.

Guttman, L. (1947). Scale an intensive analysis for attitude, opinion, and achievement. In Kelly, G. (Ed.). *New methods in applied psychology* (pp. 173–180). Baltimore, MD: University of Maryland.

Haller, G., Haller, D., Courvoisier, D., & Lovis, C. (2009). Handheld vs laptop computers for electronic data collection in clinical research: A crossover randomized trial. *Journal of the American Medical Informatics Association, 16*(5), 651–659.

Harwood, E., & Hutchinson, E. (2009a). Data collection methods series: Part 2: Select the most feasible data collection mode. *Journal of Wound, Ostomy, and Continence Nursing, 36*(2), 129–135.

Harwood, E., & Hutchinson, E. (2009b). Data collection methods series: Part 5: Training for data collection. *Journal of Wound, Ostomy, and Continence Nursing, 36*(5), 476–481.

Hsiao, E., & Moore, D. (2009). Web-based data collection. *TechTrends, 53*(6), 56–60.

Kim, J., Dubowitz, H., Hudson-Martin, E., & Lane, W. (2008). Comparison of 3 data collection methods for gathering sensitive and less sensitive information. *Ambulatory Pediatrics, 8*(4), 255–260.

Lavrakas, P. (2008). *Encyclopedia of survey research methods.* Thousand Oaks, CA: Sage.

LeFever, S. (2007). Online data collection in academic research: Advantages and limitations. *British Journal of Educational Technology, 38*(4), 574–582.

Likert, R., & Hayes, S. (1957). *Some applications of behavioral research.* Paris: UNESCO.

Pallett, E., Rentowl, P., & Hanning D. (2009). The brief fatigue inventory: Comparison of data collection using a novel audio device with conventional paper questionnaire. *Journal of Pain and Symptom Management, 38*(3), 390–400.

Redmond, R., & Curtis, E. (2009). Focus groups: Principles and process. *Nurse Researcher, 16*(3), 57–69.

Reynolds, D., & Stiles, S. (2007). Online data collection for psychotherapy process research. *CyberPsychology and Behavior, 10*(1), 92–99.

Wu, Y., & Newfield, S. (2007). Comparing data collected by computerized and written surveys for adolescence health research. *Journal of School Health, 77*(1), 23–28.

chapter 11

Enhancing the Validity of Research

CHAPTER OBJECTIVES

The study of this chapter will help the learner to

- Define internal and external validity as applied to research.
- Discuss the critical nature of internal validity as applied to research as evidence.
- Explain why external validity is an essential component of research that is to be used as evidence.
- Compare the concept of validity in quantitative research to trustworthiness in qualitative research.
- Identify threats to internal and external validity in quantitative studies.
- Determine threats to trustworthiness of a qualitative study.
- Appraise strategies that will control threats to the validity or trustworthiness of a research study.

KEY TERMS

Applicability and transfer-ability	External validity	Population validity
	Historical threats	Replicability
Argument	Instrumentation	Subject selection
Audit trail	Internal validity	Testing
Bracketing	Maturation	Triangulation
Effect size	Member checking	Type I error
Experimental mortality	Novelty effect	Type II error
Experimenter effect	Placebo effect	

Introduction

Whether developing a research study, reading a research report, or contemplating the use of research findings, the challenge is to determine if the intervention or manipulation of the variables actually causes the desired outcome or result. Internal validity refers specifically to whether the researcher and reader can be confident that an experimental treatment or condition made a difference—and whether rival explanations for the difference can be systematically ruled out. Internal validity is about the strength of the design and the controls that were placed on the experimental situation. External validity refers to how generalizable the results are and to whom. External validity is about applicability and usefulness of the findings.

For example, we might want to know if a particular exercise and diet program actually results in a significant weight loss, and that no other reasons accounted for the weight loss except the exercise and diet program. If the findings are credible and trustworthy, we will also want to know if the results can be generalized to a different or larger population.

Before determining if there is causal relationship between the outcome and the intervention, three conditions must be met:

1. *Changes in the presumed cause must be related to changes in the presumed effect.* If the treatment is changed in any way, the outcome will change. In the example, if the exercise and dietary program are changed in any way, the weight loss will change.
2. *The presumed cause must occur before the presumed effect.* In other words, the treatment or intervention must occur before the outcome. The weight loss must occur after the exercise and dietary program is introduced.
3. *There are no plausible alternative explanations.* No other factors could be responsible for the outcomes. In the example, there is nothing that has occurred that could have caused the weight loss except the prescribed exercise and dietary intervention. (Hartung & Touchette, 2009)

Good research designs reduce the possibility of alternative explanations for the hypothesized relationship. These alternative explanations for the outcome are often referred to as threats to internal validity. Several methods can be used to minimize threats to internal validity:

- Argument
- Measurement or observation
- Use of appropriate design
- Control of bias
  - Statistical analysis

Argument

A simple and straightforward way to rule out a potential threat to validity is to argue that the threat in question is not a reasonable one. For example, a study is

❝❝ *Voices from the Field* ❞❞

As part of my graduate work, I participated on a research grant that examined the role of risk-taking in work-based injury. The eventual goal was to figure out a public health intervention to reduce risky behaviors. We designed a descriptive study; the study was planned by an interdisciplinary group of mental health therapists, public health nurses, and occupational health physicians. Phase I of the study involved recruiting men and women to assess their attraction to risk behaviors so that we could establish a baseline of typical behaviors. The baseline measures, then, would become the basis for determining if an intervention had an effect in Phase II of the study. The first study was just to gather a descriptive baseline, so it seemed pretty straightforward.

Subjects were recruited through a newspaper ad. We were offering a small stipend in exchange for about an hour of time with noninvasive data collection, so we expected we would get a pretty good response, and we did. We were a bit concerned that a compensated subject may not be representative, but we hoped to get a big sample size to overcome that drawback. We had good funding, and so we were more concerned about Type II error than we were about sampling error. We scheduled more than 200 individuals for 20 different time slots over a 5-day period. We planned to accomplish the data collection in "stations," where the subject would progress from one spot to the next to provide all of the necessary data. With this process, we still needed five data collectors present at any given time. The assessment was pretty thorough and required the presence of a trained data collector, so it was quite the feat to choreograph.

On the day of the first planned data collection, it began to snow. It snowed so hard that the snowplows could not keep up, and businesses and schools were closing left and right. We managed to keep our data collectors around all day, but the subjects started trickling in after lunch. We got a lot of cancellation calls. We talked about canceling the next day, but put off a decision until the morning. We figured if we could get here, then clients could get here too.

Only about half our data collectors made it in, and we were actually pretty busy. It was clear, though, as the day progressed we were not getting a representative population. We were obviously not collecting a baseline of risk-taking behavior in a public health population. We were collecting data from young adult males who owned four-wheel-drive vehicles and really needed 25 bucks. We were studying risk-taking behaviors in a population most likely to take risks.

The team had a quick consult and decided to stop the study, even though resources had already been expended. They decided that flawed results were unlikely to warrant funding for Phase II and would not serve to inform the following study. It was a terrible pain to set it all up again, to back up and essentially start over. I thought what bad luck. It was a really well-designed study that was totally derailed by the weather.

Glenna Andrews, RN, DrPH

conducted to determine the effects of social support on job stress in nurses. One criticism of this study might be that nurse–patient ratios may have affected job stress as well. If the nurse–patient ratios did not change during the course of the study, one could argue that the impact on job stress would reasonably have remained constant. This method, however, is a weak approach and should not, except in unusual cases, be the only way to rule out threats to validity.

Measurement or Observation

Measurement or observation is another possible method to rule out threats to internal validity. This method can demonstrate that the threat either does not occur at all or occurs so infrequently that it is not a significant alternative explanation. In a study designed to determine the effects of music on agitation in a sample of hospitalized patients with dementia, the music did reduce agitation. An alternative explanation for this outcome may have been the effect of visitors on these patients. However, observation and measurement of the number and frequency of visitors revealed that this was a rare to never-occurring event for this sample.

Use of Appropriate Design

Most research questions can be examined using various designs. However, some designs are not appropriate for dealing with the specific requirements of a research problem. If the researcher wishes to determine if music is effective in reducing anxiety in patients undergoing radiation therapy, a repeated-measures design might be effective, whereas a survey design might not reveal any significant effects of the music intervention. An observational study might be appropriate if the researcher is concerned about the effects of ibuprofen on activity levels in a population of senior citizens; however, the same study will not be appropriate if the researcher is concerned with the subjects' perceptions of pain with activity. Choosing the correct design to answer the research questions is fundamentally necessary to control the threats to internal and external validity.

Control of Bias

Good design is also dependent on the absence of bias. Bias can occur in the recruitment of subjects, assignment of subjects into groups, or actions of the researcher. In tightly controlled experimental research, double-blind procedures will help to limit researcher bias (Hulley, Cummings, Browner, & Grady, 2006). However, blinding is not always possible, and its application should be considered carefully. Using more than one observer or interventionist can help control for this bias, but it can also produce experimenter or interrater reliability effects. This is a common problem that threatens the internal validity of research—protecting against one type of bias has the associated effect of creating another. Balancing the risk becomes a task for the principal investigator.

Self-selection bias can be a threat to a good design and can produce misleading results. Differences exist between subjects who volunteer to participate in a research study and those who are randomly selected, and these differences may not be immediately apparent (Portney & Watkins, 2008). The results of a study to determine the effects of prayer on anxiety in presurgical patients might be skewed by individuals who pray regularly. A carefully constructed demographic questionnaire might help to reduce this threat.

A similar concern arises if subjects self-select into the control and intervention groups. For example, subjects who believe that massage will benefit their joint pain might choose to have the treatment, running the risk of a placebo effect. Subjects who are skeptical of the effects of massage might elect to avoid the treatment, creating artificially negative results. Randomization into groups greatly reduces this risk.

There is a broad range of potential methods and designs, and each provides protections against some kinds of bias (Bordens & Barrington, 2007). Although randomized controlled trials are commonly held up as the strongest in terms of controlling bias, even these have potential sources of bias that must be accounted for. When threats to validity cannot be eliminated or controlled, then their effects must be quantified. Statistical analyses can help determine the amount of error and variability that is introduced by uncontrolled threats to validity.

Statistical Analysis

The following list gives some of the many ways to rule out alternative explanations for outcomes by using statistical analyses:

- Testing null hypotheses
- Determining the probability of Type I and Type II error
- Calculating and reporting tests of effect size
- Ensuring data meet the fundamental assumptions of the statistical tests

Testing Null Hypotheses

When attempting to determine if an outcome is related to a cause, it is necessary to know if the outcomes or results could have occurred by chance alone. This cannot be done with certainty, but researchers can determine the probability that the hypothesis is true. Understanding the definition of a null hypothesis is antecedent to this discussion.

In Chapter 4, the hypothesis was defined as "a restatement of the research question in a way that can be analyzed statistically for significance." The null hypothesis (H_0) states that there are no differences or there is no actual relationship between variables. Any observed or measured relationship happened by chance or because of sampling variations. This is based on the concept of probability or the question, "How likely is it the results are just a matter of chance?" Rejecting a null hypothesis is a statement that the intervention had an effect on the outcome. Accepting a null hypothesis is a statement that there are no differences in the outcomes based on the intervention or observation (that is, there is no cause-and-effect relationship). Using a null hypothesis enables the researcher to quantify and report the probability that the outcome was due to random error.

For example, the null hypothesis in a study states that the level of suffering in a sample of women with breast cancer will not be affected by the presence of a support system. The results of the study indicate that married women report less suffering than women who are not married. In this example, the null hypothesis has been rejected. In fact, the presence of a support system seems to predict less suffering in this sample.

Determining the Probability of Type I and Type II Error

Before accepting these results as evidence for practice, however, the probability that an error was made should be evaluated. This, coupled with the results of the hypothesis test, enables the researcher to quantify the role of error in the outcome. There are two types of error. Type I error is the rejection of a true null hypothesis; in other words, the researcher draws a conclusion that the intervention had an effect, when in fact it did not. Type I error usually occurs as a result of weaknesses in design, because the cause of Type I error is usually an uncontrolled extraneous variable. Type I error is considered a serious flaw and threatens the overall internal validity of a study. An example of a Type I error is the following:

> Two groups of students were taught statistics using two different methods. The data indicate that Group A achieved significantly higher scores than Group B. The null hypothesis (H_0) is rejected. However, Group A had subjects with higher math ability, and the teaching methods did not make a difference. Rejecting the H_0 in this case is a Type I error. The differences in the scores were not based on the teaching methods, but were caused by extraneous variables (previous math ability).

Type I error: Often called alpha (α) and referred to as the level of significance, this error is the rejection of a true null hypothesis; the researcher erroneously draws a conclusion that the intervention had an effect.

Type II error: Often called beta (β) and related to the power of a statistical test, this error is the acceptance of a false hypothesis; the researcher erroneously draws a conclusion that the intervention had no effect.

A **Type I error** is called alpha (α). The term *level of significance* is simply the phrase used to indicate the probability of committing a Type I error. The maximum acceptable level of alpha in scientific research is generally 0.05; however, 0.01 may be chosen if the decision has important consequences for treatment. Alpha is set by the researcher *a priori*, meaning before the experiment begins. The level of alpha is set based on a thoughtful consideration of the stakes of being wrong. For example, an intervention that is intended to improve self-esteem may have an acceptable error rate of 5 percent; a test of a tumor-killing drug may be more appropriate at 1 percent. Alpha is used as a standard for comparison for the p value, or the probability of a Type I error, that is yielded from most inferential statistical tests. When the calculated probability of a Type I error (the p value) is less than the acceptable level of a Type I error (alpha), then the test is considered to be statistically significant. Type I error is quantified, then, by the p value.

A **Type II error** is the acceptance of a false null hypothesis or stating there are no differences in the outcome when in fact there are differences. An example of a Type II error is as follows:

> A study was conducted to determine whether breastfeeding or bottle feeding contributed to greater maternal fatigue in the first 30 days after birth. The researchers were able to recruit 30 breastfeeding mothers into the study, but only 6 bottle-feeding mothers consented to participate. No differences were found between the groups. The research reflects a Type II error in that a difference may have been present, but the small sample did not enable the researchers to discover it.

A Type II error is called beta (β). The probability of obtaining a significant result is called the power of a statistical test. A more powerful test is one that is more likely to detect an outcome of interest. Type II error can occur when an experiment has insufficient power. Type II error means that a treatment was effective, but the experiment did not reveal it. The best way to control Type II error is to ensure that the sample is large enough to provide sufficient power to the experiment to illuminate the findings. Type II error is calculated as 1-beta, or 1-power. If the sample enables the researcher to document 90 percent power, then the probability of Type II error affecting the outcome is 10 percent.

The nurse may consider the question, "Which type of error is worse?" In health care, Type I error is generally considered more serious; a Type I error will lead the researcher to believe an intervention is effective when it is not. But focusing solely on tight controls of Type I error means that significant findings may be overlooked. The relationship between Type I and Type II error is paradoxical—as one is controlled, the risk of the other increases (Forthofer, Lee, & Hernandez, 2007). Both types of error should be avoided. Missing the opportunity for an effective treatment because its effects cannot be detected is unfortunate for patients and researchers alike. The best approach is to carefully consider and control sources of bias, set the alpha level appropriately, use an effective sampling strategy, and select a solid design for the question. Getting all these elements aligned requires a balancing of risks and benefits that is the task of the primary researcher. **Table 11.1** contrasts Type I and II errors and gives examples of each.

Calculating and Reporting Tests of Effect Size

Effect size must also be considered when evaluating the validity of a study. **Effect size** refers to how much impact the intervention or variable is expected to have on the outcome. Even though an experiment might yield statistically significant results, these may not translate into clinically important findings. An example of the impact of effect size is the following:

> **Effect size:** The magnitude of the impact that the intervention or variable is expected to have on the outcome.

> Researchers want to determine the effects of aerobic exercise on heart rate in a sample of subjects with chronic supraventricular tachycardia (SVT). The researchers are specifically measuring the relationship between aerobic exercise and heart rate. If the relationship is strong, an effect will be detected even with a small sample size. On the other hand, if it was determined that exercise has little effect on heart rate in patients with chronic SVT, a much larger sample would be needed to find any significant changes in heart rate in this study.

Large effect sizes enhance the confidence in findings. When a treatment exerts a dramatic effect, then the validity of the findings is not called into question. On the other hand, when effect sizes are very small, the potential for effects from extraneous variables is more likely, and the results may have less validity (Hulley et al., 2006).

Ensuring Fundamental Assumptions Are Met

Data analysis is based on many assumptions about the nature of the data, the statistical procedures that are used to conduct the analysis, and the match between the data and the procedures. Erroneous conclusions can be made about relationships if the assumptions

Table 11.1

A Contrast of Type I and Type II Errors

	A Type I Error	A Type II Error
A study is designed to test the effects of hydrotherapy on anxiety during the first stage of labor. All women who present to a single birthing center are invited to participate. Women are allowed to choose whether they use hydrotherapy or not.	Anxiety is reduced in the treatment group. **BUT:** All the women who choose hydrotherapy have a birth coach present. Is the reduction due to the hydrotherapy or to another cause (for example, having a birth coach)?	Anxiety is not reduced in the treatment group. **BUT:** All the women who choose hydrotherapy have a higher level of anxiety prior to labor. Is the lack of response because the hydrotherapy does not work, or because the mothers had more anxiety to begin with?
A researcher tests the effects of a virtual preoperative tour of the surgical suite on postoperative length of stay in the postanesthesia care unit (PACU). During preadmission testing, patients are given Internet access code to get into a virtual tour site. On admission, the subjects are assigned to a treatment group or a comparison group based on their self-report of completing the tour.	Length of stay in the PACU is shorter in the group that used the virtual preoperative tour. **BUT:** All the parents who used the virtual tour have personal computers and a higher level of socioeconomic resources than the control group. Is the shorter length of stay due to the virtual tour or to factors related to increased health because of socioeconomic advantage?	Length of stay in the PACU is no shorter in the group that used the virtual preoperative tour. **BUT:** All the patients who did not use the tour experienced previous surgery and so were already familiar with the surgical suite. Is the length of stay no shorter because the tour did not have an effect or because the control group did not really need it?
A nurse evaluates the effects of an evening backrub on the use of sleeping aids. Patients are randomly assigned to an experimental or control group. Patients in the experimental group are given a nightly backrub; patients in the control group are not.	Patients who receive the backrubs need fewer sleep medications. **BUT:** During the 10 minutes that the backrub is given, the nurses interact quietly with the patients about their concerns and treatment issues. Is the difference due to the backrub or the extra attention and counseling of the nurse?	Patients who receive the backrubs do not need fewer sleep medications. **BUT:** Only 10 patients assigned to the control group stayed more than one night, and so the overall sample size was less than 25 subjects. Was the lack of a difference because the backrub had no effect or due to inadequate power to detect a difference?

of the statistical tests are violated. For instance, many statistical analyses assume that the data obtained are distributed normally, that is, that the population is distributed according to a normal or bell-shaped curve. If that assumption is violated, the result can be an inaccurate estimate of the real relationship. Inaccurate conclusions lead to error, which in turn affects the validity of a study.

The researcher must be familiar with the assumptions of the tests so data are collected that have the best chance of meeting those assumptions. If assumptions are violated, tests may not run well and will yield misleading results. To maintain a rigorous approach to statistical testing, it is best to choose the appropriate statistical test when the study is designed. Selecting statistical tests *a priori* ensures that data will meet statistical assumptions, and that the choice of tests is not influenced by reviewing the data.

Factors That Jeopardize Internal Validity

A good research design controls for factors that jeopardize validity. A host of events and actions can threaten the capacity of the researcher to draw accurate conclusions about the effects of interventions. If these are measurable, then they may be called extraneous variables. Many times, however, the effects of factors that affect the trustworthiness of results are not even detected until after the experiment is complete, and they cannot be controlled or quantified (Cook, 2005).

The presence of factors that jeopardize internal validity does not necessarily mean the study is a weak one; virtually all studies have some rival explanations for results. However, the rigorous researcher attempts to predict those that might logically be expected to affect the outcome of the study and takes action to prevent as many as possible.

Historical Effects

Historical threats refer to events or circumstances that occur around the time of the introduction of the intervention, or they may occur at any time during data collection. Although the event itself may be entirely unpredictable, it can be expected to exert an effect on the subjects and, as a result, the study conclusions.

Consider a study that was designed to measure and compare the levels of stress and anxiety in individuals who commute to Manhattan via public transportation with individuals who commute to Manhattan in privately owned vehicles. The study was started on September 1, 2001. It can be safely assumed that the stress and anxiety levels of anyone working in Manhattan were considerably different after the September 11, 2001, World Trade Center terrorist attacks. Although this may be an extreme example, it demonstrates how an event can change the data or results of a study.

> **gray matter**
>
> Threats to internal validity may include the following:
> - History
> - Maturation
> - Testing
> - Instrumentation
> - Subject selection
> - Experimental mortality

Maturation Effects

Maturation in a research study is related to changes that occur in subjects over time that do not occur as a result of the intervention or attribute being studied. Subjects can change because of normal aging, physical growth, acquisition of knowledge and skills outside the study variables, or physical changes related to a disease process. For example, when studying the effects of relaxation techniques on the management of pain in patients with bony metastasis, the effects of the techniques will be minimized as the disease worsens.

Maturation is a particular concern in populations that are expected to change over time and in longitudinal studies. For example, populations that include children, individuals with chronic diseases, or the elderly are prone to the effects of maturation, particularly if measures are taken over an extended period of time.

> **Historical threats:** Threaten validity because of events or circumstances that occur during data collection.
>
> **Maturation:** Threatens validity because the changes that occur in subjects do not occur as a result of the intervention, but because time has passed.

Testing Effects

Testing: Threatens validity due to the familiarity of the subjects with the testing, particularly when retesting is used in a study.

The threat of testing is related to the effects of taking a test and then retesting the subject. Subjects can become more proficient at test taking based on repeated experiences. For example, the effects of different types of educational methods on the retention of skills necessary to manage central lines in the intensive care unit could be measured with a knowledge test. If the test were administered immediately following the instruction and then repeated within 2 weeks, results may indicate there is no difference in the retention of knowledge and skills based on the educational method. The results may be due to having seen the test before, rather than the effects of the teaching method. One method to reduce the risk of this threat is to schedule the retesting at longer intervals or retest using a different test.

Instrumentation Effects

Instrumentation: Threatens validity because the instrument or data collection procedure has changed in some way.

Instrumentation effects may occur because the instrument or data collection device has changed in some way. This can also be a threat when the data are collected by multiple individuals. In a study designed to determine if 3-year-old males exhibit aggressive behavior more frequently than 3-year-old females in a playgroup, the observers needed to use specific criteria to score or count aggressive behaviors. If Observer #1 scores any physical contact as aggressive but Observer #2 considers only hitting and kicking as aggressive, the resulting data will not be valid. This threat can be reduced by training the observers carefully, using very specific protocols, and testing interrater reliability.

Treatment Effects

Placebo effect: Threatens validity because subjects may perform differently because they are aware they are in a study or as a reaction to being treated.

Subjects may react to the treatment itself, even if it does not exert a therapeutic effect. Also called the placebo effect, the treatment itself may elicit a response that cannot be differentiated from a physiological response. This threat to internal validity is the primary reason for the use of randomly assigned control groups and comparison groups.

Subjects in a study may perform differently because they know they are in a study. Changes occur in the subjects not because of the intervention but because the subjects behave differently than they would normally. This is also referred to as the Hawthorne effect. Changes occur in all the groups, even those that do not receive the treatment or intervention.

Consider an intervention designed to increase self-efficacy in patients who receive chemotherapy. All subjects were recruited into the study and randomized into the intervention or control group. A pretest measure of self-efficacy was administered to all the subjects. All the subjects met with the researcher. However, the control group received written literature about chemotherapy and the experimental group received a focused, structured intervention designed to increase self-efficacy. The posttest revealed that subjects in both the control and experimental group demonstrated a statistically significant increase in self-efficacy, which could have simply been related to the subject's awareness of being in a study. The Hawthorne effect is of great concern if the researcher is in a position of perceived authority—as in leadership studies or when physicians lead research teams—so that subjects act in ways they perceive are desirable.

Because of ethical concerns, it is difficult to control for this threat. Subjects need to be informed they are in a study. However, it is possible, with IRB approval, to inform subjects they are in a study but to be less explicit about what is being studied. In a study to determine the correlation among suffering, self-transcendence, and social support in women with breast cancer, the instrument used to measure suffering was called the Life Experience Index rather than a measure of suffering. The concern was that calling it "suffering" might influence the responses.

Multiple Treatment Effects

When multiple treatments are applied at the same time, it is difficult to determine how well each of the treatments works individually. It might be the combination of the treatments that is effective. Another concern is the effect of the order in which the treatments or interventions occur. This concern about the sequence of events is particularly worrisome in interventional studies, where confirmation that the independent variable precedes the dependent one is important.

For example, a researcher may study the effects of a skin cream applied manually to prevent skin breakdown. The cream is applied using circular massage. Patients receiving the cream treatment have a lower pressure-ulcer rate than patients who do not. However, the difference may be due to the act of massaging the area and not simply the application of the cream. Multiple treatment effects threaten validity because they make it impossible to determine the unique contribution of each treatment to the outcome.

Selection Effects

Subject selection refers to the biases that may result in selection or assignment of subjects to groups in a way that is not objective and equitable. Selection effects can be exerted by the researcher through the sampling strategy or by subjects during the recruitment period. The more specialized the population under study, the more difficult it may be to recruit a representative pool of subjects (Fredman, Tennstedt, & Smyth, 2004). In a study to compare two smoking cessation treatment programs, if Group A has 40 females and 10 males and Group B has 56 males and 4 females, there may be gender differences in response to the treatment programs. Randomization or random assignment to study groups counters this threat.

Subject selection: Threatens validity due to the introduction of bias through selection or composition of comparison groups.

Experimental Mortality

Experimental mortality is also known as attrition and refers to the loss of subjects during a study. For example, a longitudinal study to examine the effects of different types of exercise on weight loss began with 100 subjects but ended with only 44. Those who stayed in the study may have been more motivated to exercise, or they may have been more physically active before participating in the project.

Experimental mortality: A threat to internal validity resulting from loss of subjects during a study.

Some subjects could have moved, become ill or injured, or been unable to continue the study for a host of other reasons. Some attrition is expected in any study. This type of risk becomes a concern, however, when validity is affected, such as if attrition is excessive or if the loss of subjects is systematic. This risk can be avoided by taking the following steps:

- Advising subjects of the time commitment in advance
- Screening participants who might be likely to drop out of the study (for example, those who have no telephone)
- Making it convenient to continue participating (Connolly, Schneider, & Hill, 2004)

If and when subjects do leave the study, the researcher should determine the reason. An analysis and discussion of the reasons for attrition can help the researcher determine if systematic sampling error will result from the loss from the subject pool. For example, if all the individuals who leave the study do so because their illness worsens, then the study will be focused only on those subjects who are less ill, and validity will be compromised.

Factors That Jeopardize External Validity

External validity refers to the generalizability of the findings of the research to other settings or populations. The goal of most nursing research is to uncover relationships in a population that can serve to improve the health and well-being of all humans (Crosby, DiClemente, & Salazar, 2006). The researcher should ask, "Can these findings be applied to other people or settings?" For example, a study exploring the relationship of smoking to physical activity might not be the same for a group of rural adolescents as for one from an urban setting.

Population validity: The capacity to confidently generalize the results of a study from one group of subjects to another population group.

Population validity refers to generalizing the findings from the sample to a larger group or population. If the sample is drawn from an accessible population, rather than the target population, generalizing the research results from the accessible population to the target population is risky. If the study is an experiment, it may be possible that different results might be found with subjects of different ages, ethnicities, or genders. A study of the effects of a support group on suffering in a population of women with breast cancer might reveal that subjects who attend support groups report lower levels of suffering. However, the findings might not be applicable to a population of males or even other females who are suffering due to causes other than breast cancer. The capacity to generalize from one group of subjects to others is called population validity. For example, population validity is present if a study conducted on children can be generalized to adolescents.

The extent to which the results of an experiment can be generalized from the set of environmental conditions created by the researcher to other environmental conditions is sometimes called ecological validity. This is a concern with experiments or interventional studies. Is the setting in which the study was conducted similar to or different from other settings? The setting may be different in geographical location, population characteristics, or level of care. For example, a study completed in an intensive care unit may not be generalizable to a rehabilitation unit.

Both population and ecological validity are important considerations when appraising research as evidence for nursing practice. The nurse must determine if the results are appropriate for application to a specific setting and group; this requires consideration of the effect of threats to external validity and how well they were controlled.

Selection Effects

As could be surmised, the selection of subjects is the process that will most affect external validity. External validity is enhanced when subjects represent the population closely, so using a strong sampling strategy will enhance external validity. It may be impossible, however, to gain access to a broad representation of the entire population. For example, what if a researcher studying the effects of early ambulation on nausea can only recruit subjects from a limited geographic area? The effects of the location, setting, and types of patients that are accessible will affect the breadth of generalizability of the results. The way the sample is selected, then, is a primary consideration in the evaluation of evidence for application to a specific practice.

Time and Historical Effects

Researchers should be cautious about transferring results obtained during one time period to a different time period. The conditions for the two time periods could be quite different. For example, the results of an intervention to teach new mothers how to feed a newborn in 1985 will not apply in 2010. The length of the hospital stay has been greatly reduced, and the amount of teaching time available may make the teaching method used in the older study ineffective.

Another threat to external validity is the amount of time it takes for an intervention or treatment to take effect. It is possible that the effects of the treatment or intervention will not become evident until weeks after the intervention. A posttest conducted immediately after an intervention might show no significant changes in the subjects. However, if testing is done in 3 months, significant changes may be detected. For example, an exercise intervention was introduced to a sample of seniors. Quality of life testing was conducted after 2 weeks of the exercise program. There was no significant improvement in reported quality of life. However, when the same subjects were tested 60 days after continued participation in the exercise program, self-report of quality of life was significantly higher.

> **gray matter**
>
> Threats to external validity may include the following:
> - Selection effects
> - Time and historical effects
> - Novelty effect
> - Experimenter effect

Novelty Effect

It is possible for subjects to react to something simply because it is unique or new. The treatment or intervention does not cause a change, but the subjects respond to the novelty. In a study to determine if online synchronous chat rooms were productive for clinical postconferences, the initial response of the students was very positive. However, in only a few weeks, the attendance and response dropped dramatically. Conversely, it is possible that subjects will not change

> **Novelty effect:** Threatens validity because subjects react to something because it is novel or new and not to the actual treatment or intervention itself.

because the intervention is too new, but they will adjust over time. In the same project, using asynchronous discussion groups was unsuccessful at the start of the project, but as time passed, students adjusted to this method of conferencing and participation increased significantly in both quantity and quality. The external validity of these results is compromised because it is impossible to separate out the real effects that can be expected in a population from those caused by novelty or familiarity.

Experimenter Effect

It is possible for subjects to react to the experimenter or researcher. The results could be very different if another individual conducts the study or applies the intervention. In a study of the sexual behavior of middle adolescents, the response rate was about 25 percent. The researcher was a middle-aged Caucasian female. The subjects were 15- to 17-year-old African American males in a high school in a major urban area. The surveys were incomplete, and the responses appeared to be random or uniform. When the same survey was administered by a 22-year-old African American male, the response rate was 88 percent, the surveys were completed, and the responses were appropriate. Experimenter effects are a threat to external validity because the intervention may only be effective when applied by a particular kind of individual.

Experimenter effect: Threatens validity due to the interaction with the researcher conducting the study or applying the intervention.

Balancing Internal and External Validity

It is the researcher's obligation to design and carry out studies in a way that maximizes both internal and external validity. However, just as the risks of Type I and II errors must be balanced, the researcher is also challenged to find ways to control each type of validity without compromising either one. The paradoxical relationship between the two types of validity makes this a formidable task.

Internal validity is supported by systematic, objective procedures carried out on randomly selected, large samples in tightly controlled settings. A review of the characteristics described in the previous sentence makes it clear that the more internal validity is controlled, the more artificial the study becomes. This artificiality limits external validity or generalizability. Nurse researchers function in applied settings with subjects who do not often behave in prescribed ways, and care is rarely delivered in laboratory settings. Finding a balance of control and usefulness is a constant challenge for creating research as evidence for nursing practice.

Trustworthiness in Qualitative Research

Many nursing research questions are best answered using a qualitative approach. The intent of qualitative research is to interpret, rather than to test, interventions. Qualitative research is sample-specific and is not intended for generalization. The concern for internal and external validity, then, is not as paramount in the design of qualitative research. However, qualitative researchers are still concerned with representing reality accurately and in searching for truth, and so generating confidence in the researcher's conclusions is still important.

That is where the simple comparisons end, however. Qualitative researchers use different terminology, and there is disagreement among researchers about the concept of validity in qualitative research. Some believe validity is not compatible with the philosophy of qualitative research, and others argue that efforts to produce validity increase the credibility of the findings. The terms *plausible*, *believable*, and *trustworthy* are generally used when discussing the validity of findings in qualitative studies (Creswell, 2008). These terms reflect the premise that the findings can be defended when challenged.

Some threats to the validity of quantitative studies jeopardize qualitative studies as well. The Hawthorne effect, selection effects, and historical events may affect subjects in both types of studies. There are some unique factors, however, that must be considered in judging the appropriateness of qualitative findings.

Although generalization is not a goal of qualitative research, the applicability and transferability of the findings is of great interest as evidence for practice. The researcher should provide an explicit description of the sample and setting so the reader can decide if this research can be applied to other samples. There is no test of significance in qualitative research. The in-depth description of the characteristics of the subject/sample being studied may allow one to conclude the extent to which it is comparable to other subjects/samples (Speziale & Carpenter, 2006). If the subjects and sample are comparable, then one would be more comfortable transferring the results to other people or places. If it can be argued that what is being observed is not dependent on the context or setting, then it might be transferred to other contexts. This enables the nurse to use the results as evidence in a dissimilar setting with more confidence.

> **Applicability and transferability:** The ability of qualitative research findings to be applied to other samples and other settings.
> **Replicability:** The likelihood that qualitative research outcomes or events will happen again given the same circumstances.

Replicability enhances the trustworthiness of the results. The credibility of qualitative studies is supported if findings are confirmed by others, much like any other kind of research. However, this is not a simple process. Replicating a qualitative study is very difficult to accomplish because the original study is conducted in the natural setting, which will invariably change if carried out with other populations or in other places (Munhall, 2006). Replications should be accompanied by thorough discussion of the similarities and discrepancies between the two study settings and populations.

The qualitative researcher can take specific action to enhance the trustworthiness of results and conclusions. A thoughtful consideration of potential threats to credibility can help the researcher plan reasonable methods to minimize their effects.

Strategies to Promote the Validity of Qualitative Research

Just as threats to validity must be considered and dealt with in quantitative design, factors that may jeopardize the credibility of qualitative studies should be recognized and addressed. Qualitative research design is usually an emergent process, however, so many decisions are made as the study unfolds that will strengthen the reader's confidence in the findings. Certain characteristics are shared by all strong qualitative studies regardless of the specific type of qualitative design.

The following methods promote the validity of qualitative research:

- Prolonged or varied field experience
- Use of verbatim accounts
- Triangulation
- Participant feedback
- Bracketing
- Audit trail

Prolonged or Varied Field Experiences

Whenever possible, qualitative researchers should collect data over an extended period of time to allow the researcher to get an accurate picture of the phenomenon being studied. For example, a study examining the work environment in a critical care unit should account for the fact that the atmosphere may vary from day to day and over time during a 24-hour period, as well as from nurse to nurse. Interviews to understand the experience of working in critical care should be done at many different times, on different days, and with different nurses to capture these variations.

Verbatim Accounts

Qualitative researchers should be careful to keep accurate field notes and to report results as direct quotes to avoid making inferences. Descriptions should be as close as possible to the participants' accounts. This ensures that the meaning that is captured is the respondents', not the researcher's interpretation of it.

Triangulation

Triangulation is the researcher's use of multiple sources to confirm a finding. In other words, isolated incidents and perceptions should not be the basis for drawing conclusions, but rather patterns of responses that appear frequently. This means the themes will be identified in the words of several respondents or identified in multiple ways (for example, words, documents, and observations). Cross-checking information and conclusions using multiple data sources to increase understanding, use of multiple research methods to study a phenomenon, and the use of multiple researchers can increase the credibility of the results (Creswell, 2008).

Participant Feedback or Member Checking

The procedure for participant feedback is also called member checking, and it involves discussing interpretations and conclusions with the participants. Checking the accuracy of the observations directly with subjects ensures that the researcher's interpretations and observations reflect what the participants actually meant. This step is essential to determine that the researcher has captured the real meaning of the data and has not interjected bias into the conclusions.

Triangulation: Cross-checking conclusions using multiple data sources, methods, or researchers to study the phenomenon.
Member checking: Checking the accuracy of the observations and conclusions directly with subjects.
Bracketing: The process of explicitly reflecting on and documenting the researcher's biases.

Bracketing the Researcher's Bias

Qualitative researchers are less concerned with bias than quantitative researchers are. Research conducted in an interpretive manner in a natural setting has inherent bias that is expected and accepted in qualitative research as long as it is not careless or excessive. However, the researcher should still critically examine personal biases and inclinations that might affect interpretation of the data. Bracketing is a strategy used to control bias. A researcher who is aware of his or her own biases and makes them explicit is less likely to succumb to them—in other words, the effects of the bias are "put in brackets" so they can be set aside. The researcher must also bracket any presumed knowledge about a subject or topic during data collection and data analysis (Munhall, 2006). The researcher needs to be open to ways in which gender, age, ethnicity, religion, politics, and other factors might affect the interview, observations, or participation in the project. A qualitative study by nature is unlikely to be 100 percent objective; however, efforts should be made to convince readers that a high level of objectivity has been maintained.

Documentation of an Audit Trail

Documentation in qualitative research includes field notes and reports, interpretations, and thorough descriptions and reports of feedback. Careful records must be kept of each of these sources of information. In addition, the emergent nature of the design requires constant decision making, with a record of the rationale for each choice. This record of data and decisions is an audit trail that allows the researcher to describe procedures and defend the results. A conscientious audit trail can also aid in replication of the research in other settings or populations. Records should be accurate, thorough, and complete. Strategies include writing early and often,

Audit trail: Detailed documentation of sources of information, data, and design decisions related to a qualitative research study.

Checklist for Evaluating the Validity of a Research Study

If the effects of an intervention are tested
✔ Changes in the outcome are associated with changes in the intervention.
✔ The researchers clearly demonstrate that the intervention preceded the outcome.
✔ The researchers identified potential rival explanations and eliminated, controlled, or accounted for them.

To assess the role of bias
✔ The researcher was blinded to group assignment.
✔ The primary researcher did not collect data.
✔ Subjects were selected using objective criteria and assigned to groups randomly.
✔ If a qualitative study, the author explicitly described a bracketing process.

Threats to internal validity/trustworthiness
✔ Extraneous variables were identified and controlled.
✔ Historical events did not occur during the study that would affect the outcome.
✔ Maturation was not an alternative explanation for the results.
✔ If testing and retesting were involved, the time interval between tests was adequate to avoid a testing effect.
✔ Attrition from the study was not excessive or systematic.
✔ If a qualitative study, the author demonstrated:
  • Prolonged contact
  • Use of verbatim accounts
  • Triangulation
  • An audit trail

Threats to external validity/transferability
✔ The sample was selected to maximize representativeness.
✔ The setting in which the study was done is adequately described to determine applicability.

including primary data in the final report, using rich descriptions, and getting frequent feedback on the documentation.

Reading a Research Study to Determine Validity

Unfortunately, there is no section of a research report labeled "validity." The reader must evaluate the validity of the design and determine if the results obtained are believable. However, it is possible to analyze a report in a systematic manner to determine potential threats to validity, what the researcher did to control the threats, and, finally, if the efforts were successful.

Two places where the reader can find information about the primary controls for validity are in the methods and procedures sections, where sampling, measurement, and analysis are described. The way samples are selected, responses are measured, and data are managed can all inhibit or enhance validity.

Most authors will describe the factors that jeopardized validity from their point of view. This description is usually found in the "discussion" or "conclusions" section, but it may be in a separate section labeled "strengths and limitations." The list may not be all-inclusive and is often subjective. Ultimately, it is the readers' obligation to determine if the results apply to their patients and setting. Some studies will have very few threats that affect them; others will have multiple threats. There is no magic number of "acceptable threats." Some are more important or have more damaging effects than others.

Replication of studies compensates for threats to internal validity. Studies that have been replicated many times with similar results have the highest level of validity and, thus, are very strong evidence for practice. Studies that aggregate and review multiple studies, such as meta-analyses, systematic reviews, and integrative reviews, compensate for many threats to internal validity and form the strongest evidence for practice.

Determining whether the researcher has controlled threats to validity can be a matter of judgment. Validity is an inexact concept and involves balancing controls with the risks of making errors. Achieving this balance is demanding, and so weaknesses are inevitably discovered when a study is scrutinized. Validity is one of the key characteristics of a study that makes it strong evidence for practice, however, and so a critical eye is required. Internal validity enables confidence that an intervention will produce an effect; external validity means it can be used for the greater good; trustworthiness means findings can be applied to broader groups. All are critical as evidence for effective nursing practices.

Using Valid Studies as Evidence for Nursing Practice

Determining if the results reported in a research study can, or should, be applied to nursing practice involves careful consideration of the validity of the study. If a study is not valid, then the results that were reported cannot reasonably be expected to occur in every setting. There are many questions to ask to determine if the independent variable actually caused or affected the desired outcome. Given an affirmative answer, the nurse must still determine if the results are applicable to a specific population. In effect, these are ultimately the critical questions used to determine what research findings should be used as evidence for practice.

When appropriate studies have been identified to support a change in practice, the nurse must critically review the research methods to determine the appropriate use of the results. The first order of critical analysis should be a systematic review of internal validity in a quantitative study or credibility in a qualitative one. If a study has poor internal validity, then external validity cannot be achieved. Using a systematic approach, the study is reviewed for threats to internal validity and their effective controls. If a study is determined to have acceptable internal reliability, then a careful consideration of external validity should precede recommendations. The type of population and the setting should be carefully reviewed, and applicability to a specific practice setting evaluated.

For example, an intervention designed to reduce the incidence of falls is implemented in a long-term care facility. Fall data have been carefully documented before and after the intervention. The data reveal a statistically significant decline in falls on the study unit. However, the patient age and level of infirmity were reduced at the time and the number of unlicensed assistive personnel (UAP) was increased. The threat to the validity of the study is obvious: A multiple treatment effect makes it impossible to determine which intervention had the result. Were patients less likely to fall because they were not as sick? Were more UAPs available to provide assistance? Or was the intervention alone responsible for the change? The threats to validity in this study mean its application to practice is limited until the study is replicated under more controlled circumstances.

If the study findings were, indeed, replicated several times, the nurse must still determine if the population and setting are similar enough to apply the findings to practice. This study, conducted in a long-term care facility, may not apply to a medical–surgical unit. Results that were generated from a population of infirm elderly in a nursing home may not apply to outpatient surgical patients. Even studies that are internally valid and replicated may not be useful as evidence if the population and setting are so specific as to have limited applicability.

Considering the internal and external validity of studies is a key step in appraising research for use as evidence in practice. Evaluating threats to internal and external validity makes up a large part of the assessment process for determining the quality of a research study.

Creating a Valid Research Study

Designing a study that has strong validity or credibility is a challenge, even for experienced researchers. The nature of applied nursing research means human beings are involved, introducing a level of unpredictability that makes it impossible to predict all threats to validity. However, some threats to validity have the potential to affect almost any study. The conscientious research designer reflects on the most common threats to validity and creates design elements to ensure that an appropriate level of control is achieved. Table 11.2 describes common threats to validity and methods to ensure their control. The most common threats relate to researcher effects, selection effects, and treatment

Table 11.2

Common Threats to Internal Validity and Associated Control Measures

Threat	What It Is	How It Is Controlled
History	Events occur during the study that have an influence on the outcome of the study	■ Random sampling to distribute effects across all groups
Maturation	Effects of the passage of time	■ Match subjects for age ■ Use analysis of covariance (ANCOVA) to measure effects of time
Treatment effects	Subject reactions that are due to the effect of being observed	■ Unobtrusive measures ■ Subject blinding ■ Use of sham procedures or placebos
Instrumentation	Influence on the outcome from the measurement itself, not the intervention	■ Calibration of instruments ■ Documentation of reliability ■ Analysis of interrater reliability
Experimental mortality	Subject attrition due to dropouts, loss of contact, or death	■ Project expected attrition and oversample ■ Carefully screen subjects prior to recruitment ■ Create thorough consent procedures so subjects are aware of what will be expected of them
Bias	Study is influenced by preconceived notions of the researcher or reactions of the subject	■ Blinding of researcher, data collectors, and subjects as to who is getting the experimental treatment
Selection effects	Subjects are assigned to groups in a way that does not distribute characteristics evenly across both groups	■ Random selection ■ Random assignment ■ Matching of subjects ■ Stratified samples

effects. These are also the reasons for some of the most common control mechanisms in research design.

Researcher effects are controlled in a variety of ways and can be addressed in both quantitative and qualitative study design. In either design, a period of reflection on the researcher's specific biases can help to ensure the researcher is aware of their potential effects. Every researcher has bias—there would be no passion for the research subject if the researcher did not have some preconceived notions about how the study would turn out. Making these explicit can help the researcher guard for their effects. As discussed earlier, in qualitative research, this process of reflecting on and documenting researcher bias is called bracketing, but it is a useful process regardless of the paradigm.

Blinding the researcher to specific elements of the study can help reduce the effects of bias (Hulley et al., 2006). When the researcher is unaware of the group assignment of subjects and cannot link subjects to data, then the potential for influencing the outcome becomes much more remote. It may be necessary for the researcher to completely remove him- or herself from the setting during data collection to ensure that bias is controlled.

Selection effects are controlled almost exclusively by the way subjects are recruited, selected, and assigned to groups. Paying careful attention to the development of inclusion and exclusion criteria ensures that objective rationales are available for leaving some individuals out of a study. Random sampling and/or random assignment to treatment groups also has the effect of minimizing selection effects.

Treatment effects are harder to control, particularly for ethical researchers interested in full disclosure. The Hawthorne or placebo effect may be present even in descriptive and correlation studies. The use of control groups or comparison groups can help ensure that any effects from participation in the study are spread evenly among subjects. Using sham procedures or comparing two interventions simultaneously can also control for changes brought about by treatment effects.

Other threats to validity will almost certainly occur during an experiment, no matter how well designed. The researcher has three basic ways to deal with these threats:

1. *Eliminate the threat:* If a threat emerges that can be neutralized, removal of the threat can enhance validity. For example, a researcher may ask research assistants to collect data if measures are subjective and bias is a concern. By removing him- or herself from data collection, the researcher has eliminated the effect he or she might have had on measuring a subjective trait.

2. *Control the threat:* If a threat emerges that cannot be eliminated, the researcher can employ methods to control its effects or distribute its effects across all subjects or groups equally. For example, research to examine the effects of childhood developmental delays on school success may be affected by socioeconomic status. By matching all the groups on this variable through stratified sampling, the effects of limited resources will be distributed across all the groups equally, neutralizing its effect on the outcome.

3. *Account for the threat:* If a threat occurs that cannot be eliminated or controlled, then the researcher must account for it in the write-up. All studies have weaknesses and threats to validity; it is up to the reader to determine if the weaknesses

For More Depth and Detail

For a more in-depth look at the concepts in this chapter, try these references:

Cook, L. (2005). Internal validity in rehabilitation research. *Work, 25*(3), 279–283.

DelBoca, F., & Darkes, J. (2007). Enhancing the validity and utility of randomized clinical trials in addictions treatment research: I. Treatment implementation and research design. *Addiction, 102*(7), 1047–1056.

Hulley, S., Cummings, S., Browner, W., & Grady, D. (2006). *Designing clinical research: An epidemiological approach* (3rd ed.). Philadelphia: Lippincott Williams & Wilkins.

Munhall, P. (2006). *Nursing research: A qualitative perspective* (4th ed.). Sudbury, MA: Jones & Bartlett.

Portney, L.G., & Watkins, M.P. (2008). *Foundations of clinical research: Applications to practice* (3rd ed.). Upper Saddle River, NJ: Prentice Hall.

Rolfe, G. (2006). Validity, trustworthiness, and rigour: Quality and the idea of qualitative research. *Journal of Advanced Nursing, 53*(3), 304–310.

CRITICAL APPRAISAL **EXERCISE**

Retrieve the following full text article from the Cumulative Index to Nursing and Allied Health Literature or similar search database:

Garcia, R., Jendresky, L., Colbert, L., Bailey, A., Zaman, M., & Majumder, M. (2009). Reducing ventilator-associated pneumonia through advanced oral-dental care: A 48-month study. *American Journal of Critical Care, 18*(6), 523–532.

Read the study carefully, searching for evidence of threats to internal or external validity. Pay particular attention to how the authors controlled these threats. Consider the following appraisal questions in your critical review of validity of this research article:

1. Identify and classify any major threats to internal validity in this study including:
   a. Experimenter effects
   b. Treatment effects
   c. Subject effects
2. What strategies did the researchers use to eliminate or control the effects of these threats? If they were uncontrollable, how did the authors account for them in the write-up?
3. What additional measures could these researchers have used to minimize the effects of threats to internal validity?
4. What was the population for this study? Was it a random or accessible sample? Describe groups to which these results could be generalized.
5. The results were not statistically significant. What kind of error might this represent (Type I or Type II)? How might the authors have controlled this error?
6. Describe the setting for this study. To what other settings could these results apply?

of a study outweigh its strengths. For example, a researcher was studying the attitudes of school nurses toward student violence when the Columbine High School shootings occurred. This historical event dramatically changed the responses of the school nurses. Although nothing could be done about the tragedy or its effects on the research study, the author reported the data as "before the incident" and "after the incident" and noted that it likely had an effect on the outcome.

When creating a study, the researcher must balance control of threats to internal validity with the need to maximize external validity. Generalizability is a key issue for research that is to be used as evidence. When a research study becomes too highly controlled, its artificial nature limits applicability to real-world populations. The researcher must balance each element that strengthens internal validity with a concern to maintain as broad of external validity as possible.

Summary of Key Concepts

- An internally valid research study is one in which there is sufficient evidence to support the claim that the intervention had an effect and that nothing else was responsible for the outcome.

- Specific conditions must be met to draw valid conclusions about causality: The intervention is related to the outcome; the intervention preceded the outcome; and rival explanations have been ruled out.
- Threats to internal validity can be minimized by creating a logical argument, collecting data to support the argument, using appropriate design, and controlling bias.
- Statistical analyses can be used to rule out rival explanations for an outcome through the use of hypothesis testing, minimizing Type I and II error, considering effect size, and ensuring assumptions are met.
- When a researcher makes a Type I error, he or she has concluded that the independent variable exerted an effect when in fact it did not. Type I error is controlled by careful design and control.
- A Type II error has occurred when the intervention had an effect but it went undetected. Type II error is primarily controlled with a strong sampling strategy and achieving an adequate sample size.
- Many factors can threaten internal validity, including history, maturation, testing, instrumentation, treatment effects, selection effects, and attrition.
- External validity refers to the generalizability of the findings of the study to other populations or settings.
- Threats to external validity include selection effects, time and history, novelty, and experimenter effects.
- The researcher must make decisions that balance internal and external validity. As internal validity gets more tightly controlled, it also becomes more artificial and has less applicability to broad populations.
- Qualitative research is judged by trustworthiness and credibility of the results. The extension of understanding from qualitative studies comes about through transferability and replication.
- Strategies to promote the credibility of qualitative research include prolonged contact, verbatim accounts, triangulation, member checking, bracketing, and audit trails.

For a full suite of assignments and additional learning activities, use the access code located in the front of your book to visit this exclusive website: http://go.jblearning .com/houser. If you do not have an access code, you can obtain one at the site.

References

Bordens, K., & Barrington, B. (2007). *Research design and methods: A process approach* (7th ed.). New York: McGraw-Hill.

Connolly, N., Schneider, D., & Hill, A.M. (2004). Improving enrollment in cancer clinical trials. *Oncology Nursing Forum, 31*(3), 610–614.

Cook, L. (2005). Internal validity in rehabilitation research. *Work, 25*(3), 279–283.

Creswell, J. (2008). *Research design: Qualitative, quantitative, and mixed methods* (3rd ed.). Thousand Oaks, CA: Sage.

Crosby, R., DiClemente, R., & Salazar, L. (2006). *Research methods in health promotion.* San Francisco: Jossey-Bass.

Forthofer, R., Lee, E., & Hernandez, M. (2007). *Biostatistics: A guide to design, analysis, and discovery* (2nd ed.). Boston: Elsevier.

Fredman, L., Tennstedt, S., & Smyth, K. (2004). Pragmatic and internal validity issues in sampling in caregiver studies. *Journal of Aging and Health, 16*(2), 175–203.

Hartung, D., & Touchette, D. (2009). Overview of clinical research design. *American Journal of Health System Pharmacy, 66*(15), 398–408.

Hulley, S., Cummings, S., Browner, W., & Grady, D. (2006). *Designing clinical research: An epidemiological approach* (3rd ed.). Philadelphia: Lippincott Williams & Wilkins.

Munhall, P. (2006). *Nursing research: A qualitative perspective* (4th ed.). Sudbury, MA: Jones & Bartlett.

Portney, L., & Watkins, M. (2008). *Foundations of clinical research: Applications to practice* (3rd ed.). Upper Saddle River, NJ: Prentice Hall.

Speziale, H., & Carpenter, D. (2006). *Qualitative research in nursing: Advancing the humanistic perspective.* Philadelphia: Lippincott Williams & Wilkins.

part IV

Research that Describes Populations

chapter 12

Descriptive Research Questions and Procedures

CHAPTER OBJECTIVES

The study of this chapter will help the learner to:

- Identify descriptive research designs and methods.
- Examine the importance of design decisions in descriptive studies.
- Compare the characteristics and applications of specific descriptive designs.
- Relate descriptive designs to evidence-based nursing practice.
- Appraise a descriptive study for strengths and weaknesses.
- Learn how to create a descriptive research design.

KEY TERMS

Case study	Longitudinal study	Spurious relationship
Correlation study	Prediction study	Suppressor variable
Cross-sectional design	Reversal designs	Tests of model fit
Epidemiology	Single-subject design	

Introduction

There is an age-old saying that goes, "You cannot know where you are going if you do not know where you have been." The descriptive researcher might more accurately say, "You cannot know where you are going if you do not know where you are." Experiments are the study of what may be; they are used to investigate interventions that may be effective or nursing actions that may prevent health problems. Descriptive research, on the other hand, illuminates an understanding of what is. Understanding the potential

❝ Scenes from the Field ❯❯

Violence is a problem that results in a myriad of detrimental consequences for individuals and communities. Although physical violence traditionally has been viewed as a male problem, researchers are exploring violent acts that are committed by females. One such phenomenon, acts of relational aggression, previously was not regarded as an act of violence, yet it can have dramatic effects on its victims. Examples of relational aggression include rumor spreading, gossiping, and socially isolating others; all have been linked to poor health outcomes.

Gomes, Davis, Baker, and Sevonsky (2009) set out to determine if relational aggression was correlated with the incidence of depression in a sample of African American college-age women. They used a cross-sectional descriptive design to explore this relationship. Two instruments were administered to all females in the entering freshman class of a large, historically African American college as part of a larger battery of tests. This minimized the threat of measurement bias. Data were collected about relational aggression via the Self Report of Aggression and Social Behavior Measure, consisting of 56 items rated on a Likert scale. The instrument has demonstrated reliability. The incidence of depression was measured using the Beck Depression Inventory II, an instrument that has been used in research and clinical settings for more than 35 years. It has demonstrated stable reliability and validity, and is reported as being the most widely accepted instrument for diagnosing depression in a normal nonpsychiatric population.

A power analysis indicated that 50 participants were needed, and 241 responses were received, exceeding the sample size required to detect a moderate effect size. After collecting the data, the authors screened all of the Beck instruments for responses indicating suicidal ideation. Two were found, and follow-up with a counselor indicated the students were not at risk.

The authors provided descriptive statistics about the sample, with a mean age of 18.3 years and representing 32 different locations around the world. The most common types of relational aggression expressed by these women were: "I have a friend who ignores me or gives me the cold shoulder when she is angry with me," "A friend of mine has gone behind my back and shared private information about me with other people," "I have a friend who excludes me from doing things with her and her friends when she is mad at me," and "When a friend of mine has been mad at me, other people have taken sides with her and have been mad at me too." The authors constructed a summary relational aggression score and a summary depression score, and these scores were analyzed using a Pearson's product moment correlation coefficient. There was a statistically significant, moderate, positive relationship between victimization via relational aggression and depression.

that an intervention has for improving health must be based on an understanding of the conditions and the people that will be affected by it. Often, an in-depth knowledge of the current state of affairs is necessary to hypothesize whether a change in practice is warranted or even desirable.

This study was a good example of a descriptive design in that it focused on a small number of variables and explored relationships without attempting to determine cause and effect. The study would suggest that subsequent studies could focus on the causal nature of aggression, or means by which it can be prevented or its effects mediated. Because this type of aggression is often underplayed or overlooked, this could be the subject of important work that could affect the health and well-being of young people in a lifelong way.

Source: Gomes, M., Davis, B., Baker, S., & Servonsky, E. (2009). Correlation of the experience of peer relational aggression victimization and depression among African American adolescent females. *Journal of Child and Adolescent Psychiatric Nursing, 22*(4), 175–181.

The purpose of descriptive research is the exploration and description of phenomena in real-life situations. In nursing practice, a descriptive design can be used to develop theory, identify problems, make decisions, or determine what others in similar situations are doing. Descriptive studies include a purpose and a question; these designs do not, however, have a treatment that is artificially introduced. Descriptive research is the study of phenomena as they naturally occur. Descriptive research helps nurses understand particular individuals, groups, organizations, communities, events, or situations so that they can design effective nursing interventions (Burns & Grove, 2008).

gray matter

In nursing practice, a descriptive design can be used to
- Develop theory
- Identify problems
- Make decisions
- Determine what others in similar situations are doing

Descriptive studies are designed to provide in-depth information about the characteristics of subjects or a setting within a particular field of study. The researcher may collect data as numbers or words, and data collection may be done via observation, measurement, surveys, or questionnaires. A wide variety of descriptive designs are available to the nurse researcher, but they all have one characteristic in common: no variables are manipulated in the study. When data are collected as numbers, the descriptive study is considered quantitative. Data that are collected as words are typical of qualitative studies. This chapter will focus on quantitative descriptive designs; later chapters will focus on the use of qualitative methods to answer descriptive research questions.

As the most basic research design, descriptive studies answer basic questions about what is happening in a defined population or situation. They help the nurse identify existing health conditions, perceptions about an illness or treatment, emotional or psychological responses, or the current distribution of disease in a population. Descriptive studies can also help identify relationships between variables, such as the association between a risk factor and a disease. These studies are useful in determining the current health status of a population so that effective preventive actions can be planned (Houser & Bokovoy, 2006).

Descriptive research plays an important role in nursing. Descriptive studies can be invaluable in documenting the prevalence, nature, and intensity of health-related conditions and behaviors. The results of descriptive studies are critical in the development of effective interventions. In nursing, the only way to understand the beliefs and values of different individuals and groups is to describe them. This descriptive knowledge helps develop nursing interventions that benefit individuals, families, or groups to obtain desirable and predictable outcomes.

Descriptive Research Studies

As with any research study, the first step is to select a topic of interest, review relevant literature, and formulate a research question based on the identified problem. Descriptive research studies address two basic types of questions:

- Descriptive questions are designed to describe what is going on or what exists. An example of a descriptive question is, "What percentage of school-age children are fully immunized in a school district?"
- Relational questions are designed to investigate the relationships between two or more variables or between subjects. An example of a relational question is, "What is the relationship between the immunization rate and socioeconomic status in a school district?"

The descriptive research question includes some common elements. The population of interest is specified, as well as the phenomenon of interest. If the question is relational, then two variables will be identified. Because there is no intervention, there will be no comparison group or expected outcome. As a result, descriptive research questions are simpler. It may be tempting to include several concepts in a single question, but the well-written descriptive research question focuses on a single concept. Multiple research questions may be called for when several concepts are of interest in a single study. **Table 12.1** provides some examples of descriptive research questions.

A well-structured research question is the foundation for the determination of a specific design. As with any research study, it is worth the time and effort to consider the elements of the research question carefully because the details of the study design will be guided by the question.

Characteristics of a Descriptive Design

Drawing good conclusions in a descriptive study is completely dependent on collecting data that are credible and complete. The elements of a good descriptive design are intended to improve the probability of obtaining accurate data and/or responses to questions. A strong descriptive design should

- Include procedures that enhance the probability of generating trustworthy data
- Demonstrate appropriateness for the purpose of the study
- Be feasible given the resources available to the researcher and existing constraints
- Incorporate steps that are effective in reducing threats to validity

Examples of Descriptive Research Questions and Designs

Type of Study	Typical Research Questions
Descriptive	What is nurses' knowledge about best practices related to oral care?
Survey	How are nurses involved in decision making about patient care, the work environment, and organizational practices?
Cross-sectional	What are the differences in job satisfaction among nurses working on different types of units?
Longitudinal	What is the effect of urinary incontinence on the quality of life of long-term-care residents over time?
Case study	What are the appropriate assessments and interventions for a patient experiencing paraplegia after heart surgery?
Single-subject study	What were the responses of an individual with type II diabetes to one-on-one counseling from a nurse?
Correlation	What is the relationship between patient satisfaction and the timeliness and effectiveness of pain relief in a fast-track emergency unit?
Predictive	Can feeding performance in neonates be predicted by indicators of feeding readiness?

The elements of a good design will help reassure the researcher that the results are valid and trustworthy. Even though descriptive designs are among the most basic studies, it is still important for the researcher to allow adequate time for planning prior to conducting the research. The validity and accuracy of a study depend on the strength of the research design (Polit & Beck, 2009).

A typical descriptive study is used to acquire knowledge in an area where little research has been conducted or when little is known about the condition under study. The basic descriptive design examines a characteristic or group of characteristics in a sample, but there are many variations on this theme. A basic descriptive design may be used as a pilot study or as the basis for designing more complex studies. It is useful in establishing the need for and the development of future, more intricate studies.

Fundamentally, descriptive designs can be classified as those that describe a phenomenon or population and those that describe relationships. There are, however, two additional ways to classify descriptive designs:

- *The number of subjects:* Descriptive designs may involve the study of an entire population, a sample, or multiple samples. Descriptive design may also focus on single subjects or individual cases. A case is not necessarily a single individual, but rather a single subject. A *subject* may be defined any number of ways. For example, the study of an individual person, hospital, or city may all represent data collection from a single entity.

Case in Point: A Descriptive Study

Lenz (2009) conducted a descriptive study to examine if baccalaureate students were prepared to counsel patients about smoking cessation. Data were gathered from two samples that consisted of 675 baccalaureate nursing students and the directors from 10 Minnesota baccalaureate nursing programs.

Two surveys were sent to the students. One contained knowledge questions about tobacco use, beliefs, and smoking cessation. The second questionnaire was a survey about their training experience. The education program directors were administered the training survey as well, which focused on how tobacco and smoking cessation were taught in the curriculum.

The researcher found the transfer of knowledge was not adequate in the nursing training programs throughout the state. The students who were surveyed reported a lack of confidence regarding advising patients to quit smoking, assessing a patient's readiness to quit, and helping patients set a quit date.

This descriptive study is a typical one in that it described the knowledge and attitudes of a sample without trying to determine causal relationships. A major strength of this study is its large sample size. As is often the case, the author used more than one instrument to capture complex data. These instruments were all tested and found to be reliable and valid, which is a critical determinant of the quality of descriptive conclusions. This research could be used confidently as evidence by nurse educators in ensuring they are preparing students for this important skill.

Source: Lenz, B. K. (2009). Nursing students' response to tobacco cessation curricula in Minnesota baccalaureate nursing programs. *Journal of Nursing Education, 48*(10), 566–573.

- *The time dimension:* Some studies explore data collected from a sample at a single point in time, whereas other designs follow subjects or individual cases over time.

Within each of these classifications are explicit designs that enable the researcher to answer specific questions. The researcher will gain direction for design decisions by considering the nature of the research question, the number of subjects that are appropriate and accessible, and the time span of interest.

Describing Groups Using Surveys

Of the descriptive studies, survey design is the most common. Although the term *survey design* is commonly used to describe a study, it is more accurately a data collection method used in general descriptive designs. Surveys are used to collect data directly from respondents about their characteristics, opinions, perceptions, or attitudes. This design is one in which questionnaires or personal interviews are used to gather information about a population. A survey can be an important method for gathering data and can be used as a data collection technique for both descriptive and relational studies. This design can be used to answer questions about the prevalence, distribution, and interrelationship of variables within a population. Survey designs can be applied at a single point in time, or responses can be gathered over an extended time span. To strengthen the survey the researcher must focus on obtaining an adequate sample representative of the target population (Brown, 2009).

The purpose of asking questions is to find out what is going on in the minds of the subjects: their perceptions, attitudes, beliefs, feelings, motives, and past events. Surveys are used to discover characteristics of people and find out what they believe and how they think. The survey is a method designed to collect primary self-reported data.

There are two categories of questions. One type of question focuses on facts, allowing the researcher to obtain information about events or people. Another focuses on perceptions or feelings, in which the participant shares feelings about people, events, or things (Woods & Kerr, 2006).

Survey Study Methods and Procedures

Designing a general descriptive survey consists of four major stages:

1. Selecting an appropriate sample
2. Planning and developing instrumentation
3. Administering the instrument and data collection
4. Analyzing the findings

The planning phase includes choice of a survey mode, which may be a questionnaire or an interview. During this phase, the instrument is selected or developed; in the latter case, it is also pilot tested for reliability and validity. The procedure for administration of the instrument is described in a detailed protocol so the subjects receive instructions that are consistent and unambiguous. Data are collected in an identical way from each subject so differences in responses can be attributed to differences in the subjects, not in the administration method. Analysis of findings is accomplished through the application of descriptive statistics, which are described in detail in Chapter 13.

> **gray matter**
>
> The following are the four major steps in designing a general descriptive survey:
> - Select an appropriate sample.
> - Plan and develop instrumentation.
> - Administer the instrument and collect data.
> - Analyze the findings.

A survey is a widely used method of descriptive data collection. Its use is popular because it is a relatively simple design that enables a wide range of topics to be covered. Surveys offer a systematic method for standardizing questions and collecting data and can be an efficient means of gathering data from a large number of subjects. The Internet has provided an additional way of reaching subjects and is a very effective method for soliciting feedback from large numbers of people in a way that is convenient to them (Sapsford, 2006).

Strengths of Survey Studies

The use of a survey design offers many advantages for the researcher, including the following:

- Survey content is flexible and its scope is broad.
- Surveys are cost-effective methods for reaching large populations.

Case in Point: A Survey Design

Drennan, Goodman, Norton, and Wells (2010) explored the extent and management of bladder problems among women prisoners. Adults who are incontinent often have feelings of shame and the desire to hide their condition from others. Women prisoners as a group may feel that they need to hide information about stigmatizing conditions more closely than most women. These authors used a self-report survey to collect data directly from women prisoners. The authors had to develop their own questionnaire, because it required a reading level below 11 years and sensitivity to a variety of cultures. One hundred forty-eight women returned the questionnaire for a response rate of 60%.

Forty-three percent of the women reported symptoms of urinary incontinence. More than half reported nocturia and 5% had experienced nocturnal enuresis (bedwetting); 12% reported pain when passing urine; 43% of the women reported these conditions had started after their imprisonment. The widespread incidence of symptoms in this population demonstrates that prison nurses and nurse practitioners should routinely assess for bladder problems using direct but sensitive questions.

This survey design was typical in that data were collected directly from participants using a validated instrument. The questionnaire was self-report to minimize embarrassment and to enhance response rate. A unique aspect of this study was the extensive process used to gain ethical approval, as prisoners are considered a vulnerable population, and so the approval of multiple review boards was necessary. The authors did not overinterpret the findings, but noted that the results of this exploratory study demonstrated that the subject warranted further research using designs that focus on prevention and treatment.

Source: Dernnan, V., Goodman, C., Norton, C., & Wells, A. (2010). Incontinence in women prisoners: An exploration of the issues. *Journal of Advanced Nursing, 66*(9), 1953–1967.

- Subjects have a greater sense of anonymity and may respond with more honesty.
- Questions are predetermined and standardized for all subjects, minimizing researcher bias.
- Large sample sizes are possible.
- A large volume of data can be collected.

Limitations of Survey Studies

Although surveys offer many advantages, some of the disadvantages associated with the use of this method include the following:

- The information obtained may be superficial and limited to standard responses.
- A survey cannot probe deeply into complexities of human behavior or explore contradictions.
- Content is often limited by subject recall, self-knowledge, and willingness to respond honestly.
- Questions may be misinterpreted by subjects, resulting in unreliable conclusions.
- Respondents may respond with socially acceptable responses to sensitive questions instead of honest answers.

The application of good design decisions can help maximize the advantages and minimize the disadvantages of survey designs. The use of reliable, valid instruments applied to large, randomly selected samples will result in the most credible results from a survey design.

Describing Groups Relative to Time

Descriptive studies may focus on the characteristics of a population at a single point in time or on changes within a population over time. Time-dimension designs are most closely associated with the discipline of epidemiology, which is the investigation of the distribution and determinants of disease within populations. These populations are often referred to as cohorts in epidemiology. Cohort studies examine sequences, patterns of change, growth, or trends over time. By describing the characteristics of groups of people at specific time periods, the researcher attempts to identify risk factors for particular diseases, health conditions, or behaviors.

> **Epidemiology:** The investigation of the distribution and determinants of disease within populations or cohorts.

When the cohort is studied at a single point in time, it is called a cross-sectional study. If data are collected from the cohort at specific time periods over a span of months or years, it is called a longitudinal study.

Cross-Sectional Designs

The cross-sectional design is used to examine simultaneously groups of subjects who are in various stages of development; the intent is to describe differences among them. This type of study is based on the assumption that the stages that are identified in different subjects at the single point in time are representative of a process that progresses over time. For example, a researcher may select subjects who have risk factors but have not yet developed disease, subjects who have the disease in early stages, and subjects who have the disease in chronic form. Other common ways to group subjects are by age or some demographic characteristic. This design is appropriate for describing the characteristics or status of a disease in a population or for describing relationships among risk factors and conditions at a fixed point in time (Crosby, DiClemente, & Salazar, 2006). Cross-sectional designs can be used to infer the association between the characteristics of individuals and their health status. They are also used to answer questions about the way a condition progresses over time when the researcher has access to a population with individuals at various stages of disease or when longitudinal studies are not realistic. Cross-sectional designs are used for samples and by definition involve more than single subjects.

> **Cross-sectional design:** Study conducted by examining a single phenomenon across multiple populations at a single point in time with no intent for follow-up in the design.

Cross-Sectional Study Methods and Procedures

The population of interest is carefully described. The phenomenon under study is captured during one period of data collection. Protocols guide the specific way in which data are collected to minimize bias and enhance the reliability of the data. Variables must be carefully defined and valid measures identified for each variable. Stratified random samples may be used to ensure that individuals who have specific characteristics or who are in various stages of disease are represented in proportion to their prevalence in the general population.

> **gray matter**
>
> Cohort studies examine the following variables:
> - Sequences
> - Patterns of change
> - Growth or trends over time

Case in Point: A Cross-Sectional Design

Tsai and others (2010) used a cross-sectional design to explore the reasons that nurses address alcohol abuse in their patients, and the barriers for them doing so. Excessive alcohol use has been associated with physical and social problems, and healthcare providers often come in contact with them in healthcare settings. Nurses may be in a critical position to suggest interventions for this problem, and yet often do not. By studying all of the 741 nurses at 10 hospitals at a single point in time, these authors were able to determine a range of facilitators and barriers to intervening in cases of alcohol abuse.

The nurses were most comfortable intervening when the disease that caused the hospitalization was related to the alcohol abuse. In addition, nurses were more likely to intervene if they believed their patients' use of alcohol could alter the course of their disease. Most nurses suggested interventions when the patient and/or their family indicated a desire to quit drinking. The most common barrier to intervention was a perception that the patient lacked motivation to change or expressed no interest in receiving an intervention. Nurses often felt unprepared to deal with alcohol addiction issues and lacked knowledge about how to do so. These authors suggested that learning about effective interventions could improve nurses' comfort with providing counseling about alcohol abuse.

This was a typical cross-sectional study in that data were gathered from all of the subjects in a population at a single point in time. One could assume that there were inexperienced and experienced nurses in this sample, and so information was gathered about a range of nurses with a single study.

Source: Tsai, Y., Tsai, M., Lin, Y., Weng, C., Chen, C., & Chen, M. (2010). Facilitators and barriers to intervening for problem alcohol use. *Journal of Advanced Nursing, 66*(7), 1459–1468.

Strengths of Cross-Sectional Studies

The use of a cross-sectional design provides the researcher with many advantages, including the following:

- Cross-sectional designs are practical and economical.
- There is no waiting for the outcome of interest to occur.
- These studies enable the exploration of health conditions that are affected by human development.
- The procedures are reasonably simple to design and carry out.
- Data are collected at one point in time so results can be timely and relevant.
- Large samples are relatively inexpensive to obtain.
- There is no loss of subjects due to study attrition.

Limitations of Cross-Sectional Studies

Although cross-sectional studies have many advantages, some of the drawbacks associated with this design include the following:

- The transitory nature of data collection makes causal association difficult.
- Cross-sectional studies do not capture changes that occur as a result of environmental or other events that occur over time.
- It may be difficult to locate individuals at varying stages of a disease or condition.
- Cross-sectional designs are impractical for the study of rare diseases or uncommon conditions.

Many of these limitations are overcome when a population is studied over time, rather than at a single point in time. Cross-sectional studies are often used as a starting point for a subsequent study carried out over time or as a pilot study for a more complex longitudinal design.

Longitudinal Designs

A longitudinal study follows one or more cohorts over an extended period of time. These designs are powerful ways to assess the effects of risk factors or the consequences of health behaviors. Longitudinal designs may answer questions about the way that characteristics of populations change over time, or they may serve the purpose of quantifying relationships between risk factors and disease. Longitudinal designs are often exploratory, seeking to answer questions about the nature of health conditions at various stages of human development. By their very nature, they are useful in answering questions about the long-term effects of exposures, treatments, or events (Haynes, Sackett, Guyatt, & Tugwell, 2006). This design is often called simply a cohort design, but it may also be known as a panel design. Longitudinal designs by definition involve repeated measures over time taken from a group of subjects.

> Longitudinal study: Study conducted by following subjects over a period of time, with data collection occurring at prescribed intervals.

Longitudinal Study Methods and Procedures

The first step in conducting a longitudinal study is to specify an appropriate population and sampling procedures. An appropriate population is described in detail, and a sample that has adequate power is selected from the population. Power must be determined based not on the number that enter the study but on the number required to complete it because substantial attrition is expected over the extended time periods involved in

---

Case in Point: A Longitudinal Design

The study of body image among breast cancer survivors is hampered by the lack of information about how a woman's idea of self changes over time. Moreira and Canavarro (2010) conducted a longitudinal study of 87 women post-breast cancer to determine how their body image changed over time. Women were asked to complete assessments of self-consciousness, shame, satisfaction with appearance, quality of life, and emotional adjustment immediately after their treatment and six months later.

In general, only shame increased over time. Having a mastectomy was associated with the greatest level of shame and lower satisfaction with appearance. Initial body image did not appear to play a role over time, although pre-existing depression did significantly increase dissatisfaction with appearance.

This study is a typical longitudinal one in that a single population was followed over time to determine symptoms that emerged long-term. This was a bit unusual in that nearly 85% of the sample remained through the study; a much higher rate of attrition is common in longitudinal studies. The authors note that understanding how symptoms play out over time can help the nurse design effective interventions applied early in the patient's course of treatment.

Source: Moreira, H., & Canavarro, M. (2010). A longitudinal study about the body image and psychosocial adjustment of breast cancer patients during the course of the disease. *European Journal of Oncology Nursing, 14*, 263–270.

longitudinal studies. The best longitudinal studies represent the population through random selection, although this is rarely a practical reality. Large samples represent the population best, provide the highest level of confidence in the findings, and compensate for the substantial attrition that is expected in longitudinal studies.

Variables must be clearly identified and valid measures identified for each. Reliable measures are extremely important in longitudinal studies because the data will be collected repeatedly. Both internal consistency and test–retest reliability are key considerations in the choice of instrumentation for longitudinal studies to ensure consistency over time.

Researchers can use two strategies to collect longitudinal data: retrospective or prospective methods. Retrospective studies are used to examine a potential causal relationship that may have already occurred. In a retrospective study, secondary data are used to obtain baseline measurements and information about periodic follow-ups and outcomes of interest. The stages of a retrospective longitudinal study are shown in **FIGURE 12.1**. The researcher performs the following steps:

1. Identifies a suitable cohort that has been evaluated in the past
2. Collects data on the expected causal variables from past records
3. Obtains data about the hypothesized outcome from past or current measures

The data are analyzed to determine if there is a predictive relationship between the past event and the outcome of interest. If a research question is written in past tense, it is generally a retrospective study. Exploratory research questions about causal events can be answered using a retrospective study method. An effective retrospective study is dependent on access to accurate and complete data about a suitable cohort. This may be difficult because retrospective longitudinal studies often rely on data that have been collected for other purposes (Szklo & Nieto, 2000).

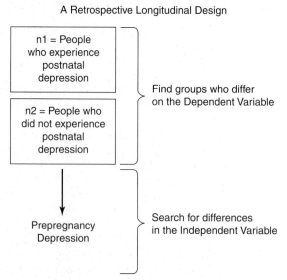

A Retrospective Longitudinal Design

FIGURE 12.1 Stages of a Retrospective Longitudinal Design

Prospective studies answer research questions written in future tense. These are considered the most powerful studies for defining the incidence and investigating the potential causes of a condition (Hulley et al., 2001). Interventions, data collection, and outcomes occur after the subjects are enrolled. The researcher recruits an appropriate cohort and measures characteristics or behaviors that might predict subsequent outcomes. As in retrospective studies, reliability of measures is critical, as are procedures to reduce attrition of subjects. Specific actions should be built into the design to maximize retention of subjects over time, such as computerized tracking systems, convenience of data collection, and periodic reporting of results to subjects (Haynes et al., 2006). The time periods at which data are collected are predetermined and based on a solid rationale. FIGURE 12.2 depicts the stages of a prospective cohort design. The researcher performs the following steps:

1. Recruits a sample from an identified population
2. Measures the hypothesized predictor variables
3. Measures outcomes at predetermined follow-up times

The researcher can expect that a large volume of data will be collected over the life of the study, and so procedures for data management should be considered in study planning.

Strengths of Longitudinal Studies

The use of a longitudinal design provides the researcher with many advantages, including the following:

- Longitudinal studies can capture historical trends and explore causal associations.
- Retrospective longitudinal studies are cost-effective and cost-efficient.

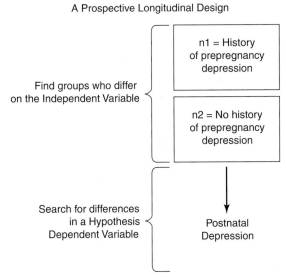

A Prospective Longitudinal Design

Find groups who differ on the Independent Variable
- n1 = History of prepregnancy depression
- n2 = No history of prepregnancy depression

Search for differences in a Hypothesis Dependent Variable
- Postnatal Depression

FIGURE 12.2 Stages of a Prospective Longitudinal Design

- Prospective longitudinal studies can document that a causal factor precedes an outcome, strengthening hypotheses about causality.
- Prospective studies provide the opportunity to measure characteristics and events accurately and do not rely on recall.

Limitations of Longitudinal Studies

Longitudinal studies also have significant limitations:

- The principal disadvantages are attrition rates and the potential loss of subjects over time.
- Retrospective longitudinal studies are dependent on accurate, complete secondary data or the subject's ability to recall past events.
- Once a longitudinal study is begun, it cannot be changed without affecting the overall validity of the conclusions.
- Prospective longitudinal studies are expensive to conduct and require time and commitment from both subjects and researchers.
- Conclusions may be based on a limited number of observations.
- Large sample sizes are expensive to access.
- Systematic attrition of subjects is possible due to the long-term commitment required.

Substantial effort must go into the planning and execution of a longitudinal study—whether retrospective or prospective—to draw valid conclusions about the relationships between variables. Longitudinal studies are quite useful in assessing potential causal relationships, but they are limited in application due to the difficulty of implementing them effectively.

Describing the Responses of Single Subjects

General descriptive designs involve evaluating the characteristics of groups of individuals or the way that whole populations respond to events. These designs result in conclusions about typical or average responses. But typical responses do not tell the nurse how a single, unique individual may respond to a condition or a treatment. The study of a single subject can be an effective means for discovering the ways that individual people react to nursing practices and health conditions.

The purpose of studying single subjects is to assess individuals, with the expectation of generalizing to other individuals in similar situations or conditions. Single-subject designs may answer exploratory questions or serve as pilot tests for later experimental designs. Questions that focus on individual responses to treatments or health conditions over time are well served with single-subject designs. These designs attempt to explore real changes in the individual, which may be obscured in traditional analyses of group comparisons. Single-subject designs reflect what happens in clinical practice because nurses focus on an individual and not a group. A single-subject design may be the only approach possible for answering questions about patients with rare diseases. These designs usually involve data collected over time, and, although they may actually include a small number of subjects, they are by definition not representative of entire populations.

> **Case study:** The meticulous descriptive exploration of a single unit of study such as a person, family group, community, or other entity.

There are two methods for studying individual subjects: case study and single-subject designs. The case study is the meticulous exploration of a single unit of study such as a person, family, group, community, or other entity. It is purely descriptive, relying on a depth of detail to reveal the characteristics and responses of the single case. The single-subject design is essentially an experimental investigation using a single case or single subject. Baseline data are collected, an intervention is applied, and the responses of the individual are tracked over time. In essence, the individual subject is serving as his or her own control.

> **Single-subject design:** An investigation using a single case or subject in which baseline data are collected, an intervention is applied, and the responses are tracked over time.

Case Study Designs

A case study is the thorough assessment of an individual case over time. This assessment may involve observation, interaction, or measurement of variables. When the data collection methods are limited to observation and interviews, the resulting data are expressed in words and the design is qualitative; qualitative designs will be discussed in a later chapter. Often the data that are collected are direct or indirect measures gathered via instrumentation or questionnaires. In this type of study, the data are numbers that are analyzed using quantitative methods. It is not unusual for a case study to involve a mixture of data collection methods that are both qualitative and quantitative. In fact, a characteristic of case study designs is that the number of subjects is small but the number of variables measured is large (Yin, 2002).

Case study designs are effective for answering questions about how individuals respond to treatment or react to health conditions. Questions related to the effects of specific therapeutic measures can be addressed with a case study, and this design is often used to demonstrate the value of a therapy to others in the professional community. The results of case study investigations are often a teaching vehicle; a common method is the use of "grand rounds" to introduce a practice via a demonstrated case. A case study approach can illustrate life-changing events by giving them meaning and creating understanding about the subject's experience. These strategies can result in a great depth of understanding about the phenomenon under study.

A case study is not intended to represent a population but to test theory or demonstrate effectiveness of a practice from a unique and individual perspective. Often, the findings of a case study generate hypotheses that can subsequently be tested in generalizable ways.

Case Study Methods and Procedures

The first step in a case study is obviously to identify an appropriate case. A "case" may be defined in a number of ways. The most common case is an individual, but a case also may be defined as a family, an organization, a county, a department, or any number of other delineations. Case study designs are often the result of opportunity; a unique or unusual case presents itself to the nurse, who takes advantage of the opportunity to conduct an in-depth study over time. Case study designs may also come about through

---

Case in Point: A Case Study

Lineham (2010) provided a reflective account of working with a 16-year-old female with congenital muscular dystrophy. The girl had been removed from her home and was institutionalized; the author cared for her over a one-year period and documented the experience. The author shared an in-depth history of the girl's social and physical challenges. The case included extensive physical assessment results, including lung function and mental health measures. The author provided a detailed description of the subject's transition from pediatric to adult health services and described the interventions that were used by various healthcare providers to help her manage her illness. This in-depth, detailed description of a single case over time is typical of case study research. By establishing a relationship with the subject, the author was able to provide a detailed account of her experience over a lengthy period of time. This author does not overinterpret the findings from this single case, but rather shares insights about caring for this single, unique subject.

Source: Lineham, K. (2010). Caring for young people with chronic illness: A case study. *Paediatric Nursing, 22*(1), 20–23.

---

careful consideration of the criteria that should be present in a subject to test a theory, evaluate an intervention, or appraise responses to a condition over time. Case study designs require commitment on the part of both researcher and subject because these designs are longitudinal, and the subject is followed for a lengthy time period. This extended contact is necessary to draw accurate conclusions about the natural state of the individual (Yin, 2002).

The key variables that are of interest are identified, defined, and captured through appropriate measures. It is important that these measures be stable and reliable over time because they will be applied repeatedly over the life of the study. On initiating the study, the nurse researcher obtains a thorough history so that observations can be compared to previous behaviors and experiences. It is important to study as many variables in the situation as possible to determine which might have an effect on the subject's responses and actions. Large amounts of data are generated, and so a conscientious data management plan is critical in the design of case study procedures. Analysis is time-consuming; it requires meticulous effort and can be difficult. Measured changes must be quantified. In the most thorough case studies, the themes and responses of the individual are reported in a holistic context. This last element is one of the reasons these studies often use a mix of methods.

Strengths of Case Studies

Some of the advantages of using a case study design include the following:

- Case studies can provide in-depth information about the unique nature of individuals.
- Responses and changes that emerge over time can be captured and appraised.
- New insights can be obtained that can potentially generate additional studies.

Limitations of Case Studies

Disadvantages associated with using a case study approach include the following:

- There is no baseline measurement to provide comparison with the intervention outcome.
- It is difficult to determine whether there is an improvement in outcome because causation cannot be inferred.
- Researcher objectivity is required when drawing conclusions because interpretation potentially can be biased.
- Results cannot be generalized to larger populations.

Single-Subject Designs

Single-subject designs are the experimental version of a case study. These designs are used—as are case studies—to evaluate the unique responses of individuals to treatments or conditions. Single-subject designs are unlike case studies in that they are always quantitative in nature and involve distinct phases of data collection. Graphic analysis techniques are used to assess the data and draw conclusions. The organization of a single-subject design is also more structured than a case study in that there is a specific sequence for measuring the baseline, introducing an intervention, and evaluating its effects.

Single-subject designs are effective for answering questions about how a particular therapy will affect a single individual. The patient response to a therapy or nursing practice can be evaluated without involving large-scale experimental designs or recruiting big samples.

Single-Subject Study Methods and Procedures

A single-subject design has three basic requirements:

1. Continuous assessment of the variable of interest
2. Assessment during a baseline period before the intervention
3. Continuing assessment of the responses of the individual after the intervention

The length of the baseline measurement period is unique to each subject; baseline measurements continue until the condition of the patient is stable. Because changes in the subject must be attributable to the intervention instead of random variability, stability in the measured variable is required during the baseline phase before the intervention is initiated. Once the intervention is initiated, measurement continues over an extended period of time to capture trends or patterns that are in response to the intervention (Barlow, Andrasik, & Hersen, 2006).

There are a number of different single-subject case designs, most of which use a baseline phase and an intervention phase known, respectively, as A and B. Measurements are captured repeatedly before and after the intervention. The most common single-subject design is referred to as the "AB" design. In the AB design, a baseline period of measures is captured (A) until the variable of interest stabilizes. Then

gray matter

Single-subject designs include the following requirements:
- Continuous assessment of the variable of interest
- Assessment during a baseline period before the intervention
- Continuing assessment of the responses of the individual after the intervention

Case in Point: A Single-Subject Design

Shaken baby syndrome often results in a variety of health problems, developmental delays, and behavioral issues. Moore et al. (2010) were interested in determining if functional analysis could be used to identify effective interventions for severe problem behavior in a very young child with traumatic brain injury from being shaken. A baby who was severely shaken at 6 months of age by a babysitter was studied over a period of 12 months. The baby was initially in a coma. After awakening, the child had severe irritability, seizures, and behavioral problems, including self-injurious behavior. One such problematic behavior was poking himself in the eye, which threatened his long-term sight. The behavior was measured in 10-second intervals in the child's home by the researchers. After a baseline from several visits was collected, the authors implemented an intervention based on functional assessment and aimed at redirecting the eye-pressing behavior to a socially acceptable form of communication. The authors used an A-B-A reversal design, in which they implemented the intervention, measured a response, withdrew the intervention, measured a response, and then re-introduced the intervention, measuring a final time. The response clearly demonstrated that the intervention reduced the self-injurious behavior to nearly zero, which increased without reinforcement and declined again with re-introduction of treatment.

This design is typical of single-subject designs in that the child served as his own control. In these studies, establishing a stable baseline of behavior is essential so that any changes as a result of the intervention can be detected. The reversal design is particularly strong in that the responses can be linked to presence or absence of the intervention. The extended time to complete the study is also typical, and one reason why these designs are difficult to implement.

Source: Moore, T., Gilles, E., McComas, J., & Symons, F. (2010). Functional analysis and treatment of self-injurious behavior in a young child with traumatic brain injury. *Brain Injury, 24*(12), 1511–1518.

an intervention (B) is introduced and measures are continued for a prescribed period of time. Changes in the subject during the B phase are then considered attributable to the intervention. In other words, the subject serves as his or her own control.

Reversal designs: Single-subject designs that continue to measure the response of the individual as the intervention is withdrawn or withdrawn and reinitiated.

Because single-subject designs suffer from many threats to internal validity, other designs can help mediate these threats. **Reversal designs** continue to measure the individual's responses as the intervention is withdrawn or withdrawn and then reinitiated. The design includes a reversal phase following the intervention. In the reversal phase, the intervention is withdrawn and conditions revert to what they were prior to the intervention. If a trend is identified in which a baseline is established, a change is noted after the intervention, and the change reverts to baseline after the intervention is withdrawn, then the researcher's conclusions about the effects of the intervention are strengthened. These reversal designs may be identified as "ABA" or "ABAB."

The analysis of single-subject data is primarily through visualization and interpretation of the trends and patterns recognized in the subject's data over time. FIGURE 12.3 depicts a single-subject graph that demonstrates an individual's response to treatment.

Strengths of Single-Subject Studies

Single-subject designs have some advantages over population-based studies when evaluating the effects of interventions:

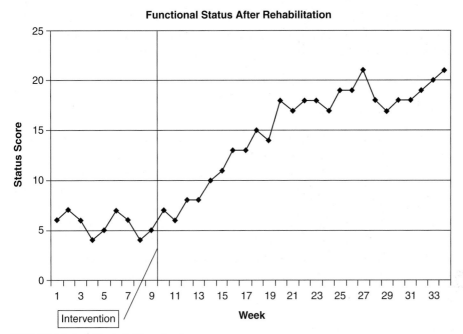

FIGURE 12.3 A Single-Subject Graph

- Single-subject designs are especially useful in exploring behavioral responses to treatment that might affect a patient's preferences and compliance.
- The unique responses of individuals can help the nurse determine whether a particular therapy will be effective for a specific kind of patient.
- These designs are flexible and involve multiple variations that may answer an assortment of questions.
- Single-subject designs explore real changes in the individual and can simultaneously serve as feedback about progress for the patient.
- Single-subject designs are easier to implement than longitudinal designs that require large samples.

Limitations of Single-Subject Studies

Although single-subject designs have many advantages, they also have significant limitations:

- Single-subject designs are not generalizable to larger populations.
- Single-subject designs are not considered sufficient evidence for a practice change.
- Both researcher and subject must be committed to measures over time.
- The subject must be informed about the risks and benefits of treatment, and the experiment must have ethical review equal to that of a larger study (Logan, Hickman, Harris, & Heriza, 2008).

Even with these limitations, single-subject designs are important in nursing research. Although nursing practice often affects the health of entire populations, it is also a profession that deals with people at their most vulnerable—people who need to be treated as the individuals they are. Understanding their distinctive responses, needs, and conditions can help the nurse identify evidence for practice that is relevant from both a scientific and a humanistic perspective.

Designs that Describe Relationships

By definition, descriptive research studies are focused on describing conditions as they exist. Many descriptive studies focus on a single characteristic, phenomenon, or group of variables. This does not, however, preclude describing the relationships between variables. Descriptive designs may be used to examine the relationships between variables in a single population or the relationship of a single variable among several populations. When these relationships are described in a quantitative way, this is referred to as a correlation study.

Correlation study: Designs that involve the analysis of two variables to describe the strength and direction of the relationship between them.
Prediction study: Research designed to search for variables measured at one point in time that may forecast an outcome that is measured at a different point in time.
Tests of model fit: Tests of association used to determine whether a set of relationships fits in the real world in the way the relationships are hypothesized in the researcher's model of reality.

Correlation studies may simply examine relationships among variables, or they may focus on the use of one variable to predict another. The latter type of study is called a prediction study. Tests of relationship or association may also be used to determine whether a theoretical model fits reality. In other words, does a set of relationships exist in the real world in the way they are hypothesized in a researcher's model of reality? These are the most complex descriptive designs and often blur the line between descriptive and causal studies. In fact, these tests of model fit are often described as "causal models." Correlation and prediction studies are quite common in nursing research, and they are valuable approaches for generating evidence for practice. Tests of model fit are less common due to their complex nature and the need for large samples.

Descriptive Correlation Designs

Correlation studies are used to answer questions about relationships or associations. Correlation studies attempt to describe the strength and nature of the relationship between two variables without clarifying the underlying causes of that relationship. These designs cannot lead to a conclusion of causality, but they are still quite helpful in nursing research. Correlation methods may be used to explore relationships to determine hypotheses and to discover associations in a data set; these studies are often precursors to experimental or quasi-experimental designs (Woods & Kerr, 2006).

Most commonly, a correlation study is used to quantify the relationship between two variables in a single data set; for example, a correlation study might be used to establish if there is a relationship between waiting room time and patient satisfaction. Correlation can also be used to determine if there is an association between a single variable in two populations; for example, a correlation study would be appropriate to determine if there is a relationship between satisfaction scores of patients and their families. In either case, the design involves selection of an appropriate sample, measuring variables in a reliable and valid way, and analyzing the results using the correlation coefficient.

Correlation Study Methods and Procedures

A correlation study is relatively simple to conduct. Criteria are developed that guide selection of the sample, and then the variables of interest are measured. In a correlation design, it is particularly important to have a representative sample, so random samples are superior to convenience samples. To obtain a true reflection of the variables being measured, large samples are needed. Relying on small samples may result in limitation in the size of a correlation coefficient, underestimating the strength of the relationship.

Data collection may be prospective or retrospective. Prospective data collection gives the researcher greater control over the reliability and validity of measures, but it can be difficult and costly to implement. Retrospective data collection from secondary sources is efficient, but the data may not be reliable or the data may only approximate the variables of interest. Determining whether to collect data prospectively or to gather it from secondary sources requires the researcher to consider the balance between validity and efficiency.

Strengths of Correlation Studies

Correlation studies are common in nursing research because they have significant advantages:

- Correlation studies are relatively uncomplicated to plan and implement.
- The researcher has flexibility in exploring relationships among two or more variables.

Case in Point: A Correlation Design

Palhares and others (2010) used a correlation design to determine if there was a relationship between quality of life and left ventricular cardiac function, which is an underlying element of hypertension. A measure of health-related quality of life was administered to 98 patients with hypertension. Left ventricular function was measured by echocardiogram. The patients were split into two groups based on the presence or absence of dyspnea, and correlations were measured across both groups.

Correlations were statistically significant but weak for quality of life and left ventricular function; the r value was –.22. However, when those with dyspnea were considered separately, the correlation between left ventricular function and quality of life was moderately strong (0.50) as well as significant.

This correlation study was typical of these designs in that a limited number of variables were measured and the relationship among them determined. These correlations were examples of weak and moderately strong correlations that were both statistically significant; it is up to the reader to determine if these findings are clinically important. The authors do not overinterpret the relationship as a causal one, but do note that this exploratory study would suggest that further study is warranted.

Source: Palhares, L., Gallani, M., Gemignani, T., Matos-Souza, J., Ubaid-Girioli, U., Moreno, H., et al. (2010). Quality of life, dyspnea, and ventricular function in patients with hypertension. *Journal of Advanced Nursing, 66*(10), 2287–2296.

- The outcomes of correlation studies often have practical application in nursing practice.
- Correlation studies provide a framework for examining relationships between variables that cannot be manipulated for practical or ethical reasons.

Limitations of Correlation Studies

Correlation studies have some distinct limitations that have implications for their use as evidence for practice:

> **Suppressor variable:** A variable that is not measured but is related to each variable in the relationship and may affect the correlation of the data.

- The researcher cannot manipulate variables of interest, so causality cannot be established.
- Correlation designs lack control and randomization between the variables, so rival explanations may be posed for relationships.
- The correlation that is measured may be the result of a suppressor variable: one that is not measured but is related to each variable in the relationship.

> **Spurious relationship:** A condition in which two variables have an appearance of causality where none exists. This link is invalid when objectively examined.

This last limitation is one of the most significant; demonstration of a correlation is not evidence of anything other than a linear association between two variables. Researchers often make the mistake of attempting to establish causality through a correlation study, reasoning that if two variables are related, one must have an effect on the other. Correlation studies only reveal if there is a relationship between two variables; these studies cannot reveal which variables occurred first and cannot isolate the effects of one variable on another—both conditions are required for causality. For example, there is a correlation between the malnutrition level of children and the time they spend in the Head Start program. Does this mean spending time in Head Start causes malnutrition? Of course not; this relationship is a reflection of a spurious relationship. In other words, some third variable—in this case, poverty—is the likely source of causality of both variables, giving the appearance of causality where none exists.

Despite their limitations, correlation designs are common and quite useful for clinical research studies. They offer a realistic set of options for researchers because many of the phenomena of clinical practice cannot be manipulated, controlled, or randomized. When applied and interpreted appropriately, correlation designs can provide a solid basis for further experimental testing. Although correlation cannot be used to determine causality, it can serve as the foundation for designs about prediction. In other words, if one variable is associated with an outcome in a consistent way, is it possible to predict the outcome if given a value for the variable? Answering this question is quite useful as evidence for practice and is the basis for a specific type of descriptive design called a predictive study.

Predictive Designs

Predictive designs attempt to explore what factors may influence an outcome. These studies may be used when a researcher is interested in determining whether knowing a previously documented characteristic (or set of characteristics) can lead to the prediction of a later characteristic (or set of characteristics). Predictive studies are sometimes called regression studies, based on the statistical test that is used for analysis.

Predictive studies are useful for questions that concern the ability to predict a given outcome with single or multiple predictor variables. These studies are tremendously useful in nursing practice because their results can be used to identify early indicators of complications, disease, or other negative outcomes so that preventive actions can be taken. Specific statistics that are generated from these studies can be used to predict an outcome for a single individual, given some specific data collected about that individual. The tests used in predictive studies yield a statistic that enables the researcher to determine how well the predictive model works in explaining the outcome. Predictive studies can also be used to establish the predictive validity of measurement scales. Therefore, predictive study methods are suitable for use with a variety of clinical questions.

gray matter

Correlation designs are useful and realistic for clinical research studies because

- These methods can be used to study phenomena or clinical practices that cannot be manipulated, controlled, or randomized.
- Data can provide a solid base for further experimental testing.
- Results can serve as the foundation for designs about prediction.

Predictive Study Methods and Procedures

Predictive studies are very similar in design to correlation studies. The population is clearly identified, variables are defined, measures are captured with reliable and valid tools, and the data are analyzed and interpreted appropriately. The primary distinction between correlation and predictive designs is the type of analytic tool applied to the data and the interpretation of the outcome. Predictive designs are analyzed using regression analysis, which tests the predictive model for statistical significance and for explanatory capacity. Predictive studies are also distinct from correlation studies in that multiple predictors may be tested against a single numerical outcome, and these predictors may be a mix of ordinal- and interval-level measures. Even nominal data may be used

Case in Point: A Predictive Study

Patients with heart failure often have trouble sleeping; lying supine produces distressing symptoms, and staying asleep is reportedly difficult as well. These sleep disturbances often affect a patient's quality of life. Wang, Lee, Tsay, and Tung (2010) used a predictive design to describe the factors that influence sleep quality in patients with congestive heart failure.

Patients with heart failure were recruited for the study, and 101 completed a questionnaire about their sleep quality and other demographic characteristics. More than 80% reported poor sleep quality. The most common reason for sleep disturbance was the need to urinate during the night. Using a regression model, these authors were able to identify the most common predictors of sleep problems: gender, perception of overall health, depression, and the number of co-morbid conditions. These four variables explained nearly a third of the variability in sleep disturbances.

This study was a typical predictive model in that a range of variables was measured for each subject, and statistical techniques were used to determine the best predictors. The authors note that further study of these elements could lead to early detection and the development of effective interventions to manage these sleep problems.

Source: Wang, T., Lee, S., Tsay, S., & Tung, H. (2010). Factors influencing heart failure patients' sleep quality. *Journal of Advanced Nursing, 66*(8), 1730–1740.

if it is specially treated and coded in the analysis procedure. This makes the predictive study one of the most useful designs for clinical practice.

Strengths of Predictive Studies

Predictive studies are quite useful as evidence for nursing practice because they have significant advantages:

- A great deal of information is yielded from a single set of data.
- The results of the study can provide information about whole samples or can be applied to individual cases.
- A variety of levels of measurement may be used in the predictive model.
- The studies are relatively simple to design and implement, and they are cost-effective.
- The data that are used may be prospective or retrospective.

Limitations of Predictive Studies

Despite their significant strengths, predictive studies have several drawbacks that researchers must consider when applying them as evidence for nursing practice:

- Although prediction can be quantified, there is no assurance of causality; suppressor variables may exist.
- The researcher may "go fishing," or explore large numbers of variables without a rational hypothesis, resulting in an increased error rate.
- Regression analysis requires relatively large sample sizes, the need for which amplifies as the number of variables increases.

Predictive studies have the advantage of helping nurses identify patients at risk for subsequent health problems so that preventive strategies can be implemented. Predictive studies can quantify the relationships between variables and outcomes and so are very useful as evidence for nursing practice. When multiple predictors and outcomes are suspected, the nurse researcher may hypothesize an overall model or a picture of relationships and interrelationships between variables. These models can be evaluated using descriptive methods and procedures, and they are some of the most sophisticated descriptive studies used as evidence for practice.

Model-Testing Designs

An extension of predictive designs is the model-testing design. Although predictive designs quantify the relationship of a predictor and an outcome, model-testing designs quantify the accuracy of a hypothesized model of relationships and interrelationships. Model testing is the process of hypothesizing how various elements in the patient care environment interact, how these elements can be measured, and the paths of direct and indirect effects from variables to outcomes. The model-testing design requires that all variables relevant to the model be identified and measured. It requires a large sample size and very precise measurement of variables. It is necessary to identify all paths expressing relationships and to develop a conceptual map (Newman, Vance, & Moneyham, 2010). The analysis examines whether the data are consistent with the model. Model-testing designs represent the complexity of patient care realistically and thoroughly. **FIGURE 12.4** demonstrates an example of a model representing environmental demands on the nurse.

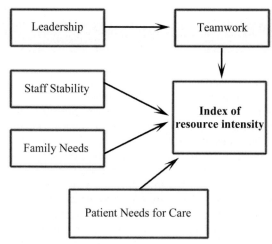

FIGURE 12.4 A Test of Model Fit

Model-testing designs are quite complicated to plan and implement, and analysis requires specialized software. The interpretation of model-testing designs requires substantial statistical expertise, and very large samples are required to achieve adequate power. For these reasons, they are not commonly used research methods for nursing evidence. Model-testing designs are complex designs for testing hypotheses about complex relationships in the patient care environment.

Reading Descriptive Research

The first step in the critique of the methods and procedures of a descriptive study is to determine the specific type of design used in the study. The design is usually specified generically as "descriptive" in the abstract and introduction of the study, and the specific type of descriptive design may appear there as well. If sufficient detail is not given in the early parts of the research report to determine the specifics of the descriptive design, the particulars should be provided in the methods and procedures section. Enough detail should be provided that the reader can judge the researcher's decisions related to the specific design that was chosen. The type of design should answer the research question and meet the intent of the researchers. A rationale for selection of the specific type of study for this question is helpful; there should be a clear link between the purpose of the study and the type of design used to achieve it.

If detail about the type of study is lacking, then the reader may need to closely examine the article for evidence of the type of design that was employed. Clues to the specific design may be present in the research question or objectives. Words such as *describe*, *explore*, *observe*, or *document* may indicate that a straightforward descriptive design was used. When individuals are referred to in the question, the study is likely a case study or single-subject design; these are always descriptive and are not considered experimental designs (regardless of how the author describes the design). If the research question uses

Where to Look for Information About Descriptive Methods

- A descriptive study is usually explicitly identified as such in the abstract and early in the introduction of the article. It should be described early enough that the reader can evaluate the information that follows in the context of a descriptive study. If it is not in the introduction, then it should appear in the first paragraph of the methods and procedures section.
- The specification of the descriptive design should be easily identifiable and a major part of the research study write-up. The explanation may be concise, but it should have enough detail that an informed reader could replicate the study.
- The specific type of descriptive design (for example, cross-sectional, correlation, or single subject) should be detailed in the methods and procedures section, even if the study has been identified generically as descriptive earlier in the study.

- Research reports may not explicitly portray a study as retrospective, even though these designs are very common in nursing research. On the other hand, a researcher will generally be explicit if a prospective study was accomplished. The reader has to scrutinize the data collection procedure to determine if any of the variables were collected from secondary sources. Look for words such as *ex post facto*, which is commonly used to describe retrospective designs.
- If the measurement process is complex, there may be a separate section for procedures, which may be labeled as such, or called "protocols." This section may describe variables in detail as well as the measurement procedures.

words such as *relationship*, *association*, *prediction*, or *test for fit*, then a correlation design is likely. The design should have a clear link to the research question, and the specifics of the methods and procedures should match both the question and the stated design.

Other clues can be deduced from the description of the sources of data and the measurement procedures. If the only statistics that are reported are descriptive (e.g., mean, median, standard deviation), correlation (e.g., correlation coefficient, Pearson, rho), or for regression (e.g., r-squared, beta), then the study is descriptive, regardless of the author's designation. If the protocol for measurement involves record retrieval, abstracting data from patient charts, or access to databases, then the design is almost certainly retrospective. If the protocol calls for recruiting subjects, then the study is prospective. Scrutinize measures for documentation of the timing of data collection. Collecting data at a single point in time clearly means the study is a general descriptive, correlation, or cross-sectional study. References to periodic data collection mean the study is either a case study, single-subject design, or a longitudinal one. Predictive studies may be of either type; it is not uncommon for researchers to collect predictor variables at a single point in time and outcome variables at some future point in time. These studies, however, are revealed by their almost exclusive reliance on regression analytic techniques, so they should be identifiable from the type of statistics that are reported.

Although space restrictions in journals may limit the amount of information the researcher can provide about the study methods and procedures, a reasonably informed researcher should be able to replicate the study from the information provided. A descriptive study—although considered a basic design—should still demonstrate a systematic

Checklist for Evaluation of Descriptive Methods and Procedures

✔ The design is identified as descriptive in the abstract and/or the introduction.
✔ The specific type of descriptive design is specified in the methods and procedures section.
✔ There is a clear and appropriate link between the research question and the descriptive design.
✔ The rationale for selection of a descriptive study is specific and appropriate.
✔ The primary variables of interest are clearly identified and defined.
✔ The interpretation and conclusions are congruent with description and do not imply causality.
✔ If the study is longitudinal, a rationale is provided for the timing of data collection.

and rigorous approach to implementation. The population of interest should be defined, with inclusion and exclusion criteria specified for sample eligibility. Methods for recruiting and/or selecting subjects should be clear and unbiased; the reader needs to be watchful for signs of researcher bias or selection effects. Confidence in the conclusions of the researchers and the capacity for generalizability are both dependent on a strong sampling strategy.

Scrutinize the measurement procedure to ensure that reliable and valid instruments were used to collect the data. The type of reliability that is documented should be specific to the descriptive design. For example, cross-sectional measures should have strong internal reliability because consistency across subjects is most important. Conversely, test–retest reliability is a bigger concern in longitudinal studies because stability over time is critical for drawing valid conclusions. If data are collected retrospectively, look for operational definitions that ensure consistency in data retrieval. Mention should be made of training for data collectors and checks for interrater reliability if multiple data collectors were involved.

Finally, examine the conclusions section to ensure that the authors do not over-interpret or make inferences that go beyond what the results can support. Descriptive studies, at their most fundamental, can only describe. Descriptive studies may suggest or imply causal relationships, but no descriptive study can confirm a causal relationship. This is particularly tempting for the authors of correlation studies. This reasoning is understandable: If two variables are strongly related, then it is enticing to conclude that one affects or causes the other. But without the controls that are inherent in an experimental design, and without a randomly chosen comparison group, it is impossible to confirm all the conditions necessary for causality. The correlation documents the strength of a relationship, not which came first. Correlation studies do not allow the researcher to rule out rival explanations for the relationship through the control of internal validity. A correlation between two variables may represent the mutual effects of some completely different variable.

Descriptive studies are some of the most common research studies undertaken. With the preceding cautions in mind, they can be some of the most useful research studies for providing evidence for nursing

gray matter

Though not considered the strongest evidence for a change in nursing practice, findings from descriptive studies can be used to support the following:

- Assessment of patients and patient care
- Diagnosis of patient care conditions
- Care planning
- Nursing interventions
- Evaluation of outcomes

practice. An understanding of the patient care situation as it exists can help the nurse plan strategies that meet existing needs with a high likelihood of acceptance. Knowing what is can be a powerful means for creating innovative solutions to achieve what can be.

Using Descriptive Research in Evidence-Based Nursing Practice

Descriptive research is not considered strong evidence for a change in nursing practice. Without the controls provided by experimental designs and control groups, these types of studies cannot provide strong conclusions about causality—a condition necessary for support of a nursing intervention. On the other hand, evidence-based practice in nursing relies on expert judgment and an understanding of patient preferences to design appropriate and acceptable interventions, and this is where descriptive research provides a great deal of value. Evidence-based research in nursing practice uses research findings to guide decisions about actions, interventions, and policies in a number of ways.

There are many uses for descriptive evidence in nursing practice: Assessment, diagnosis, care planning, intervention, and evaluation of outcomes all rely on accurate description of phenomena, patient responses to care and conditions, and the acceptability of treatments.

Assessment of Patients and Patient Care

Descriptive studies can help the nurse determine the distribution of risk factors and disease in the populations of interest to his or her specific practice. Of particular value is assessment of the signs and symptoms that patients exhibit as they react to treatments or respond to their health conditions. Predictive studies in particular can help the nurse identify early signals that a patient may be at risk for a health condition or complication, so that preventive steps can be initiated. Case studies and single-subject designs aid the nurse in understanding how individual patients may respond to treatment and clarify the unique aspects of individuals that may affect their response to an intervention.

Diagnosis of Patient Care Conditions

Descriptive studies familiarize the nurse with the kinds of conditions that may present in a particular patient population, so he or she can achieve more accurate diagnoses of their nursing conditions. Cross-sectional and longitudinal studies help document the health needs of populations; model tests may also illuminate the relationship between conditions and nursing diagnoses.

Care Planning

Thorough description of the health needs of populations and the responses of individuals to care can help the nurse plan strategies to meet their needs. Descriptive studies are particularly helpful in the design of effective patient teaching plans and health promotion activities. Individual compliance with a teaching plan is dependent on the patient's acceptance of the need for change and willingness to incorporate new behaviors into his or her life. Understanding the ways that individuals respond to health conditions can help the nurse design plans that meet each patient's goals more effectively.

Interventions

Descriptive studies facilitate interventions that are acceptable to patients and encourage compliance. A descriptive study can also detail the difficulties a nurse might have in implementing an intervention or the barriers that exist in changing a current practice. Case studies are particularly helpful in identifying the processes a nurse might use to implement a change in evidence-based practices or how a nurse was successful in helping an individual deal with his or her health conditions.

Evaluation of Outcomes

Descriptive studies help the nurse identify the outcomes that are reasonable and appropriate to evaluate after a treatment has been initiated or a health condition identified. Evaluating patient outcomes based solely on nursing actions and interventions is difficult to quantify because other care providers are also performing treatments and interventions (Polit & Beck, 2009).

Nurses make decisions that have important implications for patient outcomes. Understanding the health problems of populations, the responses of individuals to health treatments and conditions, and the processes nurses may use to initiate change are key considerations in evidence-based nursing practice. The diversity of descriptive research is matched only by its usefulness. The nurse is well served by reviewing descriptive research prior to planning interventions to maximize the probability that actions will be effective, efficient, and acceptable to those who are served by them. Descriptive research findings enhance both nursing practice and the patient experience.

Creating Descriptive Research

Descriptive designs are common in nursing research and are some of the most easily implemented studies. As such, they are appropriate for novice researchers in both academic and clinical settings. The information generated by a descriptive study can support evidence-based nursing practice—but only if it is generated by rigorous studies that produce valid, credible results. "Descriptive" is not necessarily synonymous with "simple," and it is certainly not equal to "careless." Thoughtful consideration of the elements central to study design is needed before beginning a descriptive/correlation research study. A systematic series of decisions must be made to design a strong descriptive study.

- Clarify the purpose of the study and carefully construct a research question. It should be easy to provide a rationale for the selection of a descriptive study based on the purpose statement and the wording of the research question.
- Identify a design that will answer the question in the most efficient, effective way. The specifics of the design should be the result of careful consideration of both the strengths and limitations of the design, as well as the skills and resources of the researcher.

A Note About Pilot Studies

A pilot study is an intentionally smaller version of a study, with a limited sample size or group of measures. Its primary purpose is to test the methods and procedures of a study prior to full implementation. The processes used for research are often complex and require testing with small samples so that mistakes, errors, and inefficiencies can be corrected prior to the use of large samples.

A pilot study can assess costs, time, efficiency, and accuracy on a smaller scale. Pilot studies are likewise used to test instrumentation for reliability and validity or data collection procedures for difficulties leading to inconsistencies. Grant-making agencies prefer to see studies that have been fully or partially tested on a pilot level because it provides a level of assurance that the researcher can accomplish the research plan.

Although a pilot study is ideally a prospective part of the research plan, some researchers may wind up describing their study as a pilot because of an unacceptable response rate, a sample size with insufficient power, or a measurement that could not be verified as reliable. In this case, the author may "live and learn" from the study by using it as a case study, in effect, to plan a more effective set of research processes.

- Describe the population of interest, and determine inclusion and exclusion criteria for the sample. Devise a sampling strategy that maximizes the representativeness of the population and supports the external validity of the findings.
- Clarify the variables of interest and write operational definitions for each before selecting measurement instruments. If there are multiple raters, create a data dictionary so all the data collectors understand what each variable represents. Use the operational definitions to identify the appropriate measurement tools, not the other way around.
- Determine a measurement procedure that will generate trustworthy data. If instruments or tools are to be used, ensure that they possess the appropriate psychometric properties for the specific study design that is proposed.
- Manage the data collection process carefully. Methods should be incorporated that will ensure reliability among raters, whether they are retrieving data from records or gathering them directly from subjects. This often includes training and observation for reliability before data collectors function independently.
- Design a process for maintaining the integrity of the data set. Specific measures should be planned for restricting access and ensuring confidentiality, such as password-protected files and locked file cabinets. Incorporate periodic quality checks into the data management process.
- Use the appropriate analytic tools for the question to be answered and the types of data that are collected. Consider the level of measurement of each variable in selecting the specific statistical treatment.
- Report the analysis accurately and completely; report each test that was run, even if it did not contribute to the overall outcome of the study. This reduces the potential for selective retention of findings—a threat to validity of the study.

CRITICAL APPRAISAL EXERCISE

Retrieve the following full text article from the Cumulative Index to Nursing and Allied Health Literature or similar search database:

Hardin, S., Bernhardt-Tindal, K., Hart, A., & Henson, A. (2011). Critical-care visitations: The patients' perspective. *Dimensions of Critical Care Nursing, 30*(1), 53–61.

Review the article, focusing on the sections that report the question, design, methods, and procedures. Consider the following appraisal questions in your critical review of this research article:

1. Is the research question made explicit early in the paper? Is there a clear link between the question and the purpose of the study?
2. What elements of this question and purpose make this study appropriate for a descriptive design?
3. What is the specific descriptive design used by these authors? Is it appropriately linked to the question?
4. Was the sample adequate for the descriptive design that was selected?
5. What efforts were made to ensure reliable, valid measures (for example, operational definitions of variables, using instruments with low error)?
6. What are the strengths of the design, methods, and procedures of this study? Contrast them with its limitations.
7. How could this study be incorporated into evidence-based practice?

- Draw conclusions that are appropriate for the intent of the study and the results that were found. Although it is acceptable to note relationships that are suggested or implied by the data—and certainly to pose additional hypotheses that should be tested—descriptive studies can only describe.

Developing a design for a study will require attention to each of these elements. The fact that a descriptive design is common and basic should not lead one to the conclusion that it can be accomplished without a great deal of forethought and planning. Considering these details will result in a stronger study.

Summary of Key Concepts

- The purpose of descriptive research is the exploration and description of phenomena in real life situations.
- Descriptive research designs are used in studies that construct a picture or make an account of events as they naturally occur; the investigator does not manipulate variables.
- A descriptive design can be used to develop theory, identify problems, provide information for decision making, or determine what others in similar situations are doing.
- Two basic types of questions are addressed with descriptive designs: general descriptive questions and questions about relationships.

- Additional ways to classify descriptive studies are according to whether they involve groups of subjects or individuals and whether data are collected at a point in time or periodically over time.
- Retrospective studies rely on secondary data that have been collected in the past, often for other purposes; prospective studies involve data collection in the future for the express purpose of the study.
- Survey research involves collecting data directly from respondents about their characteristics, responses, attitudes, perceptions, or beliefs.
- Cross-sectional studies describe a population at a single point in time; longitudinal studies follow a cohort of subjects over an extended period of time.
- Descriptive designs can be used to measure the responses of unique individuals, either through case study or single-subject designs.
- Correlation studies examine relationships as they exist or may use variables to predict outcomes. Correlation studies may also test models for their fit with reality.
- Descriptive research does not enable the investigator to establish cause and effect between variables, but these studies are still valuable as evidence for assessment, diagnosis, care planning, interventions, and evaluation.

For a full suite of assignments and additional learning activities, use the access code located in the front of your book to visit this exclusive website: http://go.jblearning .com/houser. If you do not have an access code, you can obtain one at the site.

References

Barlow, D., Andrasik, F., & Hersen, M. (2006). *Single case experimental design* (3rd ed.). Boston: Allyn and Bacon.

Brown, S.J. (2009). *Evidence-based nursing.* Sudbury, MA: Jones & Bartlett.

Burns, N., & Grove, S.K. (2008). *The practice of nursing research: Appraisal, synthesis, and generation of evidence* (6th ed.). St. Louis: Elsevier Saunders.

Crosby, R., DiClemente, R., & Salazar, L. (2006). *Research methods in health promotion.* San Francisco: Jossey-Bass.

Haynes, R., Sackett, D., Guyatt, G., & Tugwell, P. (2006). *Clinical epidemiology: How to do clinical practice research* (3rd ed.). Philadelphia: Lippincott Williams & Wilkins.

Houser, J., & Bokovoy, J. (2006). *Clinical research in practice. A guide for the bedside scientist.* Sudbury, MA: Jones & Bartlett.

Hulley, S., Cummings, S., Browner, W., Grady, D., Hearst, N., & Newman, T. (2001). *Designing clinical research* (2nd ed.). Philadelphia: Lippincott Williams & Wilkins.

Logan, L., Hickman, R., Harris, S., & Heriza, C. (2008). Single-subject research design: Recommendations for levels of evidence and quality rating. *Developmental Medicine and Child Neurology, 50,* 99–103.

Newman, K., Vance, D., & Moneyham, L. (2010). Interpreting evidence from structural equation modeling in nursing practice. *Journal of Research in Nursing, 15*(3), 275–284.

Polit, D., & Beck, C. (2009). *Essentials of nursing research: Appraising evidence for nursing practice* (7th ed.). Philadelphia: Wolters Kluwer Health/Lippincott Williams & Wilkins.

Sapsford, R. (2006). *Survey research.* Thousand Oaks, CA: Sage.

Szklo, M., & Nieto, F. (2000). *Epidemiology: Beyond the basics.* Gaithersburg, MD: Aspen Publications.

Woods, M., & Kerr, J. (2006). *Basic steps in planning nursing research from question to proposal* (6th ed.). Sudbury, MA: Jones & Bartlett.

Yin, R. (2002). *Case study research: Design and methods.* Thousand Oaks, CA: Sage.

chapter *13*

Summarizing and Reporting Descriptive Data

 CHAPTER OBJECTIVES

The study of this chapter will help the learner to:

- Interpret descriptive data when summarized as measures of central tendency, variability, and correlation.
- Use graphical presentations of descriptive data to understand research data.
- Critique the appropriateness of statistics used to summarize descriptive data.
- Select appropriate statistical techniques to summarize and present descriptive data.

KEY TERMS

Bar chart	Histogram	Rate
Box plot	Line graph	Scatter plot
Coefficient of variation (CV)	Mean	Standard deviation
Correlation analysis	Median	Standardized score
Derived variable	Mode	Standard normal distribution
Descriptive data	Range	Variance
Frequency		

Introduction

Summarizing descriptive data is the first step in the analysis of quantitative research data. Because it is the first step, other steps depend on its careful completion. When descriptive data are summarized correctly, they provide useful information about participants in the sample, their answers to survey questions, and their responses to study inquiries.

> **Descriptive data:** Numbers in a data set that are collected to represent research variables.

311

❝❝ Scenes from the Field ❞❞

The lack of privacy in the emergency department is the subject of many a joke. A combination of factors—hospital gowns with scant coverage, curtains instead of doors between beds, hallway consultations over care—may mean this particular stereotype is real. Two nurses measured patient perceptions of privacy in three busy emergency departments. Their findings indicate that most patients feel their privacy is violated while in emergency care.

Questionnaire data were collected from more than 360 patients over various dates and shifts. One section of the questionnaire focused on demographic characteristics, one section focused on privacy and personal space, and a final section was related to satisfaction. All of the privacy and satisfaction data were collected via a four-point Likert scale. The demographic data were a mix of interval (e.g., age) and nominal variables (e.g., ethnicity).

The demographic characteristics were reported in a table. Only two of the variables were interval (age and length of hospitalization), and these were represented by the mean and standard deviation. The remaining demographic variables were categorical and were reported with both the number of occurrences and their relative percentage.

All of the Likert scale responses were ordinal, and so were reported by response. In other words, the percentage reporting "high" was depicted in a table next to the number reporting "average" and "low." The authors, appropriately, did not report means for these ordinal data. The final table showed the correlation between each aspect of privacy and patient satisfaction. For these correlations, the r values and p values were reported. The presentation of the data in tables made it easy to pick out the final results and how they related to each of the other variables.

It is not surprising that most of the respondents did not feel their privacy was respected while in the emergency department. The element of privacy most violated was "informational," followed by "physical" and "psychosocial." There was a strong (more than 0.7) and statistically significant relationship between the perceptions about privacy and patient satisfaction.

These authors note that the data suggest that a demonstrated respect for privacy may help improve the satisfaction of patients. Addressing this issue from a clinical and practical standpoint is the challenge.

Source: Nayeri, N., & Aghajani, M. (2010). Patients' privacy and satisfaction in the emergency department: A descriptive analytical study. *Nursing Ethics, 17*(2), 167–177.

Analysis of descriptive data entails the use of simple mathematical procedures or calculations, many of which are straightforward enough to be done with a calculator. Yet, these simple numerical techniques provide essential information in a research study. When it comes to descriptive analysis, readers of research have different needs than do those who conduct research studies. The purposes of summarizing descriptive data for readers of research include the following:

- Giving the reader a quick grasp of the characteristics of the sample and the variables in the study

- Providing basic information on how variables in a study are alike (measures of central tendency) and how they are different (measures of variability)
- Conveying information about the study in numerical and graphical methods to enhance understanding of the findings (Lang & Secic, 2003)

The purposes of summarizing descriptive data for researchers include the following:

- Reviewing the data set using frequency tables to check for coding or data entry errors
- Visualizing the descriptive data, particularly the shape of distributions, to determine if statistical assumptions are met for the selection of appropriate statistical analysis
- Understanding the characteristics of the participants in the study and their performance on variables of interest in the study
- Gaining an in-depth understanding of the data before inferential analysis

In quantitative research, a summary of descriptive data can be accomplished using statistical techniques such as measures of central tendency, variance, frequency distributions, and correlation. These statistics provide a method to summarize large amounts of data from a research study into meaningful numbers.

Care must be taken by researchers who create descriptive reports; correct statistical techniques must be selected for the data that have been collected. The level of measurement of a variable is a primary consideration when deciding which statistical technique to use to summarize descriptive data. In addition, the report of descriptive data needs to be presented in the most meaningful way—in other words, in a way that readers comprehend and cannot easily misunderstand. The same principles apply to nurses who use statistical techniques to summarize descriptive data in the clinical setting—descriptive data must be analyzed appropriately and reported in meaningful ways to others in the clinical setting.

When reading the analysis of descriptive data, the appropriateness of the statistical technique should be appraised. Even more critical, the summarization of the data and the nurse researcher's interpretation of the data are critiqued by the reader to determine confidence in the findings.

An Overview of Descriptive Data Analysis

Statistical analysis of descriptive data is conducted to provide a summary of data in published research reports. Descriptive data are numbers in a data set that are collected to represent research variables and do not involve generalization to a larger set of data such as the population. For example, a data set could contain variables including ages of participants, years of experience as a nurse, and scores on a job satisfaction instrument. These data could be analyzed for the purpose of summarizing information about this sample—not comparing groups within a study to infer findings to the population. Simply put, descriptive statistics use numbers or graphic displays to organize and describe the characteristics of a sample (Fisher & Marshall, 2008).

Descriptive statistics involve a range of complexity, from simple counts of data to analyses of relationships. The most common descriptive statistics are classified in the following ways:

- Counts of data, expressed as frequencies, frequency tables, and frequency distributions
- Measures of central tendency, expressed as the mean, median, and mode
- Measures of variability, including the range, variance, and standard deviation
- Measures of position, such as percentile ranks and standardized scores
- Graphical presentations in bar charts, line graphs, and scatter plots

The specific types of summary statistics that are applied to descriptive data are driven by the nature of the data and the level of measurement of the variable. It is important to apply as many descriptive techniques as necessary to provide an accurate picture of the variable instead of a single measure that may mislead a reader. For example, providing a percentage of 100 percent hand washing compliance for a month may look very good, but by excluding the frequency count—and that count is $n = 1$—a complete picture is not provided.

Understanding Levels of Measurement

The initial step in descriptive analysis is to choose the appropriate statistical analysis for the level of measurement of each variable. This is the responsibility of those who create descriptive studies and is an important point for critique by nurses who read research reports. These levels of measurement were described in detail in Chapter 9, but they are so important to the selection of appropriate statistical techniques that a review is warranted here. Data can be collected in one of four possible levels of measurement: nominal, ordinal, interval, or ratio. Each level has characteristics that make it unique, and each requires a particular type of statistical technique. Table 13.1 shows descriptive statistical techniques that are appropriate for each level of measurement.

Table 13.1

Levels of Measurement and Appropriate Summary Statistics

Level of Measurement	Distributions	Central Tendency	Variability	Shape
Nominal	■ Frequency ■ Percentage	■ Mode		
Ordinal	■ Frequency ■ Percentage	■ Mode ■ Median	■ Range ■ Minimum/Maximum	
Interval/Ratio		■ Mode ■ Median ■ Mean	■ Range ■ Minimum/Maximum ■ Standard Deviation ■ Variance	■ Skew ■ Kurtosis

Nominal-level data are those that denote categories; numbers given to these data are strictly for showing membership in a category and are not subject to mathematical calculations. Nominal data can be counted, not measured, so they can be summarized using statistics that represent counts. Summary statistics appropriate for this level of measurement are frequency, percentage, rates, ratios, and the mode.

Ordinal data are also categories, but have an added characteristic of rank order. The difference from nominal data is that the categories for a variable can be identified as being less than or greater than one another. However, because the level of measure is still categorical, the exact level of difference cannot be identified. Statistical techniques appropriate for ordinal data include those appropriate for nominal data plus range, median, minimum, and maximum.

Interval and ratio data are recorded on a continuous scale that has equal intervals between all entries. Data collected on interval or ratio levels result in numbers that can be subjected to many mathematical procedures including mean, standard deviation, variance, and evaluation of the distribution (skew and kurtosis).

Identifying Shape and Distribution

Initial analyses of data are meant to help the researcher identify the distribution, and therefore the shape, of the variable's data. The outcome of this analysis, coupled with the level of measurement, guides the researcher to select the appropriate statistics to present the description of the variable's center and spread.

Summarizing Data Using Frequencies

Frequency is a statistical term that means a count of the instances in which a number or category occurs in a data set. Frequencies are used commonly in clinical settings; for example, a frequency might be used to document the number of infections in a surgical department, the number of patient falls on a nursing unit, or the number of nurses who leave in the first 18 months of employment. In research, frequencies are used to count the number of times that a variable has a particular value or score. A researcher may collect data on nominal-level variables or ordinal-level variables and generate a frequency count per category to summarize the data. If information about gender were desired, two values (male and female) would be collected; the number of participants in the study who were male and the number who were female would be tallied.

Frequency: A count of the instances that an event occurs in a data set.

Frequency data can also be used to calculate percentages, rates, and derived variables. A percentage is a useful summary technique that shows the relative frequency of a variable. For example, if gender was measured as a variable and there were 180 female participants in a sample of 400, the percentage of female participants would be 45 percent. The number 45 percent is more meaningful as a summary value than the frequency count because readers can tell quickly that slightly less than half of the sample was female. To calculate the percentage in this example, the number of female participants is divided by the number of participants in the entire sample (180/400 = 0.45 or 45 percent).

Rate: A calculated count derived from dividing the frequency of an event in a given time period by all possible occurrences of the event during the same time period.

Rates that are clinically important can be calculated to provide information for data trends over time. Like percentage, a rate is calculated by dividing the frequency of an event in a given time period by all possible occurrences of the event during the same time period. The difference is that percentages by definition are "per 100," whereas rates can have a different denominator, such as per 1000 patient days. Monthly surgical infection rates are an example; the number of surgical site infections in a month is divided by the total number of surgical procedures in that month. When calculated periodically, patient outcomes expressed as rates can be monitored as a basis for action planning to improve care (Altman, 2006).

Derived variable: A new variable produced when data from other variables are combined using a simple formula.

Derived variables are created when data from other variables are put into a simple formula to produce a new piece of information—a new variable. An often-used derived variable is the hospital length of stay. It is calculated by summing the number of inpatient days on a nursing unit (a frequency) in a month and dividing it by the number of patients in the unit. Rates and derived variables may be used to represent the effects of extraneous variables or to describe baseline performance. Operational definitions of these variables are important to include to support consistency in the method of calculation.

Summarizing Data Using Frequency Tables

Interval-level data can be summarized in a frequency table, but they must be grouped into categories first. Because interval-level data can fall anywhere on a continuous scale, each data point could theoretically be a unique number; as a result, there can be many different values in the data set, which makes interpreting the data difficult. Table 13.2 contains a data set that could benefit from summary as a frequency table. To create a frequency table for interval-level data, the data are sorted from lowest value to highest value, categories are created for the data, and the number of occurrences in each category

Table 13.2

Unordered Data Set of Years as a Nurse

Years as a Nurse

13	5	23	5	3
7	5	30	20	5
8	6	17	21	11
7	6	27	5	18
2	1	9	9	16
2	1	3	5	9
1	5	30	1	28
2	2	16	3	12
5	5	20	15	17
23	20	17	9	24

Table 13.3		

Frequency Table for Years as a Nurse

Years as a Nurse	Frequency	Percentage
1–3	11	22
4–9	18	36
10–17	9	18
18–30	12	24
Total	50	100

is counted. Collapsing several years together provides an even clearer picture. **Table 13.3** represents the same data in a frequency table that includes both counts and relative frequency (percentage). Representing complex data in this way enhances interpretation and understanding of the values. Although the data in the original table did not easily reveal any patterns, review of the frequency table makes evident that most participants in the study had few years of nursing experience; in fact, the majority of participants had 9 or fewer years of experience.

Summarizing Data Using Frequency Distributions

In many ways, graphical presentation of data is easier to understand because the data are presented in summary fashion with colors, lines, and shapes that show differences and similarities in the data set. An easy chart to create is a bar chart for nominal or ordinal data. The most common way to design a bar chart is to have categories of the variable on the x-axis of the chart (horizontal) and the frequency for each on the y-axis (vertical). Bar charts provide the reader with a quick assessment of which category has the most occurrences in a data set.

A bar chart showing the frequency per category enables evaluation of the shape of the distribution of values. These graphs are called frequency distributions or histograms. For example, the values of subjects' ages can vary theoretically from less than one year to a little over 100 years. These values can be represented in a graph with the value (age) placed on the x-axis and the number of cases on the y-axis. Histograms are also the most common graph used with interval or ratio data. **FIGURE 13.1** depicts a histogram of interval-level data. The histogram shows categories for values of the variable across the horizontal dimension, and frequencies are displayed on the vertical dimension. In this histogram, the reader can see that most of the values of the variable "age" were between 14 and 17 in this data set.

Another useful feature of the histogram is that it shows the curve of the data. The researcher can see whether the data in the study are normal, skewed, or have an abnormal kurtosis. Based on the distribution of the data the researcher will then select the statistic for describing the center and spread of the data. Figure 13.1 depicts an approximately normal distribution. A normal distribution, often called a bell curve, has

Histogram: A type of frequency distribution in which variables with different values are plotted as a graph on x-axes and y-axes, and the shape can be visualized.

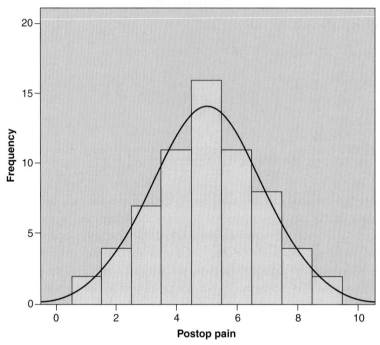

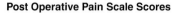

FIGURE 13.1 A Normal Distribution

a large proportion of values of the variable in the middle of the distribution and smaller proportions on the ends (tails). The shape of the distribution is symmetrical, meaning that the right and left sides of the distribution are mirror images. The shape of the distribution of a variable in a research study is important because many statistical procedures require a normal distribution to yield reliable results (Norman & Streiner, 2008).

Some variables are not symmetric and so do not have a normal distribution. Asymmetric distributions may be described as demonstrating skew or kurtosis. A skewed distribution has a disproportionate number of occurrences in either the right or left tail of the distribution. Describing the type of distribution can be counterintuitive; the skew is described by the direction of the tail. For example, distributions with more values in the positive end of the distribution trail out to the negative end and so are described as negative skew; those with more values on the lower end of the scale will trail out to the positive end and so are called positive skew. FIGURES 13.2 and 13.3 demonstrate skewed distributions. Kurtosis refers to an unusual accumulation of values in some part of the distribution, particularly in the size of the tails. Those with large tails are called leptokurtic and those with small tails are called platykurtic. A leptokurtic distribution is depicted by the histogram in FIGURE 13.4.

Researchers who create data have a responsibility to check the descriptive data for compliance with underlying assumptions of the planned statistical techniques. These

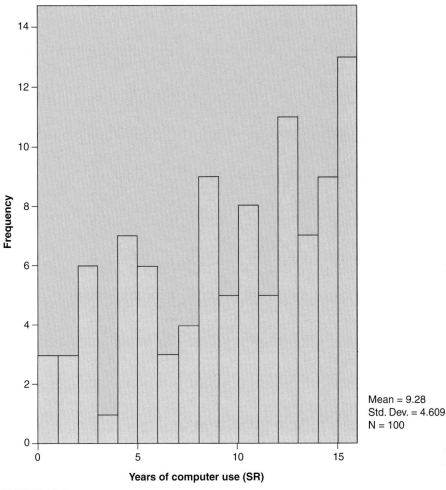

FIGURE 13.2 A Negatively Skewed Distribution

assumptions often include a requirement for variables to have a normal distribution (not skewed or kurtotic) and to have equal variances (similar spread of scores around the mean). A visual inspection of the graphical display of values of a variable via a histogram can give a researcher a quick indication of whether the variable meets the requirements for distribution.

Describing the Center and Spread

By first checking the shape of the distribution of data in a variable, the researcher has the ability to appropriately select statistics to describe the variable's center and spread. Measures of central tendency are used to describe the variable's center and include the

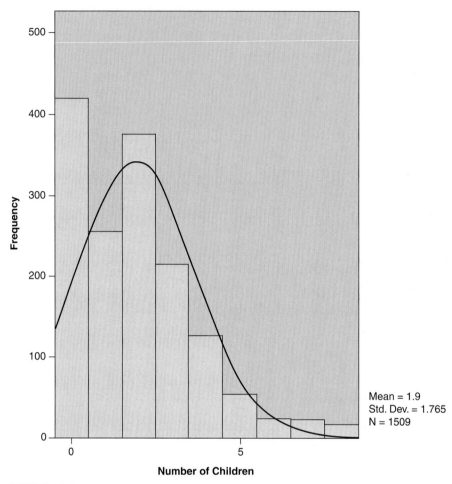

FIGURE 13.3 A Positively Skewed Distribution

mean, median, and mode. The spread, or variability, of the variable's data is calculated via standard deviation, range, and percentiles.

Summarizing Data Using Measures of Central Tendency

A measure of central tendency is the name given for a single number that summarizes values for a variable. These measures represent the way the data tend toward the center; they reflect what may be a typical response in the data set. For example, age of participants in a sample might be an important variable in a study. Instead of listing all the ages of participants, a researcher can summarize the data using a measure of central tendency such as the average (mean) age of participants in the sample. If, for example, the mean age were 25 rather than 75, the reader would know that participants were young adults rather than elderly participants. Other measures of central tendency include the median and the mode.

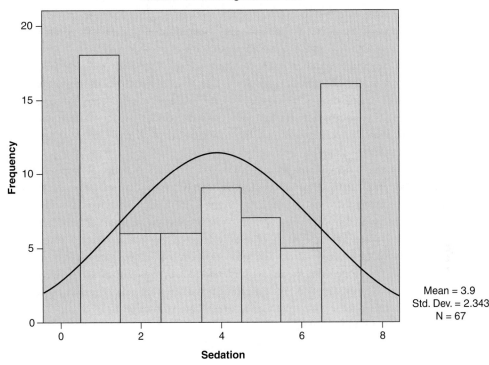

FIGURE 13.4 A Distribution with Kurtosis

The mean is commonly called the average. This number is calculated by adding all scores in the data set and dividing the sum by the number of scores in the data set. The mean is an easily recognized and interpreted measure of central tendency. It is familiar to most readers and easy to calculate. On the other hand, the mean is disproportionately affected by extreme values. For example, the mean salary in an organization would be $20,000 if five employees were each paid $20,000 a year, or if four employees were paid $5,000 a year and one were paid $80,000. This sensitivity to extreme scores is a weakness of the mean; thus data that are normally distributed are most appropriate to submit to the calculation of a mean score. Only data measured at the interval and ratio levels are appropriate for calculating a mean score.

Mean: The average; a measure of central tendency.

The median is another measure of central tendency, but it is not a calculation; it is a location. Whereas the mean takes every number in the data set into the calculation, the median requires the data set to be arranged in numerical order so the value in the middle of the data set can be determined. The values of a data set are arranged in sequence from smallest to largest, and the center of the data set is determined by finding the exact midpoint of the data. When there is an even number of values in the data set, the two most central values are averaged to obtain the median. The median can be used with normal, skewed, or kurtotic distributions because it is

Median: A measure of central tendency that is the exact midpoint of the numbers of the data set.

not influenced by extreme values in the data set. The median can be used with ordinal, interval, or ratio data, but its usefulness in inferential statistical procedures is limited. Its primary weakness is that it represents only the middle of the data set and can be used in only a narrow range of statistical procedures.

Mode: A measure of central tendency that is the most frequently occurring value in the data set.

An additional measure of central tendency is the mode, the most frequently occurring value in the data set. Some data sets will not have a mode, or they may have multiple modes. It is an easy statistic to determine, but it has limited usefulness. The mode is not used in inferential statistics and provides little information about a data set. It is, however, the only measure of central tendency that can be applied to nominal data.

The mean is a dependable measure of the center of the distribution because it uses all numbers in the data set for its calculation; however, when extreme values exist in the data set, the mean is drawn toward that extreme score. Thus, researchers should use the mean statistic with caution in distributions that are badly skewed, particularly those with small sample sizes. The median is the middle point of the data set; it is not sensitive to extremes, making it a good choice as a measure of central tendency in distributions that are skewed. The mode helps the reader understand if any value occurs more frequently than others. The minimum and maximum help assess the spread of the data. How these numbers come together to depict a data set is demonstrated in Table 13.4. These last numbers give an indication of the breadth of variability in the data set, but more sensitive statistics are needed to evaluate the way individual values vary from the typical case.

Summarizing the Variability of a Data Set

Although a typical case can be described statistically, values for individual subjects will differ, sometimes substantially. Statistical techniques can demonstrate variability in ways that enhance understanding of the nature of the individual values represented by the variable scores. For skewed data, a researcher can use a variable's range as well as percentiles to appropriately represent the variability of the data. To calculate the range, the analyst would first identify minimum and maximum values in the data set. The minimum value is the smallest number in the data set, and the maximum value is the largest. The range is determined by subtracting the minimum value from the maximum value of the variable, and is the simplest way to represent the spread of the data. This single number provides an indication about the distance between the two most extreme values in the data set. The range is easy to calculate, which makes it useful for getting a quick understanding of the spread of scores. However, more powerful measures use every number in the data set to show the spread of the individual values from the middle of the data set.

Range: A measure of variability that is the distance between the two most extreme values in the data set.

Variance: A measure of variability that gives information about the spread of scores around the mean.

Variance and standard deviation are the most commonly used statistics for measuring the dispersion of values from the mean. Just as the mean is used to represent the center of normally distributed data, the standard deviation and variance are representations of variability of data. The variance and standard deviation provide information about the average distance of values from the mean of a variable. Variance can be calculated using a calculator, a spreadsheet, or statistical

Table 13.4

Interpreting Measures of Central Tendency

The variable of length of inpatient stay for adult community-acquired pneumonia has values of:
- Mean: 1.4 days
- Median: 0.78 days
- Minimum: 0.5 days
- Maximum: 12.3 days

Meaning:
The median is smaller than the mean; this indicates a positively skewed distribution, because more scores will be in the lower half of the distribution. This indicates that most people stay shorter than this mean value, and that some extreme values are likely artificially inflating the mean length of stay. The broad range between minimum and maximum reflects that the scores are spread out.

The variable of length of inpatient stay for pediatric community-acquired pneumonia has values of:
- Mean: 2.2 days
- Median: 2.4 days
- Minimum: 0.5 days
- Maximum: 4.6 days

Meaning:
The median and the mean are roughly equal; this indicates the distribution is likely a normal one. The range between minimum and maximum is not large, and the similarity between the measures of central tendency is a sign that extreme values are unlikely to have an effect on these statistics.

The variable of length of inpatient stay for aspiration pneumonia has values of:
- Mean: 4.3 days
- Median: 5.6 days
- Minimum: 0.8 days
- Maximum: 8.9 days

Meaning:
The median is larger than the mean; this indicates a negatively skewed distribution because more scores are in the upper half of the distribution. This means that more of these patients stay longer than average. There is a moderate range between the minimum and maximum, and a moderate difference between the measures of central tendency, indicating there may be only a few extreme values in the data set.

software. The calculation of variance and standard deviation is explained in the box that follows; it is illustrated here to provide an understanding of the concept.

The calculation results in a single score that provides information about the spread of scores around the mean. When the variance increases, the distance of scores from the mean is larger and the distribution is spread away from the mean. The distribution will appear flat and spread out, as demonstrated by the distribution in FIGURE 13.5. Likewise, when the variance decreases, the distance of scores from the mean is smaller, meaning more scores are clustered around the mean, and the distribution is taller, as depicted in FIGURE 13.6. The distribution will appear tall and thin. The variance is based on a

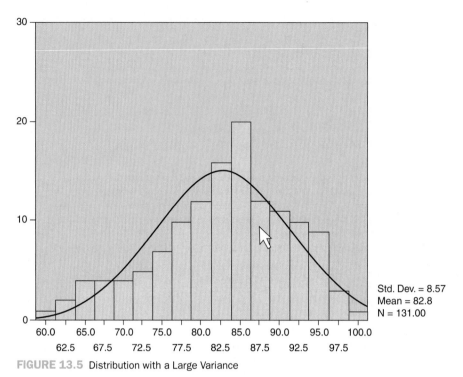

Std. Dev. = 8.57
Mean = 82.8
N = 131.00

FIGURE 13.5 Distribution with a Large Variance

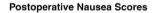

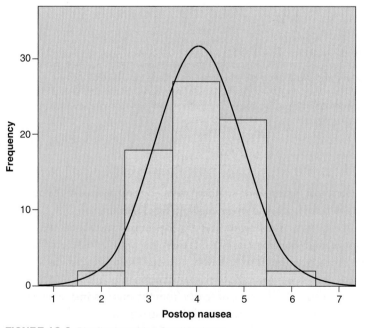

Mean = 4.06
Std. Dev. = 0.893
N = 71

FIGURE 13.6 Distribution with a Small Variance

Calculating the Variance and Standard Deviation

Step:	Demonstrated on sample X_i:	This step:
	2 4 4 5 5 6 7 7	
	8 8 9 9 9 10 10 12	
1. Calculate a sample mean.	Sum(X_i) / n 115 / 16 = 7.19	Provides the value of the "typical" case.

2. Subtract the mean from each score.

Value	Minus the mean =		Identifies the distance of each individual data point from the typical case.
2	7.1875	–5.1875	
4	7.1875	–3.1875	
4	7.1875	–3.1875	
5	7.1875	–2.1875	
5	7.1875	–2.1875	Each individual distance is called a
6	7.1875	–1.1875	*deviation score* or a *residual*.
7	7.1875	–0.1875	
7	7.1875	–0.1875	
8	7.1875	–.8125	
8	7.1875	0.8125	
9	7.1875	1.8125	
9	7.1875	1.8125	
9	7.1875	1.8125	
10	7.1875	2.8125	
10	7.1875	2.8125	
12	7.1875	4.8125	

3. Square each deviation score.

Square the deviation:

			If the deviation scores are summed, they will always equal 0— the distances above the mean will be equal to those below.
-5.1875^2	=	26.9102	
-3.1875^2	=	10.1602	
-3.1875^2	=	10.1602	
-2.1875^2	=	4.78516	Squaring the deviations eliminates the sign and gives us the absolute distance without identifying them as positive or negative.
-2.1875^2	=	4.78516	
-1.1875^2	=	1.41016	
-0.1875^2	=	0.03516	
-0.1875^2	=	0.03516	
0.8125^2	=	0.66016	This is called the squared distances from the mean.
0.8125^2	=	0.66016	
1.8125^2	=	3.28516	
1.8125^2	=	3.28516	
1.8125^2	=	3.28516	
2.8125^2	=	7.91016	
2.8125^2	=	7.91016	
4.8125^2	=	23.1602	

(continued)

Calculating the Variance and Standard Deviation *(Continued)*

4. Sum the squared deviation scores.	Sum (deviation scores) = 108.438	We are interested in the average distance from the mean. An average is a sum of the values divided by sample size. This step is analogous to the first step of this process, summing the values.
		This value is called the sum of squares; it represents the sum of squared deviations from the mean.
5. Divide by the sample size − 1.	108.438/(n − 1) = 108.438/(16 − 1) = 7.229	This is the *variance*, or the average squared distance from the mean.
6. Identify the square root.	Square root (7.229) = 2.6887	This is the *standard deviation*, or the average distance from the mean of the values in this data set.

Standard deviation: The most easily interpreted measure of variability of scores around the mean; represents the average amount of variation of data points about the mean.

squared value, so it may be difficult to interpret. The square root of the variance, the standard deviation, is a more easily interpreted measure of the distance (spread) of scores around the mean because its scale is proportional to the original set of numbers. The standard deviation represents data in the same way as the variance. Large standard deviation scores relative to the mean indicate that values in the data set are spread out from the mean, and small standard deviation scores relative to the mean indicate that values are close to the mean. The standard deviation is more frequently reported in research reports than is variance because it is more easily interpreted (Horton, 2009). The variance, on the other hand, is more commonly used in the calculation of other statistics, such as those used to determine standard error and the differences between groups. It is helpful to calculate at least one standard deviation value manually to understand its underlying conceptual meaning.

Variance and standard deviation are subject to the same limitations as the mean because all scores in the data set are used in the calculation, and the mean is used in the calculation. Thus, extreme scores in the data set will affect the variance and standard deviation. When it is appropriate to use a mean to describe the data set (fairly normal distribution without extreme skew), it will be appropriate to use variance and standard deviation.

Coefficient of variation (CV): A calculation that produces a number that depicts the standard deviation relative to the mean [CV = $100(SD/\bar{X})$].

The mean and standard deviation are powerful as building blocks to other statistical techniques because they can be manipulated algebraically. In some cases, readers of research reports want to compare the variability of a variable across different groups or even different studies. The coefficient of variation (CV) is

> **Table 13.5**

Interpreting Measures of Variability

The Variable of Length of Inpatient Stay:	Has Values Of:	Resulting in a Coefficient of Variation:	Meaning:
Adult community-acquired pneumonia	▪ Mean: 1.4 days ▪ Standard deviation: 0.8 days	$(0.8 / 1.4) \times 100 = 0.571 \times 100 = 57.1$	A moderately large amount of variability
Pediatric community-acquired pneumonia	▪ Mean: 2.2 days ▪ Standard deviation: 0.2 days	$(0.2/2.2) \times 100 = 0.090 \times 100 = 9.0$	A very small amount of variability
Aspiration pneumonia	▪ Mean: 4.3 days ▪ Standard deviation: 1.1 days	$(1.1/4.3) \times 100 = 0.256 \times 100 = 25.6$	A small amount of variability

a calculation that produces a number that depicts the standard deviation relative to the mean, allowing for the comparison of the variability of different variables measured with different scales. The formula for the coefficient of variation is $CV = 100(SD/\bar{X})$. Table 13.5 depicts data with their associated measures of variability and an interpretation of these statistics.

A review of these descriptive statistics shows how the variance and standard deviation help the reader understand a data set in terms of both the "typical" response (mean and

A Note About Scale

The word *scale* is used frequently when talking about descriptive data. Scale refers to the units of measurement of the variable. For example, height is commonly measured with a scale of inches, and weight is commonly measured with a scale of pounds. Scale is also used with respect to the potential range of the data. Height has limitations of scale in that people are not taller than 7.5 feet, so if height were measured in inches, its scale would be restricted to the range of 0 to 90 inches. Weight in people, on the other hand, has been measured as high as 1000 pounds. So height will never have as many possible "units" as weight. If we try to compare these two scales—if we wanted to compare their means, for example, to see if a person of average height is also of average weight—the scale size means the average number of units of weight will always be several times

as big as the average number of units of height. Is an individual who is 15 pounds above average in weight and 2.5 inches above average in height an overweight person? It is hard to tell using the raw values. Using percentiles or standardized scores to represent numbers eliminates this problem. Instead of expressing a value in terms of its absolute number of units, the value is expressed by its relative position on the scale. This enables us to compare where each value falls relative to its specific scale, in a standard way, so that unit to unit comparisons are possible. So if an individual is 1 standard deviation above the mean in weight and also 1 standard deviation above the mean in height, he or she is not overweight. Measures of relative position enable the comparison of values across variables, regardless of the scale with which they are originally represented.

median) and how individual subjects are different from that typical response (variance and standard deviation).

Summarizing Data Using Measures of Position

Values from a data set can be divided into parts so that readers can understand where a particular value lies in relation to all other values in the data set. The percentile rank is the most commonly used statistical technique for this purpose. A percentile is not synonymous with a percentage; a percentile represents the percentage of values that lie below the particular value of interest. For example, a score of 92 percent on an exam may be at the 100th percentile if it is the highest score in the class. Conversely, it may be at the 0 percentile if it is the lowest score in the class. The minimum score in a data set is always at the 0 percentile, the maximum score is always at the 100th percentile, and the median is always the 50th percentile (given that 50 percent of the scores are always below the median). Percentiles are common ways to represent healthcare numbers such as patient satisfaction and scores on standardized tests, when a fairly narrow range of scores is expected.

Quartiles are identified by dividing the data set into four equal parts. The first quartile contains the 0 to 25th percentile rank (that is, the lowest 25 percent of the scores), the second quartile contains scores in the 26th to 50th percentile rank, the third quartile contains scores in the 51st to 75th percentile rank, and the fourth quartile contains all scores above the 76th percentile rank. This technique is particularly helpful when the researcher is examining achievement or when performance against others in the study is important. It is also a useful technique for dividing scores on interval-level variables into logical groups to study differences between them.

Sometimes a researcher may want to transform scores gathered in a research study to standardized scores, which express the distance from the mean for a single score. Just as the standard deviation represents the spread of scores around the mean for an entire data set, a standardized score represents the distance of a single point from the mean. This distance is represented by the standard deviation so that standardized scores can be compared across variables, even if the scale of measurement is radically different. The most commonly used standardized score is the z-score. The z-score is calculated by finding the difference between the individual value and the mean, then dividing that number by the standard deviation. The resulting score depicts the variable in terms of its relative position in the overall data set.

When all of the scores in a data set have been converted to a z-score and depicted as a histogram, the result is called a standard normal distribution. A standard normal distribution has a mean of 0 and a standard deviation of 1. This transformed distribution retains its original shape, and the z-scores can be used to determine in which percentile a given score would fall. This is helpful in determining the probability that an individual score would fall in a specific place in the distribution. Distributions with a bell shape have approximately 68 percent of scores between +1 or –1 standard deviation and 95 percent of scores between +2 or –2 standard deviations, as shown in FIGURE 13.7. These characteristics of a standard normal distribution are very

Standardized scores: A measure of position that expresses the distance from the mean of a single score in standard terms.

Standard normal distribution: A bell-shaped distribution in which the mean is set at zero and a standard deviation at one.

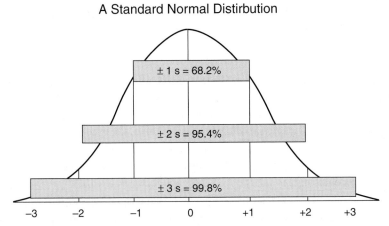

FIGURE 13.7 The Standard Normal Distribution

useful as a basis for determining the probability that a specific statistical finding is due to standard error and will become the basis for judging random chance in inferential analyses, discussed in later chapters.

All of the descriptive statistics presented thus far are considered univariate, meaning they are used to study a single variable at a time. These statistics are appropriate for analysis of data collected for general descriptive studies. Descriptive statistics can also be applied to describe bivariate relationships, or the study of two variables at a time.

Summarizing Scores Using Measures of Relationship

Bivariate descriptive statistics can be very useful in describing the strength and nature of relationships between variables and are the appropriate tests to use for analysis in correlation studies. Correlation analysis examines the values of two variables in relation to each other. Correlation analysis can be used to examine the relationship between two variables in a single sample or between a single variable in two samples. For example, one would expect that census in a hospital and the number of laboratory tests ordered have a relationship—as the values for census increase, the values for number of tests ordered increase. This type of relationship is called a positive correlation. A different example may show a negative correlation such as scores on a quality-of-life scale and stages of a chronic disease. In this example, as the stage of chronic disease progresses, the quality of life for the client may decrease. These are both examples of a correlation between two variables in a single sample. The values of a single variable may also be appraised for its relationship between two samples; for example, there may likely be a positive correlation between the adult weight of mothers and their daughters.

Correlation statistics can be shown numerically and in graphic forms. The notation of rho or r is used to represent a bivariate correlation in a sample. The most common correlation coefficients are the Pearson product moment correlation and the Spearman's rank order correlation. The former is used for interval- or ratio-level data, and the latter

> **Correlation analysis:** A measure that depicts the strength and nature of the relationship between two variables.

for ranked or ordinal data. In either form, the correlation can be positive or negative with values between –1 and +1, inclusive. Values of exactly –1 or +1 are known as perfect correlations, reflecting a perfect linear relationship in which a change in a variable of one unit is accompanied by a change in exactly one unit in the other variable. A correlation coefficient with a value of 0 has no correlation. The direction of the relationship is interpreted from the sign; a negative correlation coefficient reflects an inverse relationship (as one variable increases, the other decreases) and a positive correlation coefficient reflects a positive relationship (as one variable increases, the other variable increases as well). The strength of the relationship is interpreted based on the absolute value of the coefficient itself, regardless of its sign (Kremelberg, 2010). An example of interpretation of correlation coefficients for a set of variables appears in Table 13.6.

An advantage of the correlation coefficient is that it can be an efficient way to determine both the strength and direction of a relationship with a single statistic. On the other hand, a correlation coefficient only reflects a linear relationship; in other words, the relationship has to be proportional at all levels of each variable before it will be depicted accurately with a correlation coefficient (Motulsky, 2010). There are important relationships in health care that are curved, rather than linear, and are not represented well by

---

Table 13.6

Interpreting Measures of Correlation

Variable 1	Variable 2	Correlation Coefficient	The Sign Means	The Number Means
Pneumonia length of stay in days	Results of pulmonary function tests	–0.850	The negative sign indicates an inverse relationship; as results of pulmonary function tests improve, length of stay in days decreases.	0.8 to 1.0 absolute value indicates a strong relationship.
Pneumonia length of stay in days	Number of co-morbid conditions	+0.678	The positive sign indicates a positive relationship; as the number of co-morbid conditions increases, the length of stay also increases.	0.6 to 0.8 absolute value indicates a moderately strong relationship.
Pneumonia length of stay in days	Nutritional status	–0.488	The negative sign indicates a negative relationship; as the quality of nutritional status improves, the length of stay in days decreases.	0.4 to 0.6 absolute value indicates a moderate relationship.
Pneumonia length of stay in days	Annual days absent from work	+0.213	The positive sign indicates a positive relationship; as annual days absent from work increase, the length of stay in days increases.	0.2 to 0.4 absolute value indicates a weak relationship; less than 0.2 indicates no relationship.

a correlation coefficient. For example, a dose–response curve will follow a curvilinear trajectory, but it is still a very important relationship in nursing care.

A note is in order about correlation coefficients and statistical significance. Often, a p value, indicating the probability of chance, is reported with the correlation coefficient. It is often erroneously interpreted as evidence that the relationship is a significant one. In reality, the p value represents the probability that the measured relationship is due to standard error, and even very weak correlation coefficients can be statistically significant. The strength and direction of the correlation coefficient are the characteristics that determine if it is clinically significant, and this can only be determined by the application of the expert judgment of the clinician (Fawcett, 2009).

A correlation coefficient is an efficient and easily interpreted way to describe the degree and direction of a linear relationship between variables. These relationships can also be represented graphically using a scatter plot. Scatter plots are effective means for evaluating relationships and determining if those relationships are linear. They are one of a group of graphical presentations that can illustrate statistical results in a visual way, which are often more easily interpreted and understood by readers.

Summarizing Data in Graphical Presentations

It is just as important to use the correct graphical technique as it is to use the correct statistical technique to summarize descriptive data. In some ways, graphical presentation of data is easier to understand because the data are presented in summary fashion with the colors, lines, and shapes to show differences and similarities in the data set. An easy chart to create is a bar chart for nominal or ordinal data. The most common way to design a bar chart is to have the categories of the variable on the x-axis of the chart (horizontal) and the frequency on the y-axis (vertical). Bar charts provide the reader with a quick assessment of which category has the most occurrences in a data set.

> Bar chart: A graphic presentation for nominal or ordinal data that represents the categories on the horizontal axis and frequency on the vertical axis.

The most common graph used with interval or ratio data is the histogram. FIGURE 13.8 depicts a histogram of interval-level data. The histogram shows categories for values of the variable across the horizontal dimension, and frequencies are displayed on the vertical dimension. In this histogram, the reader can see that most of the values of the variable were between 14.0 and 17.0 in this data set. Another useful feature of the histogram is that it shows the curve of the data. The researcher can see whether the data in the study are normal, skewed, or have an abnormal kurtosis. The histogram pictured in Figure 13.8 has a normal distribution.

Line graphs are used to show change over time. Values for the variable are summarized using a mean, and the mean is then followed over some period of time, such as monthly for a year. Line graphs are used in time-series designs, single-subject designs, or to determine the effectiveness of a new intervention or research protocol. Line graphs are easy to read and quickly show results over time.

Sometimes the best way to display the data is to illustrate where the majority of the scores lie in the data set. A box plot provides a good method to show this,

> Line graphs: A graphic presentation that plots means for a variable over a period of time.
> Box plot: A graphic presentation that marks the median of the values in the middle of the box and the 25th and 75th percentiles as the lower and upper edges of the box. It indicates the relative position of the data for each group and the spread of the data for comparison.

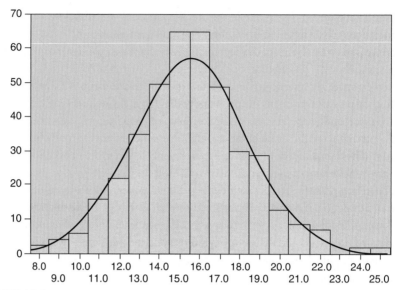

FIGURE 13.8 An Example of a Histogram

particularly when a variable is measured in different groups. The box plot is a visual representation of measures of position. The median of the values for a variable in all groups of participants is marked in the middle of the box. The 25th and 75th percentiles for each group form the lower and upper edges of the box, respectively. Scores contained within the box are those between the 25th and 75th percentiles and represent the middle 50 percent of the values for each group. The minimum and maximum values are marked with an *x* or connected by a line to the box. The resulting chart is sometimes called a "box and whiskers," referring to the box with lines extending from the top and bottom; it shows a side-by-side comparison of the relative position of data for each group. It gives the reader a picture of the spread of the data (minimum and maximum values) and where 50 percent of the values lie (within the box). FIGURE 13.9 represents a box-and-whiskers plot for a measure of postoperative pain in the hours after surgery. Inspection of the graph shows the reader that hour 4 is the point at which pain reaches its peak, after which it gradually declines.

Scatter plot: A graphic presentation that indicates the nature of the relationship between two variables.

The most common use of scatter plots is to show the nature of the relationship between two variables. Scatter plots require graphing two variables measured from the same subject at the same time. When all data in the set have been plotted, the graph shows whether the points are closely grouped (associated) or scattered (no association). The closer the dots are to forming a discernible, straight line, the more associated the variables are to one another. FIGURE 13.10 demonstrates three data sets containing two variables displayed as scatter plots. The scatter plot on the left shows two variables that have a positive relationship to each other, the center scatter plot shows two variables that have a negative association, and the scatter plot on the right shows no association between the two variables.

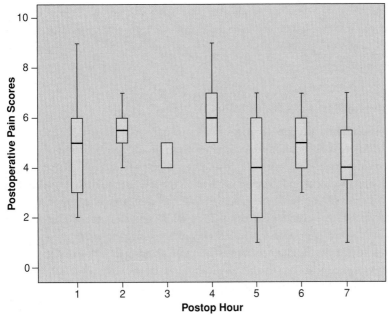

FIGURE 13.9 A Box-and-Whiskers Plot

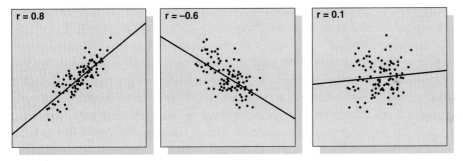

FIGURE 13.10 Scatter Plots

Charts and graphs provide useful information to readers when used appropriately. Bar graphs are easy to create for nominal and ordinal data. Frequency data from different groups can be compared using bar graphs so a reader can quickly see which group has the highest number of instances of a particular variable. Histograms are used in a similar manner for interval-level or ratio-level data. The bars in histograms are connected, which denotes a variable that has continuous numbers. Histograms have an added feature of showing the shape of the distribution of a variable. Line graphs are usually created to show the mean value of a variable over some period of time. This graph is particularly helpful when a change in the mean (either higher or lower) might signal the need to change a nursing practice. Whereas the line graph typically shows the mean over time, the box plot shows the distribution over time. Each box contains the 25th to 75th percentiles of the distribution. Watching trends over time using a box plot is helpful if the median point or the middle 50 percent of the distribution is important. Finally, a scatter plot is an effective way to visually represent the strength and direction of a relationship between two variables.

Common Errors in Summarizing Data

The most elementary error is made when an inappropriate statistic is used to summarize data. There is never an instance when a mean should be calculated on race, gender, or other categorical data. However, those new to statistical analysis may forget these levels of measurement and, seeing numbers on the screen, run descriptive analysis. The statistical analysis computer package will calculate a mean when provided the correct commands, but this number is meaningless. What would a mean of 5.6 on the variable race indicate—an error! Other problems occur when data are entered incorrectly; this is addressed later in the chapter in the section on creating descriptive data.

Erroneous conclusions can be drawn about variables when some data are presented without the benefit of seeing all appropriate descriptive data. Descriptive data analysis of a variable should always include measures of central tendency and variability. For example, a variable measured for two different groups can have approximately the same mean, but a different spread of scores around the mean. The interpretation of the performance of the groups is dependent on knowing both the values of a typical case and how far individual data points deviate from the typical case.

Researchers should always disclose frequency and percentage information in research reports so that a reader can understand whether a change in percentage over time is a function of sample size or change in the values of the variable. For example, a researcher studying the development of pressure ulcers within the first month of admission to a nursing home over a 3-month period of time reported the following percentages: 8 percent, 7.5 percent, and 0 percent. The reader might logically believe that the last month was a breakthrough in preventing new ulcers. However, the percentage is calculated by taking number of ulcers and dividing by total admissions for the month. When these data are also presented as 6/75, 6/80, and 0/20, a different conclusion can be drawn: The number of admissions has declined.

A common error in the interpretation of descriptive data is the overinterpretation of the results. In other words, the researcher interprets the data in a way that goes beyond what the statistics were intended to reflect. This is most common with the correlation coefficient. Although the correlation coefficient is an excellent way to represent the strength and direction of a relationship between two variables, it is limited to description of that relationship. Because the variables are measured simultaneously, the researcher cannot draw conclusions about causality. It is not uncommon, however, for a researcher to interpret a strong correlation as evidence that one variable has an effect on,

gray matter

The following are common errors in summarizing descriptive data:

- Inappropriate statistics
- Incorrectly entered data
- Selected data presented without the context of the whole data set
- Lack of disclosure of frequency and percentage information
- Overinterpretation of results
- Inconsistent presentation of data
- Graphic representation that hides important aspects of the data set

causes, or in some way influences the other. Correlation is evidence only of a relationship, not of causation, and overstating the relationship should be avoided (Rosner, 2010).

When a researcher has a command of statistical techniques, it can be tempting to present data in complicated ways that are sophisticated enough to amaze fellow researchers. However, the point of reporting descriptive analyses is to inform, not to impress. The readers of research that is intended as evidence for nursing practice are generally practitioners, not statisticians. If it requires the help of a statistician to interpret the results section of an article, then the author has not presented the findings well. Descriptive data should be presented in the most uncomplicated fashion that accurately and completely represents the findings so that understanding and application to practice are maximized.

A final pitfall to avoid is presenting data graphically in a way that hides important aspects of the data set. This is generally unintentional, but it can limit the reader's understanding of the research results. For example, showing only the mean values will hide the distribution of the variable. The researcher needs to create different types of charts to determine which one best displays the meaning of the data. Descriptive analysis is reported in the best way when it is reported in the most accurate, complete, and understandable way that is not easily misinterpreted.

Reading the Descriptive Data Section in a Research Study

Descriptive statistics are the most common statistics the reader of nursing research will encounter. Studies that have more sophisticated and complex intentions will still present descriptive data about the sample and the individual variables. A thorough understanding of descriptive statistical concepts will assist the reader in determining the fundamental characteristics of the subjects and variables in a study, helping to determine if the study will apply in a particular setting (Garden & Kabacoff, 2010). Reading the descriptive statistics can be confusing, however, because of the technical jargon associated with statistical analysis and the Greek letters that are used as symbols. Table 13.7 summarizes the notations that are used to represent descriptive statistics for populations and samples. The most commonly used symbols are those that represent statistics within a sample and include n, x, s, and s^2, which represent data set size, mean, standard deviation, and variance, respectively.

Table 13.7

Summary of Symbols Used for Descriptive Statistics

	Symbol for Population	Symbol for Sample
Data set size	N	n
Mean	μ (mu)	x
Standard deviation	σ (sigma)	s
Variance	σ^2 (sigma squared)	s^2
Correlation	ρ (rho)	r

Where to Look

Where to look for descriptive results:
- The report of descriptive data is typically the third or fourth major heading in a research report and may be called "Results" or "Findings."
- Statistics that describe the size, composition, and characteristics of the sample are often presented first in this section, or they may appear with the description of the sampling procedure.
- The report typically includes descriptive reports for each individual variable and each scale or summary score; these may be presented in tables, figures, graphs, or narrative form.

The report of descriptive data analysis usually follows the methods section, although descriptive statistics may appear in the description of the sample and research variables. The report of descriptive data is typically the third or fourth major heading in a research report and is often called "Results" or "Findings." Readers of research reports will often see the sample described first. Following the description of the sample, descriptive data for variables used in the study are presented. Some authors use narrative descriptions of the scores for variables, whereas others use tables to display data. Likewise, readers of research reports are more likely to see descriptive data about variables by group membership. An example of descriptive statistics by group membership appears in Table 13.8. These data represent a study of three groups—two intervention groups and a control—that have test anxiety measured at pretest and posttest periods. The reader can see that test anxiety scores decreased in both the cognitive-behavioral and the hypnosis groups, whereas the control group stayed essentially unchanged.

Readers of research reports should not accept the results without an appraisal of the appropriateness of data analyses. The reader can systematically evaluate whether appropriate decisions have been made for data analysis and reporting by asking a series of guiding questions:

Checklist for Evaluating Descriptive Results

✔ The descriptive report of the sample provides enough details to judge the adequacy and characteristics of the sample.

✔ The presentation of descriptive statistics is understandable and clear.

✔ Complete descriptive statistics are presented for each variable (for example, measures of both central tendency and variability).

✔ The tables, graphs, or charts complement the text and enhance understanding.

✔ Graphical representations are consistent in scale and orientation.

✔ The descriptive statistics are not misleading, open to misinterpretation, or confusing.

✔ The descriptive results give a full and clear picture of the variables under study.

✔ The data have not been overinterpreted and conclusions do not go beyond what the statistics can support.

Table 13.8

Means of Test Anxiety Score by Group and Time

	N	Mean	SD
Pretest			
Control	38	25	8.38
Cognitive–behavioral	38	27.33	10.21
Hypnosis	38	23.63	8.52
Posttest			
Control	36	24.58	10.12
Cognitive–behavioral	34	19.25	10.44
Hypnosis	35	18.20	7.05

- What variables were included in the study?
- What was the level of measurement for each variable?
- Were the descriptive statistics appropriate for the level of measurement of each variable?
- Were the descriptive statistics appropriate for the research question (that is, descriptive or correlation)?
- Were the descriptive results presented in the appropriate form for maximum understanding?

With patience and persistence, most readers should be able to comprehend the meaning of the findings from a descriptive research study. Descriptive data provide the reader with an understanding of the sample and variables through measures of central tendency and variability. This information is the foundation for more complex statistical analysis such as inferential statistics.

Using Descriptive Data Analysis in Practice

When considering the use of descriptive results, nurses should determine whether the report makes sense in light of the kinds of patients and outcomes that are found in their specific practice. In other words, can the results be generalized to the setting in which the reader is practicing? For example, if a study investigated functional status of patients who have undergone coronary bypass surgery, it might not be advisable to apply the results to a facility whose patients have had medical treatment of myocardial infarctions.

Nurses use descriptive data in clinical practice every day. Descriptive analysis is used when nurses check trends in vital signs (minimum and maximum values, line graphs), when they review infection rates for a clinical unit (number of patients with infections divided by all patients), or calculate average length of stay for clients with certain diagnoses (sum of inpatient days in a month divided by number of patients in the unit). Descriptive data can inform nursing practice in relation to the way diseases, complications, and health issues are distributed in the population of patients. Moreover, nurses who conduct quality improvement studies use descriptive data to develop evidence about clinical outcomes. Even though this type of evidence is lower on the hierarchy of evidence, it provides data that can guide clinical nurses to improve nursing practice and clinical outcomes. Descriptive analyses are often the first step in designing an intervention study that will provide conclusive evidence for a practice change.

When considering the types of descriptive data that would be useful in practice, nurses might ask the following questions:

- What type of data would be useful to track clinical outcomes?
- What are the operational definitions for data to be collected when tracking clinical outcomes?
- What is the appropriate level of measurement for the data?
- What types of descriptive statistics could summarize the data best?
- What graphs, charts, and tables might present the trends in clinical outcomes?

Asking these questions can lead the nurse to the development of systems to collect descriptive data and create reports that can inform their own practice as well as communicate the need for practice change to others.

Creating Descriptive Data Summaries for a Research Study

Researchers who report descriptive data from a research study must create and follow a data analysis plan with careful attention to detail. It is only through systematic attention to the data analysis process that appropriate results are generated and errors are detected and corrected before final analysis. The first order of business is to review the research design and research questions/hypotheses. This review helps to reorient the researcher to the major aims of the study and the specific types of analyses that should be used to describe the sample and to answer research questions.

Following this review, the researcher should follow a step-by-step process of preparing the data for analysis. It is likely that preparing the data for analysis will take more time and effort than the actual analysis itself. It is not unusual to take several days to enter, inspect, and clean the data and only minutes to run descriptive statistics. The process is one that may feel laborious, but it is imperative for accurate, complete results.

In the initial stages of data collection, the researcher labels all surveys or tools with a unique number so that data from different participants can be retrieved later, if necessary, without confusion. A codebook is developed with numerical codes substituted for words that describe nominal variables. For example, the researcher may collect data on gender, race, and marital status. The researcher may label males as 1 and females as 2. The number lacks mathematical meaning; it only serves as a category so a statistical analysis computer program can count instances of data in the categories. The codebook should be stored as an electronic or paper record with the data file so the codes can be easily retrieved and referred to during analysis.

Regardless of the way the data are collected, an organized system of maintaining data integrity must be established. Data from each participant should be filed in such a way that retrieval of the data is easy. A notebook, file folder, or computer file is commonly used. Because the security of the data is the responsibility of the researcher, the data should be password protected if it is stored on a computer, or locked in a filing cabinet if a paper system is used. As data are generated in the research study, they should be reviewed for completeness and accuracy before storing.

Once the data collection phase is over, the data entry phase begins. Data must be meticulously entered into a statistical analysis computer program using the codes that were developed earlier. Verification of the data quality is completed by having a second person compare the raw data with the data that were entered for each participant in the study; these should match. The researcher next runs some initial descriptive statistics to catch any outliers or errors in coding. The minimum and maximum values are particularly helpful in finding data outliers and errors. For example, in a study on resuscitation events, a participant who reports being involved in 100 events in the past year when the next highest value is 25 would be considered an outlier on that variable. This number may be true or it may be an error. The researcher should inspect the raw data for that participant to determine the veracity of the data. Another common mistake is simple miscoding that is not caught in the earlier verification; entering a 3 as a code when the only options are 1 or 2 will be found in this initial analysis. An easy way to find this type of coding error is to run frequencies on the data set. Once outliers and errors have been found, the data are cleaned by returning to the raw data set to correct the data entry errors. The file is then saved with a name that denotes it is the cleaned data file.

The early analysis phase begins with inspecting the cleaned data file for missing values—data that were not recorded by a participant. Several options are available to the researcher in such cases, including deleting participants with missing data, deleting the variable with missing data, or substituting a value (mean or estimate) for the missing data (Marshall & Jonker, 2010). The early analysis phase also entails looking at sample characteristics of participants compared to those who started the study but did not complete it. The researcher should inspect the characteristics of the sample to see if there were differences between those who persisted in the study and those who withdrew. This comparison can help identify any attrition bias.

Next, the researcher may need to change (transform) the data to prepare it for making summative scales. Often items on research instruments are worded in reverse to reduce response set bias. Once the data are collected, the researcher needs to change the scoring of the reversed items so he or she can add them to positively worded items. This transformation is done using the statistical analysis computer program. When all transformations have been completed, items can be combined into subscales or scale scores by following the scoring directions. Finally, the researcher is ready to perform the descriptive analysis for the purpose of reporting results from the study.

To begin the descriptive analysis, the researcher should develop a list of variables in the study. The researcher might collect data on variables including gender, race, marital status, age, medical diagnosis, conditions, length of stay in the hospital, and other characteristics. The researcher may have independent and dependent variables that correspond to research questions such as blood pressure, pulse, quality of life, and others. The researcher should list each variable, the level of measurement, and appropriate descriptive statistics for that level of measurement. If data have been numerically coded—for example, if "male" is coded as "1" and "female" as "2"—then a permanent codebook should be created for later reference during interpretation of the results.

Once the researcher has developed the list of appropriate descriptive statistics for variables, then the data analysis procedures can be run. Descriptive analysis can be completed using a variety of methods. Simple descriptive analyses can be calculated by hand, using an electronic calculator. Although laborious, and subject to error, it is possible to complete most descriptive statistics without complex software. Common spreadsheet programs can also be used to calculate descriptive statistics, including measures of central tendency, variability, relative position, and correlation. Advantages of spreadsheet software are their wide availability and the capacity to produce graphical representations of data as well as numerical ones. Specific statistical software is the fastest and most efficient way to complete a descriptive analysis. Statistical software can yield both numerical and graphical summaries of data and can be used to analyze and compare measures for subgroups as well as the entire sample. The advantage of using statistical software for descriptive analysis is that the data are prepared and ready for more complex analyses if needed.

Reporting Descriptive Results

Although descriptive results are reported in a myriad of ways, there are standards for the way descriptive results are reported. The goal of descriptive reporting is to convey the most complete information in the most straightforward and concise way. Thebane and Akhtar-Danesh (2008) developed a set of standards for reporting descriptive results for nursing research, and these can serve as a guide when writing this section of a report.

Demographic and outcome data will be measured as nominal, ordinal, or interval. The appropriate report for each includes:

- *Interval:* Report the mean, followed by the standard deviation in parentheses, e.g., mean age was 38.6 ($s = 2.4$).
- *Ordinal:* Report the median, with the minimum and maximum scores following in parentheses, e.g., median pain score was 4 (min = 1, max = 7).
- *Nominal:* Report the number for each category followed by the percentage in parentheses, e.g., number of females was 25 (51%).

When outliers exist, a box plot should also be provided for reference. Any methods that were used to deal with missing data or to normalize data should be described in enough detail that the reader can determine the effect these procedures may have had on the results.

A common question is how accurately to depict the data, that is, how many decimals should be reported. Guidelines developed by Lang and Secic (2003) have set the standard for reporting precision as:

- *The mean:* To, at most, one decimal place more than the original data.
- *Standard deviation:* To, at most, two decimal places more than the original data.
- *Percentages:* For sample size over 100, report to one decimal place. For between 20 and 100 subjects, report percentages as whole numbers. For fewer than 20 subjects, report the actual raw number.

Tables and graphs are helpful in visually understanding the data and condensing large amounts of information into smaller sections.

Summary of Key Concepts

- Summarizing descriptive data is the first step in the analysis of quantitative research data.
- Descriptive data are numbers in a data set that are calculated to represent research variables and do not involve generalization to larger populations.

 CRITICAL APPRAISAL **EXERCISE**

Retrieve the following full text article from the Cumulative Index to Nursing and Allied Health Literature or similar search database:

Natan, M., & Rais, I. (2010). Knowledge and attitudes of nurses regarding domestic violence and their effect on the identification of battered women. *Journal of Trauma Nursing, 17*(2), 112–117.

Review the article, focusing on the sections that report the results of the descriptive analyses. Think about the following appraisal questions in your critical review of this research article:

1. What are the variables that are measured?
2. Do the measures yield numbers that represent nominal-, ordinal-, or interval-level data?
3. Have the authors used the correct descriptive statistics for the level of measurement of the variables?
4. Are the statistics represented in the most understandable way? Discuss the use of tables relative to the type of information being reported. Are there graphical representations that might simplify the report?
5. Do the authors provide the right descriptive numbers about the sample, measurement instruments, and results?
6. Do the authors interpret the data appropriately, that is, they do not overinterpret?
7. Refer to the title of the article. Is this an appropriate representation for a descriptive study? Why or why not?

- Nominal and ordinal data are best represented by frequencies, percentages, and rates.
- Interval- and ratio-level data can be represented by measures of central tendency, variability, and relative position.
- Measures of central tendency include the mean, median, and mode. The mean is easily calculated and interpreted but is influenced by extreme scores. The median represents the midpoint of the data but does not reflect extremes well. The mode is the most frequently occurring value; it is of limited usefulness in descriptive analysis.
- Measures of variability include the variance, standard deviation, and coefficient of variation, all of which represent how spread out the data values are in relation to the mean.
- Measures of relative position include percentiles and standardized scores, which enable the comparison of values when the scales of measurement are different.
- The relationship between two variables in a sample is represented by a correlation coefficient.
- A frequency distribution enables the researcher to determine the shape of the variable's distribution, which may be normal, skewed, or have kurtosis.
- Data must be analyzed using the correct statistical procedure for the level of measurement of a variable.
- The data may be presented numerically and graphically in a way that conveys the most accurate information about the variables in the study.
- Some errors in reporting descriptive data include using the wrong statistics for the level of measurement; presenting incomplete, overly complicated, or misleading data; or drawing conclusions that go beyond what the data will support.
- Data must be meticulously collected, entered, checked for quality, and cleaned prior to analysis.

For a full suite of assignments and additional learning activities, use the access code located in the front of your book to visit this exclusive website: http://go.jblearning.com/houser. If you do not have an access code, you can obtain one at the site.

References

Altman, D. (2006). *Practical statistics for medical research*. London: Chapman and Hall.

Fawcett, J., & Garity, J. (2009). *Evaluating research for evidence-based nursing practice*. Philadelphia: F.A. Davis.

Fisher, M., & Marshall, A. (2008). Understanding descriptive statistics. *Australian Critical Care, 22*, 93–97.

Garden, E., & Kabacoff, R. (2010). *Evaluating research articles from start to finish*. Thousand Oaks, CA: Sage.

Horton, L. (2009). *Calculating and reporting healthcare statistics*. Chicago: American Health Information Management Association.

Kremelberg, D. (2010). *Practical statistics*. Thousand Oaks, CA: Sage.

Lang, T., & Secic, M. (2003). *How to report statistics in medicine*. Philadelphia: American College of Physicians.

Marshall, G., & Jonker, L. (2010). An introduction to descriptive statistics: A review and practical guide. *Radiography, 16*, e1–e7.

Motulsky, H. (2010). *Intuitive biostatistics: A nonmathematical guide to statistical thinking*. New York: Oxford University Press.

Norman, G., & Streiner, D. (2008). *Biostatistics: The bare essentials* (3rd ed.). Hamilton, Ontario, Canada: BC Decker.

Rosner, B. (2010). *Fundamentals of biostatistics* (7th ed.). Pacific Grove, CA: Duxbury Press.

Thebane, L., & Akhtar-Danesh, N. (2008). Guidelines for reporting descriptive statistics in health research. *Nurse Researcher, 15*(2), 72–81.

part V

Research that
Measures Effectiveness

chapter *14*

Quantitative Research Questions and Procedures

 ## CHAPTER OBJECTIVES

The study of this chapter will help the learner to:

- Examine quantitative research designs and methods.
- Describe the importance of design decisions in quantitative studies.
- Compare the characteristics and applications of specific quantitative designs.
- Relate quantitative designs to evidence-based nursing practice.
- Appraise a quantitative study for strengths and weaknesses.
- Learn how to create a quantitative research design.

 ## KEY TERMS

Case–control study	Ex post facto research	Quasi-experimental designs
Causal–comparative	Nonequivalent comparison group before/after design	Time-series designs
Comparison group		
Control group	Nonequivalent comparison group posttest only	
Experimental designs		

Introduction

Evidence for nursing practice means that nurses are able to practice based on what they know, rather than what they think. Quantitative research enables the nurse researcher to determine what is known. The purpose of quantitative research is to use measurement to determine the effectiveness of interventions and to report these effects with an identified level of confidence. Quantitative research is generally reported using numbers,

Scenes from the Field

The ability to suck is a critical ability for the premature infant. Sucking is involved in both nutritional and neurological development. Oral feeding is a complex and exhausting task for the premature newborn; supporting the infant in achieving success at sucking can make a dramatic difference in a newborn's development. Standley et al. (2010) set out to determine if music could help these babies learn to suck more effectively.

Previous research had demonstrated that a variety of stimulation techniques administered to preterm infants can offset some of the adverse neurological effects they typically experience. Music had been shown to be effective in improving weight gain, reducing stress, shortening length of hospitalization, and increasing oxygenation. There was much theoretical reason to believe that music may have broader effects.

These authors used a 3×3 block design, meaning they tested between three treatment conditions at three different times. The treatment was a pacifier-activated lullaby system. When the infant sucked on a pacifier, it triggered a recording of a woman's voice singing soothing lullabies. The outcomes measured—the dependent variables—were days of nipple feeding, discharge weight, and total weight gain. At baseline, none of the infants received treatment; this made up one block of the design. The dependent variable was measured again after one trial of the lullaby system, and again after three trials. Subgroup analysis of gestational age and gender were also included in this full factorial analysis.

The music was successful in improving sucking behavior in the more mature babies. The length of gavage feeding was reduced significantly after even one trial, but even more dramatically after three treatments. These findings were across all groups at 36 weeks gestation. However, at 32 weeks gestation, the treatment actually lengthened the amount of time required for gavage feedings. Female infants receiving the lullabies learned to nipple feed significantly faster than male infants. The lullaby babies also went home sooner after beginning to nipple feed.

This was a complex design but one that controlled a number of potential extraneous variables. Measuring over time allowed each baby to be its own "control" and meant the treatment was not withheld from any of the babies. Music is an inexpensive treatment and one that is used frequently by nurses. This evidence would support its use in helping preterm infants become independent feeders sooner.

Source: Standley, J., Cassidy, J., Grant, R., Devasco, A., Szuch, C., Adams, K., et al. (2010). The effect of music reinforcement for non-nutritive sucking on nipple feeding of premature infants. *Pediatric Nursing, 36*(3), 138–145.

which is helpful because math and statistics are universal languages. Nurse researchers are focused on detecting truth; quantitative methods and procedures allow the nurse to describe what is known in a standard, universally understandable way.

Quantitative research involves the measurement of variables of interest and subsequent statistical analysis of the data. Quantitative analysis can be used to

- Determine the effects of an intervention
- Measure the relationships between variables
- Detect changes over time

Quantitative studies provide some of the strongest evidence for nursing practice because they enable the researcher to draw conclusions about the effectiveness of interventions. These studies are designed to provide high levels of control so that confidence in the results is enhanced. If all conditions are controlled so that the effects of a variable or intervention can be isolated, then the probability is low that the outcome is due to something other than the intervention. Quantitative methods allow the researcher to measure the probability that some other factor caused the outcome, specifically things such as extraneous variables, measurement error, or sampling error. Quantitative designs are intended to isolate and evaluate the effects of an intervention, treatment, or characteristic (which are referred to as independent variables) on a specific outcome (referred to as the dependent variable).

Quantitative studies can also answer questions about relationships between a cause and an effect, but sometimes causality has to be inferred. For example, the relationship between risk factors and disease cannot be tested with a true experimental design, because it is not ethical to expose healthy individuals to risk factors they would otherwise not experience. As a result, researchers must study these variables as they naturally occur. Because these studies do not allow for control over many extraneous variables, other explanations for the outcome may arise. Subjecting these kinds of study data to quantitative analysis allows the researcher to determine the probability that a relationship was caused by something else and to express risk relationships in quantifiable ways (Haynes, Sackett, Guyatt, & Tugwell, 2006).

Quantitative studies may be applied to determine changes over time in a single group of individuals. In essence, subjects serve as their own controls. Time-series data can provide substantial information about the effectiveness of interventions because these kinds of studies yield measures of both how much difference the intervention made and how long it took to be detectable.

These studies are useful as evidence for nursing practice in multiple ways. The focus on scientific studies as a basis for evaluating the effectiveness of interventions is a cornerstone in evidence-based nursing practice. These studies can help the nurse appraise the effectiveness of an intervention, determine the relationship between actions and patient responses, and measure changes over time. Overall, quantitative studies play an important role in establishing evidence-based practices and testing new or improved interventions.

Quantitative Research Questions

Quantitative studies address a considerable number of research questions. These questions are usually focused on the effects of interventions, actions, risk factors, or events. Words such as *what* and *when* often begin these questions, which use active verbs such as *affect*, *influence*, or *change*. Overall, quantitative research studies focus on establishing a statistical relationship between variables and measuring the probability that error was responsible for the outcome (Locke, Silverman, & Spirduso, 2010). These research questions, then, will have variables that can be operationally defined and measured in a numerical way.

The quantitative research question includes some common elements. It is most amenable to the PICO approach introduced in Chapter 4. The quantitative research question identifies the following elements:

- Population of interest
- Intervention under study
- Comparison that makes up the control
- Outcome of interest

A carefully constructed research question gives the researcher guidance in research design and communicates a great deal about the study in a single statement. It is a key tool for ensuring a quantitative study has all the elements needed for a controlled trial. Table 14.1 provides some examples of quantitative research questions that are appropriate for quantitative study.

Table 14.1

Examples of Quantitative Research Questions

Research Question	Design Used to Answer It
What are the effects of early ambulation (within 24 hours) and later ambulation (after 24 hours) on the rate of postoperative pneumonia in patients undergoing gastric bypass surgery?	Experimental designs
What is the effect of focused imagery on the pain associated with chest tube removal after coronary bypass surgery when compared to patients receiving no focused imagery for chest tube removal?	Experimental designs
Does the introduction of bar coding on a patient care unit result in lower medication error rates when compared to patient care units without bar coding?	Quasi-experimental designs
Does the implementation of an evidence-based practice council in a hospital result in greater levels of research knowledge among nurses than in hospitals with no evidence-based practice council?	Quasi-experimental designs
Are symptoms of myocardial infarction recognized in a shorter period of time in men than they are in women after presentation to an emergency department?	Causal–comparative designs
Do women who have in vitro fertilization have higher levels of parenting anxiety than women who have natural pregnancies?	Causal–comparative designs
Do women who have more than three children have higher rates of chronic urinary tract infections than women who have two or fewer children?	Case–control designs
Do men with abdominal hernias have a higher rate of abdominal aneurysm than men who have not been diagnosed with abdominal hernia?	Case–control designs
Is aggressive, early pulmonary rehabilitation effective in preventing long-term complications of community-acquired pneumonia?	Time-series designs
Does participation in a nursing residency result in increased retention of new graduate nurses?	Time-series designs

Characteristics of a Quantitative Design

Several different types of studies are classified as quantitative designs, but they all have some basic characteristics in common. These studies all rely on numbers to measure effects and to quantify error. These designs are best suited to study objective characteristics and human responses that can be quantified. All these studies involve comparing groups of subjects in some way—either between groups or within a single group over time. These designs are intended to be applied to samples that represent populations so that the findings can be generalized to larger groups of people with a high level of confidence that the study's outcome will be the same. Most quantitative studies are aimed at determining effects, whether they are directly attributed to a cause or inferred because of a measured relationship (Newell & Burnard, 2010). It is the establishment of the relationship between an independent variable and a dependent one that requires the controls that are built into quantitative studies.

An Interest in Variables

Quantitative studies are focused on measuring relationships among variables. These variables may be classified as independent (an intervention) or dependent (an outcome). In this case, the researcher is interested in the effect of the independent variable on the dependent variable. Quantitative studies require quantifying the variables of interest, and so these variables are usually objective characteristics or responses that can be reported as numbers. For example, the objective characteristics of heart health can be measured as blood pressure, heart rate, serum cholesterol, and other indicators of cardiac risk. On the other hand, the responses of pain, anxiety, and nausea have to be reported by the individual, and so are often recorded on scales or other instruments. Quantitative researchers are interested in a third type of variable: the extraneous variable. Extraneous variables are not part of the central study, but they do exert an effect. Many of the design elements in quantitative studies are intended to mitigate these effects through controls.

Control over Variables

Quantitative studies exhibit a high level of control over the variables of interest. An independent variable is controlled by the researcher; it is introduced into a patient care situation and manipulated to determine its effects. The researcher then puts measures in place to identify when the dependent variable has occurred and to quantify that response. The requirement for control over variables is not limited to those variables internal to the study. A key focus of quantitative designs is to control variables that are extraneous to the study, but that may exert an effect. The quantitative researcher attempts to eliminate these variables through strong design, if possible. If the effect of the variables cannot be avoided, then the researcher must control them through sampling strategy, intervention protocols, or statistical analysis. On occasion, variables may occur that cannot be eliminated or controlled, or the

gray matter

Characteristics of all quantitative design studies include:

- Relying on numbers to measure and quantify errors
- Studying objective characteristics and responses that can be measured
- Comparing groups of subjects in some way
- Applying interventions to samples to generalize to populations
- Aiming to determine effects of an intervention through a high level of control

variables may arise during the experiment, such as an external event. In this case, the researcher accounts for their effects in the research report.

This level of control lets the researcher rule out alternative explanations for the outcome in a systematic way. It increases confidence on the part of the reader that the intervention—and nothing else—caused a given effect.

The Use of Measurement

Quantitative analysis is, at its most fundamental, based on quantifying something. It is clear, then, that variables in quantitative studies will be measured. Measurements may be direct or indirect, and values may be collected prospectively or retrospectively. Data may be gathered from primary or secondary sources. The measures themselves must be reliable and valid to rule out measurement error as an extraneous effect. Quantitative studies are characterized by data collection using instrumentation that yields numerical data. Data may be collected at a single point in time, at a baseline and after an intervention, or over time periods. Reliability of instruments, raters, and measures is a central concern.

Comparisons of Groups

Most quantitative studies focus on a comparison of groups of some kind. Comparisons may be made between the following groups:

- An intervention group and a control group
- A group with a risk factor and a matched group without
- A group at baseline and after treatment

Comparisons between groups are usually applied to test the effects of an intervention. With sufficient control and a strong sampling strategy, if differences between groups are detected, then it can be assumed the intervention was the cause. When control groups are not possible, the researcher can study the effects of a risk factor by comparing outcomes to a group without the risk factor. Comparisons within groups, such as a time-series design, can reveal both if a treatment has an effect and when it is likely to occur. Regardless of the question and intent, some comparison between or within groups is characteristic of these designs.

A Priori Selection of a Design

Quantitative designs are selected after the research question is clarified and the literature review is complete, and then they are not changed. Although some aspects of the study may necessarily need to adapt to changing conditions, the bulk of decisions about quantitative designs is made before the study begins. This minimizes the potential for introducing researcher bias or changing the study after it has begun, to alter the results. This *a priori* selection of design, protocol, and analytic method is characteristic of good quantitative designs.

The details of the design are determined by the nature of the research question and the resources of the researcher. Fundamentally, quantitative designs can be classified in the following ways:

- Experimental designs answer questions about the effectiveness of interventions.
- Quasi-experimental designs answer questions about the relationships between variables.
- Comparisons of intact groups answer questions about differences in the characteristics of groups.
- Time-series designs answer questions about the effectives of interventions over time.

A general design is selected early in the research planning stage. Within each of these designs are variations on the central theme, but each has distinctive applications and characteristics. These provide the researcher with guidance in the development of the specific research protocol and plan.

The Gold Standard: Experimental Design

Experimental designs answer questions about the effectiveness of interventions. These studies are considered the "gold standard" for evidence-based practice because they provide convincing support for the value of a treatment (Machin & Fayers, 2010). Experimental designs are often referred to as randomized controlled trials because these designs have in common random assignment of subjects and a high level of control. Subjects are randomly assigned to groups so the researcher can assume the groups are basically similar in most ways. They are sometimes referred to simply as "clinical trials." Design elements of experiments enable the researcher to control extraneous variables so the effect of an intervention can be isolated and quantified. Experimental designs also enable the researcher to measure the effects of error and calculate the probability that the results were due to random events rather than the intervention. Overall, experimental designs—particularly when they are conducted in multiple sites or when multiple studies are reviewed in aggregate—are considered the strongest evidence for practice and are at the top of the evidence pyramid.

> **Experimental designs:** Highly structured studies of cause and effect applied to determine the effectiveness of an intervention.

Experimental designs are those in which the researcher moves from passive observer and data collector to active involvement in the intervention. In other words, the researcher is not looking for relationships, but hoping to cause them. A clinical trial is the typical experiment: Subjects are randomly assigned to either an experimental or a control group, the intervention is applied to the experimental group while withheld from the control group, and differences in a specified outcome are measured. If differences are found, then they can be assumed to be attributable to the intervention because all other differences between the groups are controlled.

> **Control group:** A subgroup of the sample of an experimental study from which the intervention is withheld.

Characteristics of Experimental Designs

Experiments have some fundamental characteristics that enable researchers to draw conclusions about cause and effect. The reader will recall that three conditions must be met to draw a conclusion about cause and effect:

- The cause must precede the effect in time.
- The influence of the cause on the effect must be demonstrated.
- Rival explanations for the outcome must be ruled out.

Experimental designs also demonstrate consistent characteristics that allow the researcher to draw conclusions about causality.

The Independent Variable Is Artificially Introduced

The independent variable (the "cause" in cause and effect) is introduced and manipulated in an experiment. Although much can be deduced from studying naturally occurring phenomena, extraneous variables make it difficult, if not impossible, to isolate the effect of a single intervention (Machin & Fayers, 2010). In an experimental design, the only difference between groups is the intervention, and so its effects can be isolated and quantified. Manipulating the independent variable also enables the researcher to sequence the treatment so a subsequent outcome can be revealed, which is one of the conditions necessary to infer causality.

Subjects Are Randomly Assigned to Groups

A hallmark of the experimental design is random assignment to groups. When subjects are randomly assigned to groups, then it can be assumed that all their other characteristics are randomly (and equally) distributed in both groups. This feature enables the researcher to draw a conclusion that the only difference between the two groups is the intervention. Randomization means the researcher can rule out rival explanations, which is a second condition for determining causality.

Experimental Conditions Are Highly Controlled

In experimental designs, the researcher builds in controls for extraneous effects of variables or subject characteristics. Controls may be incorporated into sampling strategies, methodology, data collection, or analysis, but the most common is the use of a control group. These controls also help the researcher rule out rival explanations for the outcome.

Results Are Quantitatively Analyzed

The differences between groups are measured quantitatively and analyzed using inferential statistics. Inferential statistics yield numbers that are helpful in two ways: They allow the researcher to determine the probability that random error is responsible for the outcome, and they give the reader information about the size of the effect. Statistical analysis enables the researcher to draw a conclusion that the independent variable had an influence on the outcome, which is a third condition for concluding a cause-and-effect relationship exists.

Questions that Are Best Answered with Experimental Design

Experimental designs are best applied to answer questions about the effectiveness of interventions. The ability to introduce a treatment in a highly controlled situation enables the researcher to draw conclusions about causality, influence, and relationships. Questions that are focused on the sequence between a cause and an effect are also answered with experimental designs. Some words that appear in questions for experimental designs include *affect, cause, relate, influence,* and *change.* Examples of questions include: What is the effect of continuous, low-level zinc ingestion on the occurrence of the common cold among young adults? Does a video game introduction to the surgical suite change the level of anxiety preoperatively for children when compared to children who receive a traditional introduction? Does access to a clinical consultant influence the level of use of evidence-based practice on a patient care unit as compared to a unit that has no clinical consultant?

The research question for an experimental design is most adaptable to the PICO design. The question identifies the population, intervention, comparison, and outcome. A carefully constructed research question for an experimental study essentially provides an outline of design elements (Wood & Ross-Kerr, 2006). The methods and procedures that are used to answer the question are all linked inextricably to the elements of a well-considered question.

Experimental Design Methods and Procedures

Conducting experimental studies requires that the researcher make decisions about how the study will be carried out to demonstrate the key characteristics. Design of the methods and procedures involves a series of systematic steps based on carefully considered choices.

1. *What is the population of interest?* Objective inclusion and exclusion criteria help the researcher consider and describe the specific population that is of interest.
2. *How will subjects be assigned to groups?* Experimental designs all require random assignment to groups, but there are multiple methods for randomization. For a review, see Chapter 8.
3. *How will the intervention be applied?* Carefully considered, detailed directions for applying the intervention will minimize error associated with inconsistent application of the treatment.
4. *What will be the comparison?* For some studies, the comparison is "no treatment," a true control group. However, it is usually not ethical to withhold treatment from a patient in the name of science. So the comparison is made to a standard treatment, or in some cases, a sham treatment (to control treatment effects).
5. *How will the outcome be measured?* Reliable, valid measures are required to minimize measurement error, ensure accuracy, and measure with precision.
6. *How will differences between the groups be quantified?* The choice of statistical tests is part of the planning process. These will be covered in depth in the next chapter.

Strengths of Experimental Designs

Experimental designs are the gold standard for evidence-based practice. They are considered some of the best scientific evidence available for support of nursing practice. The use of an experimental design offers many advantages for the nurse, including the following:

- Experimental designs are considered the strongest evidence for practice.
- These designs are the only ones that allow a definitive conclusion about cause and effect, and so they are ideal for testing the effectiveness of interventions.

Case in Point: An Experimental Design

Tonsillectomy is a common procedure in pediatric patients. Standard preoperative preparation includes a period of fasting to minimize the danger of aspiration of stomach contents during surgery. However, these children often have problems with postoperative nutrition, due to throat pain after the procedure. If the child's preoperative fasting is lengthy and it lasts for several hours postoperatively, the child could have problems with fluid balance, further complicating recovery.

Klemetti et al. (2010) used a prospective, randomized intervention study to determine the effect of the way in which families were prepared for preoperative fasting. They wanted to determine if face-to-face counseling about preoperative nutrition would be more effective in reducing postoperative thirst than the standard approach. The standard approach was to provide the parents with written instructions without any face-to-face counseling. Of the 134 children who were scheduled for tonsillectomy and recruited for the study, 124 agreed to participate. The children were randomly assigned to the counseling group or the standard treatment group. One nurse provided all of the counseling to minimize treatment effects. The researcher was blinded as to which group received the intervention when postoperative data were collected. Postoperative hunger and thirst were scored at 2-hour periods following surgery until 24 hours postoperatively, and then again at 24 hours.

The counseling appeared to be a successful intervention. The children whose families received individual counseling had low levels of thirst and hunger up to 24 hours, whereas the control group's hunger and thirst increased until the following morning. The differences were statistically and clinically significant.

This randomized trial was a well-done example of testing a new treatment against a standard one. Randomization and blinding of the researcher minimized a host of threats to validity, and made the results stronger as evidence for practice. These data would support the benefits of spending time counseling families and children prior to surgery so that their postoperative recovery is a smooth one.

Source: Klemetti, S., Kinnunen, I., Suominen, T., Antila, H., Vahlberg, T., et al. (2010). The effect of preoperative fasting on postoperative thirst, hunger, and oral intake in paediatric ambulatory tonsillectomy. *Journal of Clinical Nursing, 19,* 341–350.

- Experimental designs are recognized and valued by other disciplines.
- Experimental designs are generally understood by the public and patients.

Limitations of Experimental Designs

Despite their clear strengths, only a small percentage of healthcare research studies are experimental designs. Additionally, of those experiments reported in the literature, many have serious flaws—groups may be assigned other than randomly, or serious errors may affect the outcome (Melnyk & Fineout-Overholt, 2010). Although experiments offer many advantages, some of the disadvantages associated with the use of this method include the following:

- Experimental designs are complex and difficult to carry out.
- These designs require substantial resources in terms of time, researcher skill, and access to subjects.
- Many aspects of health care cannot be manipulated (for example, the presence of a risk factor, the worsening of a disease).

- Increasing control also means the experiment becomes more artificial, and generalizability may be limited as a result.

More Common: Quasi-Experimental Designs

Experimental designs provide clear evidence of the effectiveness of interventions, and yet they are uncommon in nursing and health care in general. This is because of the difficulty in achieving the high levels of control that are characteristic of experiments in an applied setting. In addition, it is not always desirable—or ethical—to manipulate an independent variable or to withhold treatment, and so alternative designs must be selected. Quasi-experimental designs have many of the characteristics of experimental designs except for one key feature: Quasi-experimental studies do not randomize subjects to groups, but rather work with intact groups or convenience samples. Because of this single feature, control and generalizability are limited.

> **Quasi-experimental designs:** Studies of cause and effect similar to experimental designs but using convenience samples or existing groups to test interventions.

Characteristics of Quasi-Experimental Designs

Quasi-experimental designs have many characteristics in common with experimental designs. Specifically, the researcher identifies an independent and dependent variable of interest and strives to control as many extraneous variables as possible. Subjects are

---

Case in Point: A Quasi-Experimental Design

Dramatic increases in life expectancy combined with the increased rate of chronic disease in the older population have resulted in a larger number of elderly needing institutional help for daily living. Although nursing homes serve the physical needs of the elderly, life in long-term care can mean limitations on physical and social activity. A researcher set out to determine if an indoor gardening program for nursing home residents could affect their socialization, life satisfaction, loneliness, and activity level.

Two nursing homes were selected for the study, and baseline measures of satisfaction, loneliness, socialization, and activity level were collected. One nursing home implemented an indoor gardening program, while residents in the comparison nursing home had standard activities. Fifty-three individuals participated in the 8-week study.

There were significant improvements in life satisfaction and socialization, and a significant decrease in perceived loneliness in the gardening group. Activity level was the same for both groups. It

appears that a structured activity such as gardening may help the elderly deal with some of the challenges of long-term-care living.

This was a typical quasi-experimental design in that the subjects were not randomized to an experimental and control group, but were part of an intact group. It would be difficult to include some residents from a single facility in a gardening program and not others, and so the quasi-experimental design was more feasible than a true randomized trial. In other respects, such as measurement procedures and procedural control, this study was more like an experiment. These controls enabled the restriction of extraneous variables. Although these data cannot be assumed to generalize to the larger population of nursing home residents, this evidence is strong for application in similar settings.

Source: Tse, M. (2010). Therapeutic effects of an indoor gardening programme for older people living in nursing homes. *Journal of Clinical Nursing, 19*, 949–958.

separated into groups, and differences between the groups are measured. Data are collected numerically and analyzed statistically.

The primary difference between experimental and quasi-experimental designs is the lack of random assignment to treatment groups. This characteristic weakens quasi-experimental studies when compared to experimental ones because, without randomization, it cannot be assumed that the intervention and comparison groups are equivalent at the beginning of the study. This leaves room for the potential for other explanations for the outcome, and so a clear conclusion about cause and effect cannot be drawn.

Quasi-experimental designs often involve studying intact groups. This may be because it is impractical or impossible to deliver the intervention to some members of a group and not others. For example, a nurse educator may be interested in the effectiveness of an educational technique used on one patient care unit and compare outcomes to another patient care unit that did not receive the education. A comparison group exists, but it is not a true control group because the subjects are not assigned to groups randomly (Mitchell & Jolley, 2009).

Comparison group: A subgroup of the sample of a quasi-experimental design from which the intervention is withheld. Subjects are similar to and compared with the experimental group, but are not randomly assigned.

Quasi-experimental studies can still be strong ones because they meet two of the three conditions for inferring causality: The independent variable precedes the dependent variable, and the influence of the independent variable can be measured.

Questions that Are Best Answered with Quasi-Experimental Design

Quasi-experimental designs can be used to answer many of the same types of questions as their experimental counterparts. Questions about the effectiveness of interventions are often addressed with quasi-experimental designs. The questions often begin with *what* or *how* and use action verbs to indicate an expected effect. The variables are measurable and can be quantified using numbers.

The primary difference between the two is in the way results are interpreted, not the way the questions are worded. Quasi-experimental designs are not as strong as experimental designs because they are not controlled, and it cannot be assumed the sample represents the population. If the researcher is careful not to overinterpret the results, then quasi-experimental studies have a great deal to contribute to the body of nursing knowledge.

Quasi-Experimental Design Methods and Procedures

Quasi-experimental design decisions are made *a priori*, as are experimental ones. Although there are many similarities between experimental and quasi-experimental methods, there are some key differences.

- *The population of interest is identified:* In quasi-experimental studies, identifying the population is heavily dependent on the accessible population and the way that subjects are naturally divided into groups.
- *Group assignments are identified:* Quasi-experimental studies often rely on convenience samples made up of intact groups. As such, group membership is not

assigned so much as it is identified. The criteria for membership in a group are clearly identified, however, so the researcher controls selection effects.

- *An intervention is applied:* The independent variable is identified and applied to the treatment group using standardized, detailed procedures.
- *An outcome is measured:* Quasi-experimental studies have dependent variables, and these are measured in both groups to determine if the intervention affected an outcome.
- *Differences in groups are quantitatively analyzed:* Statistics are applied to determine the magnitude of any effects that are identified and the probability that sampling error is responsible for the outcome. Different statistics may need to be applied, however, because many inferential tests assume randomness, and adjustments in calculations are called for with convenience samples.

Nonequivalent comparison group before/after design: The strongest type of quasi-experimental design in which subject responses in two or more groups are measured before and after an intervention. **Nonequivalent comparison group posttest only:** A type of quasi-experimental design in which data are collected after the intervention is introduced. Lack of baseline data may introduce extraneous variables in the results.

The most common quasi-experimental design is the nonequivalent comparison group before/after design. In this design, subject responses in two or more groups are measured before and after an intervention. The only difference between this design and a true experiment is the lack of randomization. It is the strongest of the quasi-experimental designs and so provides good evidence for nursing practice.

On occasion, researchers are unable to collect pretest data before the intervention is introduced. In this case, serious flaws are introduced into this design, which is classified as nonequivalent comparison group posttest only. In these studies, it is impossible to determine the subject characteristics that were present when the experiment began. There is no basis for determining the baseline equivalence of the groups, and so a multitude of extraneous variables is potentially introduced.

Strengths of Quasi-Experimental Designs

The use of a quasi-experimental design offers many advantages for the researcher, including the following:

- Quasi-experimental studies are more feasible than true experiments to conduct in an applied setting.
- True experiments may not be feasible or ethical; it may be impossible to deliver an intervention to some people in a group and not others.
- Quasi-experimental studies introduce a level of control that reduces the effect of extraneous variables.
- Accessible subjects can be used for the study so that larger samples may be obtained.

Limitations of Quasi-Experimental Designs

Although quasi-experimental designs offer many advantages, some of the disadvantages associated with the use of this method include the following:

- It is inappropriate to draw firm conclusions about cause and effect without random assignment to groups.

- Groups may not be equivalent in characteristics and so extraneous variables are introduced.
- Rival explanations for the outcome exist and may weaken confidence in the results.

Designs that Focus on Intact Groups

All the designs considered thus far in this chapter have focused on studies in which the independent variable is introduced, manipulated, or added to the situation in some way. In some cases, though, the independent variable is not introduced so much as it is located. In other words, the researcher must find subjects in which the independent variable is a natural occurrence and compare these individuals to those in whom the variable is naturally absent. The researcher then measures an outcome of interest—the dependent variable—in both groups to infer causality.

These studies are sometimes called nonexperimental designs because the independent variable is not manipulated. Indeed, technically it should not be called an independent variable at all because it is not changed or introduced. It is, however, very common to use the independent/dependent terminology when referring to the variables in this group of studies.

These studies can take on one of several forms. Ex post facto research (based on a Latin phrase meaning "operating retroactively") relies on the observation of relationships between naturally occurring differences in the presumed independent

Ex post facto research: An intact group design that relies on observation of the relationships between naturally occurring differences in the intervention and outcome.

Case in Point: Ex Post Facto Design

Stress is pervasive in society and can have a myriad of physical and psychological effects. The influence of stress during pregnancy has been studied broadly, but its role in health-promoting behaviors of new mothers is poorly understood. Gill and Loh (2010) wanted to determine if stress was associated with healthy behaviors in new primiparous mothers. A second goal was to determine if such a relationship could be mediated by optimism on the part of the mother.

This study was an ex post facto cross-sectional design. A sample of 174 primiparous mothers was asked to complete a questionnaire that measured perceived stress and health-promoting lifestyle behaviors, and a test that measures optimism. Data were collected at 12 months postbirth via an online survey system. Results indicated there was a relationship between perceived stress and health-promoting behaviors among these mothers. This re-

lationship was mediated positively by the optimism of the mother.

This typical ex post facto design used data that were recalled retrospectively by subjects to measure relationships among variables. The online data collection method enhanced response rate, but the 12-month time frame could have led to gaps in recall or errors in completing the instruments. These problems are also typical of these designs. Although the findings support the relationship between stress and health-promoting behaviors, it is impossible to determine causal relationships from this study because temporality of the influencing variables cannot be verified. However, these data do suggest that including stress management in the education of new mothers could enhance health promotion after birth.

Source: Gill, R., & Loh, J. (2010). The role of optimism in health promoting behaviors in new primiparous mothers. *Nursing Research, 59*(5), 348–355.

and dependent variables (Gall, Gall, & Borg, 2007). It is so named because the data are usually collected after the fact, meaning that both the independent and dependent variables have already occurred. This weakens the capacity of these studies to support cause and effect because the researcher cannot prove temporality. In other words, the researcher is dependent on the subject's recall to determine if the independent variable preceded the dependent one.

Studies of intact groups may also be classified as causal-comparative. These nonexperimental investigations seek to identify cause-and-effect relationships by forming groups based on a categorical classification (Gall et al., 2007). In other words, groups are assigned based on certain characteristics that the individuals inherently possess. Groups are then assessed relative to an outcome of interest. Subjects may be assigned to groups based on any categorical classification, such as gender, ethnicity, or geographic region. An outcome of interest is then measured to determine if the groups differ. If they do, it is assumed that the differences in the outcome are due to the differences in the classification of the subject. For example, a researcher may be interested in determining if men and women express the same amount

> **Causal-comparative:** An intact group design that involves categorization of subjects into groups. An outcome of interest is measured and differences are attributed to the differences in classification of subjects.

Case in Point: Causal–Comparative Design

Case management has been demonstrated to reduce costs and hospital stays associated with chronic illness. This approach is relatively recent, and little research exists about the type of case management that is most effective. Thomas (2010) set out to determine if the type of case management model was associated with length of stay across varying specialty units and levels of care.

The author used a causal–comparative retrospective study that included more than 39,000 medical, surgical, and cardiology inpatients. Medical record data about length of stay were collected for patient stays on surgical, intermediate, and intensive care units. Two models of case management were used during the time period studied. The hospital first used a traditional model, more accurately described as utilization management, in which nurses documented patient need for care and justified stays to payers. A later model used by the hospital was called the full immersion model and included traditional utilization management, with additional focus on enhanced communication with physicians and support for a coordinated plan of care.

Statistically significant reductions in length of stay were measured using the full immersion model when compared to the traditional utilization review model. Length of stay was more than 1.5 days shorter in the full immersion model, and variability in length of stay was smaller as well.

This study is typical of causal–comparative research in that no intervention was manipulated, and data were collected retrospectively. A group was identified that experienced traditional case management and a comparison group was found that experienced the full immersion model. Comparable outcomes were measured in each group. Although not definitive for cause and effect, causal–comparative studies such as this one still provide evidence that can be applied to practice. In the case of organizational studies—in which the manipulation of a variable in an entire hospital is not feasible—this may be the strongest design available.

Source: Thomas, P. (2010). Case manager role definitions: Do they make an organizational impact? *Professional Case Management, 13*(2), 61–71.

Case-control study: An intact group design that involves observation of subjects who exhibit a characteristic matched with subjects who do not. Differences between the subjects allow study of relationships between risk and disease without subjecting healthy individuals to illness.

of anxiety prior to cardiovascular angiography. In this case, the independent variable is loosely interpreted as "gender" and the dependent variable is "anxiety."

A third type of intact group design is the case-control study. These studies are common in epidemiology and public health because they enable the study of the links between causative agents and disease (Morrow, 2010a). Case–control studies are often used to judge the relationships between risk factors and disease states or between an event and an outcome (Armenian, 2009). For example, an infection control nurse may be interested in determining the source of infections on a given patient care unit. Patients who exhibited the infection would be matched carefully with patients who did not, and both groups would be appraised for exposures to potential infectious agents. In this case, the independent variable is interpreted as "exposure" and the dependent variable is "infection." Case–control studies are always performed by looking backward in time. For this reason, they are sometimes referred to simply as retrospective studies, in contrast with longitudinal studies, which must be prospective (Morrow, 2010a).

The Kinds of Questions that Studies of Intact Groups Answer

Ex post facto research is useful for studying the effects of events that occur for some individuals and not for others. For example, the nurse may want to investigate whether patients who have medication errors have longer lengths of stay in the hospital than patients who do not. The nurse will select records from patients with medication errors and compare them to patients without errors and determine if there is a difference in their length of stay.

Case in Point: Case–Control Design

Infections make up significant morbidity in children who are hospitalized, and the most common infection is blood borne. The majority of bloodstream infections in children are associated with intravascular catheter use. Central line–associated bloodstream infections (CLABSIs) are a serious complication, and understanding the risk factors for this condition is the subject of a study by Wylie et al. (2010).

The researchers used a case–control design involving more than 600 children, with 204 cases of CLABSI matched with 406 controls without the condition. All patients had a central venous catheter and were matched by ICU admission date to rule out the effect of a unit-based infection. Independent predictors of CLABSI included a lengthy duration of ICU central access, central venous catheter placement

in the ICU, nonoperative cardiovascular disease, presence of a gastrostomy tube, and receipt of a blood transfusion.

This study is a typical case–control design in that the authors found subjects with and without the dependent variable and explored differences in the measured variables in each group. Although not definitive for causal agents, case–control studies nevertheless can guide the nurse to identify and minimize potential risk factors.

Source: Wylie, M., Graham, D., Potter-Bynoe, G., Kleinman, M., Randolph, A., Sandora, T., et al. (2010). Risk factors for central line associated bloodstream infection in pediatric intensive care units. *Infection Control and Hospital Epidemiology, 31*(10), 1049–1056.

Causal–comparative studies are useful for understanding the relationship between causal variables and their potential effects, particularly when the intervention is of a group nature. It is difficult, for example, to provide an innovative educational technique to some students in a classroom and not others. Likewise, it is nearly impossible to study changes in the way patient care units are organized or managed without using causal–comparative studies. Without huge, unwieldy samples, the researcher cannot apply the intervention randomly. These designs are useful for questions that involve the way groups react to interventions or to study the effectiveness of management strategies, educational efforts, or developmental work.

Investigating the differences between intact groups gives the nurse valuable information about the relationships between actions and responses. These designs are helpful for the study of relationships between risk factors and disease because it is not ethical to subject a healthy individual to a risk factor just to study its effects. In this case, it is necessary to find individuals with risk factors and compare their outcomes to individuals without the risk factors (Leedy, 2009). For example, the nurse may wish to determine if patients who are unable to ambulate until the second postoperative day have a higher risk of thromboemboli than patients who are able to ambulate on the first postoperative day.

These research questions often begin with "What is the difference?" or "What is the relationship between?" to reflect an expectation that the independent variable will have a demonstrable effect. Good questions for these studies will have an identified population, a variable of interest, some comparison group, and an outcome.

Methods and Procedures for Studies of Intact Groups

Studies of intact groups require a systematic approach and efforts to exert as much control as possible. Because these studies have neither random assignment nor a manipulated intervention, the evidence they provide is much weaker than experimental or quasi-experimental designs. The researcher, then, should make an effort to control as much as possible to strengthen the conclusions. A systematic approach includes the following steps:

1. *The population of interest is identified.* As in quasi-experimental studies, identifying the population is heavily dependent on the accessible population and the way subjects are naturally divided into groups. Inclusion and exclusion criteria are particularly important in these studies to minimize selection effects.
2. *Group characteristics are identified.* Group characteristics of interest are identified. The independent variable is operationally defined so the researcher will be certain that a subject possesses it; the comparison group is carefully matched on all other characteristics. This process of carefully matching subjects with the independent variable and those without is critical for case–control studies. Matching helps to control extraneous variables such as gender, age, and diagnosis.
3. *The outcome of interest is defined.* The dependent variable is operationally defined so it can be quantified and measured.
4. *Variables are measured.* The variables are measured either directly or indirectly, from either primary or secondary sources. In the case of ex post facto research,

record retrieval is often necessary. Reliability and validity of measures are important considerations to minimize measurement error.

5. *Differences in groups are quantitatively analyzed.* Statistics are applied to determine the magnitude of any effects that are identified and the probability that sampling error is responsible for the outcome.

As can be seen, many procedures in studies of intact groups are intended to minimize error associated with measures, sampling, and analysis because it is impossible to control extraneous variables. Minimizing other sources of error through adequate controls strengthens the ability to use the results as evidence for practice.

Strengths of Studies of Intact Groups

The use of studies of intact groups offers many advantages for the researcher, including the following:

- These designs are a practical way to study interventions that are of a group nature or that cannot ethically be withheld or manipulated.
- Studies of intact groups are helpful in applied settings because they provide direction for educators, managers, and group leaders.
- These designs are relatively easy to carry out and are often implemented using secondary data.

Limitations of Studies of Intact Groups

Although studies of intact groups offer many advantages, some of the disadvantages associated with the use of these methods include the following:

- The researcher cannot draw definitive conclusions about cause and effect using these studies.
- Data collection is often secondary and so is dependent on the accuracy and completeness of the record.
- The researcher forfeits control of the independent variable and so cannot ensure that extraneous variables did not affect the outcome.

Time-Series Designs

Time-series designs: A type of quasi-experimental design that involves one group that receives the intervention; an outcome is measured repeatedly over time.

A final type of experimental design has a dual focus: The researcher is interested in both the effects of an intervention and the timing of its effects. Time-series designs are sometimes categorized as quasi-experimental because they do not have randomly assigned groups. Indeed, time-series designs have only one group: the group receiving the intervention. A baseline is measured and an intervention applied, and then measures are taken periodically over a specified time period.

In these studies, subsequent measures are compared to the baseline measure, and changes that emerge are assumed to be due to the intervention. In these designs, subjects actually serve as their own comparison group, with subsequent responses each compared to the preintervention period.

The Kinds of Questions that Time-Series Designs Answer

Time-series designs answer questions about the effectiveness of interventions and the timing of responses. In some cases, the effects of an intervention may have a delayed onset or may take time to fully develop. For example, a study of functionality after total knee replacement will demonstrate an initial period of decreased functionality, followed by improvement over several months' time. These designs enable the nurse to counsel patients about what they can expect from a treatment in terms of both effects and timing (Crosby, DiClemente, & Salazar, 2006). Time-series designs are also useful when a change is being implemented and the researcher is focused on the results of that change. A unit may change its procedure manual to evidence-based practice guidelines and desire to measure the effects of the change. It is difficult, if not impossible, to construct a randomized trial focused on this type of change, but a comparison to a baseline helps the researcher infer what results were achieved.

Time-series studies often have questions such as "What is the effect over time?" or "When do effects occur?" Results of these studies are useful for practicing nurses in evaluating both what to expect from an intervention and when to expect it.

Time-Series Design Methods and Procedures

Time-series designs are carried out systematically in a way very similar to other quasi-experimental designs. Although subjects are not randomized to groups, other elements are controlled as much as possible so extraneous variables are held to a minimum. In this way, rival explanations can be considered and reasonable conclusions drawn. The following steps are involved in a time-series design:

1. *The population of interest is identified:* Because there will be only one group, describing the population of interest also describes the sample. Inclusion and exclusion criteria are important to minimize selection effects. A random sample may be drawn from an overall population, but more often an accessible sample of convenience is used.
2. *Variables are defined:* The independent variable is the intervention, as in other experimental and quasi-experimental designs, and the dependent variable is the outcome of interest. Both are operationally defined in a quantifiable way before the experiment begins.
3. *The baseline condition is measured:* The outcome of interest and subject characteristics are measured at the beginning of the study, before any intervention is applied. This may take the form of a single, point-in-time measure or multiple measures over a specified time period.
4. *The intervention is applied:* Detailed protocols for implementation are used to apply the intervention. These protocols maintain the consistency of the intervention so treatment effects can be isolated from experimenter effects.
5. *Outcome variables are measured over time:* The variables are measured at specified intervals over an extended time period.

6. *Differences in groups and time periods are quantitatively analyzed:* Statistics are applied to determine the magnitude of any effects that are identified from baseline to each time period and between time periods. Any changes are evaluated for the probability that sampling error is responsible for the outcome. In addition, the data from time-series studies are analyzed for differences over time to determine what changes can be expected at each interval.

Strengths of Time-Series Designs

The use of a time-series design offers many advantages for the researcher, including the following:

- Fewer subjects are required to achieve adequate power. Time-series studies have substantial power because there are more observations per subject.
- The effects of the intervention over time can be quantified. This is particularly helpful for interventions that take some time to have an effect, such as lifestyle changes or conquering an addiction.
- Multiple data points can be collected both before and after the intervention. The extended time period for measurement strengthens the researcher's ability to attribute change to the intervention (Portney & Watkins, 2008).
- Time-series analysis can be applied to evaluate the effects of change on groups of individuals, such as organizational changes or cultural events.

Case in Point: Time-Series Design

Sakamoto and others (2010) used a time-series design to track factors associated with the eradication of methicillin-resistant *Staphylococcus aureus* (MRSA) from a neonatal intensive care unit. Case records of more than 1200 infants admitted to a neonatal intensive care unit (NICU) over a 6-year period were studied to determine conditions that may have been associated with eradication of the cultured micro-organisms. The incidence of MRSA colonization or infection was calculated each month during the study period. The amount of alcohol-based hand sanitizers used and nurse-to-patient ratios were also collected for the study period.

A time-series analysis was conducted to identify significant predictors of MRSA incidence rates. A statistical technique was used that compensates for seasonal effects. The primary association with reduced MRSA colonization was the use of hand sanitizers. Staffing ratios and enhanced surveillance were not associated with the decline in incidence of MRSA.

This time-series design is typical in that the associations of variables are measured over time. The timing of interventions—such as the hand sanitizer use in this study—is measured relative to changes in the outcome variable. This study is unique in the span of time it covered. Six years is a lengthy study, and without retrospective data collection from complete medical records, it would be difficult to carry out. These data do provide good evidence that increasing the use of hand sanitizer can be associated with a reduction in unit infections.

Source: Sakamoto, F., Yamada, H., Suzuki, C., Sigiura, H., & Tokuda, Y. (2010). Increased use of alcohol-based hand sanitizers and successful eradication of methicillin-resistant *Staphylococcus aureus* from a neonatal intensive care unit: A multivariate time series analysis. *American Journal of Infection Control, 38*, 529–534.

Limitations of Time-Series Designs

Although time-series designs offer many advantages, some of the disadvantages associated with the use of this method include the following:

- The inability to include a meaningful control group limits the ability to determine cause and effect.
- Rival explanations may exist for observed outcomes.
- Attrition can be a particular problem because there is only a single sample. Loss of subjects over time may weaken the results of the study.

Reading Quantitative Research

The first step in the critique of the methods and procedures of a quantitative study is to determine the specific type of design used in the study. The design is generally specified in the abstract; if not, it should be explicitly identified in the beginning of the article or in the first couple of lines in the methods section. If a design is experimental, then the authors will almost certainly identify it as a randomized controlled trial, clinical trial, or experiment.

If the design is not explicit, the reader must infer the type of design by comparing its characteristics to those of a quantitative study. If the study uses numbers and measures differences between groups (or within a group over time) then it is a quantitative analysis. If these characteristics are present but the author does not specify the type of design, assume it is quasi-experimental (Girden & Kabcoff, 2010). Randomized trials are so difficult to carry out that authors are anxious to report it if they have managed to do so.

Enough detail should be provided that the reader can judge the rationale for the design decisions made by the researcher. As with other designs, the specific type of study should be clearly linked to an appropriate research question. The research question should include all the elements required for a quantitative study: the population of interest, the intervention, a relevant comparison, and an outcome. It is helpful if the author reports a rationale for selection of the specifics of the study related to the demands of the question; there should be a clear link between the purpose of the study and the type of design used to achieve it.

If detail about the type of study is not reported clearly, then the reader may need to examine the article closely for evidence of the type of design that was employed. Clues to the specific design may be present in the research question, aims, purpose statement, or objectives. Words such as *affect, influence, change,* or *improve* may indicate that a quantitative design was used.

The reader can differentiate experimental designs from quasi-experimental ones by scrutinizing the group assignment procedure. If subjects are assigned to groups randomly and an intervention is applied, then it is a true experiment. If subjects are assigned any way other than randomly, it is quasi-experimental (regardless of how the author describes it). If only one group exists and measures are taken over time, then it is a time-series design. Groups may be labeled as "convenience samples" or "accessible groups," but in either case, this indicates studies that involve intact groups rather than randomly assigned ones.

Quantitative studies often have the most detailed methods and procedures sections of any research reports. The reader should be able to follow the way samples are selected and assigned to groups, the protocol used to apply the intervention, the way outcomes were measured, and the way data were analyzed. It is not uncommon for the author to provide figures or photographs to demonstrate the intervention protocol or measurement procedures. Enough information should be provided that a reasonably informed researcher can replicate the study from that information. The authors should demonstrate a systematic and rigorous approach to controlling extraneous variables through controls of internal and external validity. A review of these strategies from Chapter 11 is helpful in assessing the adequacy of internal and external controls.

Finally, examine the conclusions section to ensure that the authors do not over-interpret or make inferences that go beyond what the results can support. Only experimental studies can result in a definitive statement about cause and effect. Although quasi-experimental, time series, and studies of intact groups may infer causality, authors should interpret these results with caution. Extraneous variables can only be controlled when subjects have been assigned to a control group in a way that ensures the baseline equivalency of treatment groups, and that requires randomization. Any other type of study yields information about the assumed effectiveness of interventions, but it cannot be considered conclusive evidence of effects. These latter studies may suggest or imply causal relationships—and the authors may use quasi-experimental studies as pilot studies for later experiments—but causal relationships are supported only through experimental design. Without the controls that are inherent in an experimental design, and without a randomly chosen comparison group, it is impossible to confirm all the conditions necessary for causality.

 Where to Look for Information About Quantitative Designs

- A quantitative design is generally identified in a straightforward way in the abstract or the introduction. If it does not appear here, then it will be in the initial statements in the "methods and procedures" section. The design should be easily identifiable and a major part of the research study write-up.
- If the study does not specify if it is an experimental design, then assume it is quasi-experimental. Experimental designs are so challenging that authors are quick to note when they have been able to carry one out.
- The specific methods and procedures should be clearly reported. The description may be concise, but it should have enough detail that an informed reader could replicate the study. If the intervention or measurement is complex, there may be a separate section for procedures, which may be labeled as such or called "protocols." This section may describe either the specific steps for applying the treatment or for measuring its effects (or both).
- What is included in the methods section is not always standard. The section should have subheadings for the sampling strategy, research design, treatment protocols, measurement, and analytic plan.

Even with all these caveats, quantitative designs produce some of the strongest evidence for nursing practice. Understanding the nature of the relationship between an intervention and its effects is a powerful way to ensure that nursing practices are, indeed, based on what is known rather than what is believed.

Using Quantitative Research in Evidence-Based Nursing Practice

Quantitative designs—particularly when they are replicated and reported in aggregate—provide some of the strongest evidence for evidence-based nursing practice. The ability to determine causality and to measure the effects of interventions provides powerful information to support practice.

There is a variety of uses for quantitative evidence in nursing practice: Assessment, interventions, and evaluation of outcomes are supported by studies that are highly controlled and that link interventions to outcomes.

- *Assessment and diagnosis of patients:* Quantitative studies can help the nurse identify if particular assessment procedures are effective in detecting patient conditions. In particular, case–control studies help determine the relationships between risk factors and disease states, and these designs are helpful in determining if the nurse can expect that a given risk factor will result in a disease state or complication.
- *Interventions:* The test of interventions is where quantitative studies really shine. Whether the interventions are planned on an individual or group basis, quantitative studies allow the reader to draw definitive conclusions about cause and effect. These studies are considered some of the strongest scientific evidence for nursing practices. Quantitative studies can help the nurse discover interventions that prevent complications, quickly address problems, and help patients attain and maintain health.
- *Evaluation of outcomes:* Quantitative studies provide strong evidence to support outcome measurement and evaluation. These studies enable the nurse to draw

Checklist for Evaluating a Quantitative Study

✔ The quantitative nature of the study is clear early in the study and the specific design is identified.
✔ A rationale is provided for the choice of a design, and it is linked to the research question.
✔ A specific procedure is described for the application of the treatment or intervention.
✔ Instruments and measurement procedures are described objectively.
✔ Reliability of the instrumentation is described and supporting statistics are provided.
✔ Validity of the instrumentation is described and supporting statistics are provided.
✔ A detailed protocol for the use of each instrument in the measurement is described.
✔ Threats to internal validity are identified and controlled.
✔ Researcher bias and treatment effects are controlled by blinding.
✔ Authors provide sufficient information to determine if findings can be generalized to other groups or settings.

conclusions about the relationships between interventions and outcomes and in the process help develop operational definitions of these variables. These definitions can be helpful in standardizing the way patient outcomes are measured, collected, and reported.

In addition, quantitative studies let the nurse determine what outcomes can be expected from specific interventions. Time-series studies have the added benefit of contributing information about the timing of responses, as well. These studies are helpful in designing patient teaching and counseling because they help the nurse provide the patient with realistic expectations from treatments and procedures.

Generalizing the Results of Quantitative Studies

Quantitative studies are intended to provide the nurse with information about how well the sample represents the population. When samples are selected randomly, the chance that the sample will represent the population increases, and so experimental designs have especially strong external validity. The description of the sample characteristics and a clear definition of the population help the nurse determine if the results could be expected to apply to his or her particular patients. Before using the results of quantitative studies in a specific population, the nurse is responsible for ensuring that the populations are similar enough that the expectation of similar results is reasonable.

The results of quantitative studies are stronger when they are in aggregate. Reviews of multiple experiments enable the nurse to draw strong inferences about the usefulness of an intervention. Experimental designs conducted in multiple sites provide some of the strongest evidence for nursing practice. It is rare that a practice change is warranted after a single study. If the study has been replicated many times in various settings and with multiple populations, then the nurse can use the results more confidently.

Creating Quantitative Research

Quantitative research is a common research method because it provides strong information about the effectiveness of interventions. It is difficult, however, to achieve the level of control that is required to rule out rival explanations for an outcome. It is because of this complexity of control that pure experimental designs are uncommon. However, quasi-experimental studies, studies of intact groups, and time-series designs can still provide compelling evidence for practice, particularly when they are replicated and reported in aggregate. The means to achieving control is to use a systematic approach to consider the design decisions inherent in quantitative study.

- *Clarify the research question.* The question should have all the elements represented by the PICO approach: an identified population, an intervention of interest, a comparison, and an outcome.
- *Identify a specific design that will answer the question in the most efficient, effective way.* This depends on several factors: whether the independent variable can be manipulated, whether it can be delivered to individuals, if it will be possible to

randomly assign subjects to groups, and whether the outcome will be measured at a single point in time or over time. By clarifying these aspects of the question, the correct design will generally become evident.

- *Describe the population of interest, and determine inclusion and exclusion criteria for the sample.* Devise a sampling strategy that maximizes representativeness of the population and will support the external validity of the findings.

- *Determine the way subjects will be assigned to groups.* If random assignment to groups is possible at all, the researcher should take advantage of it, even if it requires extra efforts. Random assignment strengthens a study in so many ways that it is worth extra time and energy.

- *Clarify the variables of interest and write operational definitions for each before selecting measurement instruments.* Identify which variable is the independent variable and which is the dependent variable. Brainstorm potential extraneous variables, and build in methods to control the foreseeable ones.

- *Devise a description of the intervention and write a protocol that is objective and detailed and that provides direction to the nurses who will apply it.* Use photographs or video recordings if these are appropriate. The protocol should include when the treatment is applied, how it is applied, to which patients, and how often. Step-by-step directions for each element of the treatment should be provided in detail. Have nurses who are not involved in the research read the protocol to uncover confusing or misleading sections. Control of variability in treatments is one of the most important considerations in quantitative research design.

- *Determine a measurement procedure that will generate reliable, valid data.* If instruments or tools are to be used, ensure that they possess the appropriate psychometric properties for the specific study design that is proposed. Provide written directions for using the measurement instruments; provide word-for-word directions to read to subjects so they are consistently applied. Determine the interrater reliability of data collectors prior to beginning data collection.

- *Manage the data collection process carefully.* Data should be collected carefully to ensure accuracy and completeness. Working with a statistician to create a data collection spreadsheet or online database is helpful because it ensures that the researcher will not have to re-enter or manipulate data prior to analysis. Apply a process for maintaining the integrity of the data set. Specific measures should be planned for restricting access and ensuring confidentiality, such as password-protected files and locked file cabinets. Incorporate periodic quality checks into the data management process.

- *Use the appropriate analytic tools for the question to be answered and the type of data being collected.* Consider the level of measurement of each variable, the number of groups to be compared, and the level of confidence needed in the outcome.

gray matter

Quantitative evidence in nursing practice may be used to:
- Identify if particular assessment procedures are effective in detecting patient conditions
- Discover interventions that prevent complications, quickly address problems, and help patients attain and maintain health
- Draw conclusions about the relationship between interventions and outcomes
- Determine what outcomes can be expected from specific interventions

Statistical analysis software is widely available; in fact, most common statistical tests can be done with Excel spreadsheets, so there is no need to manually calculate statistics. If statistical analysis becomes complicated, consult a statistician from a university or medical center.

- *Report the analysis accurately and completely; report each test that was run, even if it did not contribute to the overall outcome of the study.* This reduces the potential for selective retention of findings—a threat to validity of the study. The results of statistical tests should be reported in a standard way that enhances their understanding across disciplines. The research report should include the results of each test using appropriate summary statistics in tables or figures; the meaning of each should be explained in the text of the research report as well.

Strengthen Quantitative Studies

It is difficult to conduct a pure experimental design in an applied setting. Extraneous variables abound, and it is often unethical to withhold treatment from a control group. It is complicated to ensure that the experimental group always gets the treatment exactly the same. Time constraints and availability of individuals to collect data can hinder the validity of the experiment. Although it may be challenging to conduct a true experiment in a working unit, there are still strategies to strengthen the validity of applied quantitative studies:

- Use a comparison group of some kind. Although it may be difficult to randomly assign patients to groups, the use of a comparison group does strengthen validity, even if it is a convenience sample.
- If using a nonrandom comparison group, match the groups as closely as possible on potential extraneous variables (for example, age, severity of illness, and number of co-morbid conditions).
- Clearly identify the independent and dependent variables, and write formal operational definitions of each. These definitions can help to determine criteria for inclusion in the study, treatment protocols, and measurement systems.
- Use simple, straightforward measurement methods whenever possible. Measure unobtrusively to minimize treatment effects.
- Take advantage of automated systems to capture data whenever possible, including the recording systems that are built into some patient care equipment, such as intravenous pumps, automated beds, and medication administration systems.
- If using a chart review to capture data, select a random sample of charts to limit the labor involved in data retrieval.
- Training is critical. Train those who will apply the treatment and those who will collect the data. Set up monitoring systems and random checks to ensure the treatment and measurement systems are working consistently.
- Hide the identity of the experimental and control groups from those who are collecting data whenever possible. Blinding of those who are both subjects and data collectors minimizes several threats to validity, including treatment effects and researcher bias.
- Get help when designing the study. Universities and medical centers often have consulting statisticians available. Advanced practice nurses are also good sources of research support, as is an organization's evidence-based practice council or research team.
- Replicate the studies of others whenever possible. Finding a study that reports an experiment jump-starts a study by describing procedures and measures that a subsequent researcher might be able to use.

CRITICAL APPRAISAL **EXERCISE**

Retrieve the following full text article from the Cumulative Index to Nursing and Allied Health Literature or similar search database:

Huang, S., Good, M., & Zauszniewki, J. (2010). The effectiveness of music in relieving pain in cancer patients: A randomized controlled trial. *International Journal of Nursing Studies, 47*, 1354–1362.

Review the article, focusing on the sections that report the question, design, methods, and procedures. Consider the following appraisal questions in your critical review of this research article:

1. Is the research question (or questions) made explicit early in the paper? Is there a hypothesis?
2. How do the authors describe the design of this study? What characteristics of the study lead you to agree or disagree with their description?
3. Why is the design appropriate for this research question?
4. Was a blinding method used in this study? What does this indicate? What kind of bias could blinding control in this study?
5. Describe the inclusion and exclusion criteria. Can you think of any other characteristics that should have been controlled using criteria?
6. What is the independent variable? Dependent variable?
7. Why did these authors include a "sham" group as a placebo? Why was this better than a single control group?
8. Was the treatment protocol described adequately for replication?
9. What are the strengths of the design, methods, and procedures of this study? Contrast them with its limitations.
10. How could this study be incorporated into evidence-based practice?

- *Draw conclusions appropriate for the intent of the study and the results that were found.* Even with experimental designs, the author should resist the urge to over-interpret the data. Only pure randomized controlled trials can draw definitive conclusions about causality. However, it is common to note the causal relationships that were indicated by the data, or suggested by the findings, as long as the appropriate cautions are noted.

Developing a design for a study requires attention to each of these elements. Decisions must be made during each step that support findings and provide a clear answer to the research question. These answers provide some of the strongest scientific evidence for effective nursing practices.

Summary of Key Concepts

- The purpose of quantitative research is to use measurement to determine the effectiveness of interventions.
- Quantitative research involves measuring objective characteristics or responses of subjects, and it is reported using numbers.

- Quantitative studies are designed to provide high levels of control so confidence in the results is enhanced.
- Quantitative methods allow the researcher to measure the probability that some other factor caused the outcome, specifically things such as extraneous variables, measurement error, or sampling error.
- These studies can help the nurse appraise the effectiveness of an intervention, determine the relationship between actions and patient responses, and measure changes over time.
- Quantitative research questions have variables that can be operationally defined and measured in a numerical way.
- The quantitative research question identifies the population of interest, the intervention under study, the comparison that makes up the control, and the outcome of interest.
- Quantitative studies have many characteristic elements, including an interest in variables, control over the experiment, the use of measurement to compare groups, and statistical data analysis.
- Quantitative studies have an *a priori* design, meaning most design decisions are made before the research begins.
- Four common classifications of quantitative research in nursing are experimental designs, quasi-experimental designs, studies of intact groups, and time-series designs.
- Experimental designs are characterized by random assignment of subjects to groups, a manipulated independent variable, and an outcome of interest. Differences between groups at the end of the experiment are assumed to be due to the intervention.
- Quasi-experimental designs are very similar to experimental ones except subjects are assigned to groups in some way other than randomly.
- Studies of intact groups include ex post facto designs, causal–comparative, and case–control. These designs involve finding subjects with the variable of interest and matching them to a comparison group to discover relationships.
- Time-series design enables the researcher to determine both the effectiveness of an intervention and the timing of its effects.
- Quantitative designs are considered some of the strongest scientific evidence for nursing practice.

For a full suite of assignments and additional learning activities, use the access code located in the front of your book to visit this exclusive website: http://go.jblearning .com/houser. If you do not have an access code, you can obtain one at the site.

References

Armenian, H. (2009). Epidemiology: A problem solving journey. *American Journal of Epidemiology, 169*(2), 127–131.

Crosby, R., DiClemente, R., & Salazar, L. (2006). *Research methods in health promotion.* San Francisco: Jossey-Bass.

Gall, M., Gall, J., & Borg, W. (2007). *Educational research: An introduction* (8th ed.). Boston: Pearson Allyn and Bacon.

Girden, E., & Kabacoff, R. (2010). *Evaluating research articles from start to finish.* Thousand Oaks, CA: Sage.

Haynes, R., Sackett, D., Guyatt, G., & Tugwell, P. (2006). *Clinical epidemiology: How to do clinical practice research* (3rd ed.). Philadelphia: Lippincott Williams & Wilkins.

Leedy, P. (2009). *Practical research: Planning and design* (9th ed.). Lebanon, IN: Prentice Hall.

Locke, L., Silverman, S., & Spirduso, W. (2010). *Reading and understanding research* (3rd ed.). Thousand Oaks, CA: Sage.

Machin, D., & Fayers, P. (2010). *Randomized clinical trials: Design, practice and reporting.* Hoboken, NJ: Wiley Blackwell.

Melnyk, B., & Fineout-Overholt, E. (2010). *Evidence-based practice in nursing and healthcare: A guide to best practice.* Philadelphia: Lippincott Williams & Wilkins.

Mitchell, M., & Jolley, J. (2009). *Research design explained* (9th ed.). Florence, KY: Wadsworth.

Morrow, B. (2010a). An overview of case–control study designs and their advantages and disadvantages. *International Journal of Therapy and Rehabilitation, 17*(11), 570–575.

Morrow, B. (2010b). Research methodology series: Cohort study designs. *International Journal of Therapy and Rehabilitation, 17*(9), 518–523.

Newell, R., & Burnard, P. (2010). *Research for evidence-based practice in healthcare.* Hoboken, NJ: Wiley Blackwell.

Portney, L., & Watkins, M. (2008). *Foundations of clinical research: Applications to practice* (3rd ed.). Upper Saddle River, NJ: Prentice Hall.

Wood, M., & Ross-Kerr, J. (2006). *Basic steps in planning nursing research from question to proposal* (6th ed.). Sudbury, MA: Jones & Bartlett.

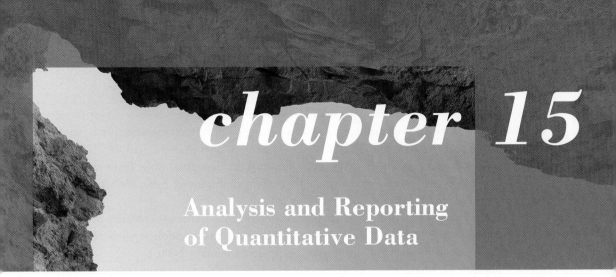

chapter 15

Analysis and Reporting of Quantitative Data

 CHAPTER OBJECTIVES

The study of this chapter will help the learner to:

- Compare inferential statistics to other types of quantitative analysis.
- Discuss the types of decisions that are made *a priori* and the rationale for making these choices prior to reviewing data.
- Describe the ways in which quantitative analyses are classified based on the goals of the analysis, assumptions of the tests, and number of variables in the study.
- Explain how sampling distributions relate to the calculation of inferential statistics and interpretation of the results.
- Summarize the usefulness of confidence intervals in interpreting quantitative data, and review characteristics of a study that affect precision of estimates.
- Relate the steps of the hypothesis-testing procedure to the way inferential analyses are conducted, interpreted, and reported.
- Differentiate the appropriate application of t tests, chi square tests, and analysis of variance.

 KEY TERMS

Alpha	Levels	Robust tests
Bivariate analysis	Magnitude of effect	Standard error
Central limit theorem	Multivariate analysis	Statistically significant
Confidence interval	Nonparametric tests	Test statistic
Effect size	Null hypothesis	Type I error
Error of multiple comparisons	Parametric tests	Type II error
Factors	Point estimate	Univariate analysis
Inferential analysis		

❝❝ *Scenes from the Field* ❞❞

Women have long believed that their food intake changes during their menstrual cycle. Studies in Western countries have found a relationship among sex hormones, the neuropeptide leptin, women's food intake, and body weight changes across the menstrual cycle. Three researchers in Taiwan replicated a study to determine if these relationships were culturally based or were demonstrated among Taiwanese women as well.

The authors recruited 46 women to participate in a cross-sectional survey design. Women were asked to keep logs of total food and macronutrient intake and their menstrual cycles. Additional data collected were serum estrogen, progesterone, and leptin.

Regardless of original body weight, women consumed more total calories and more grams of protein during the luteal phase and ovulation compared with the later follicular phase. During the follicular phase (immediately prior to menstruation) these women increased their carbohydrate intake substantially. These associations were statistically significant. However, no physiological correlates were found between appetite and hormones or leptin levels.

These data results were reported in a variety of ways that made interpretation easier. Tables were used to display demographic characteristics of the subjects. Graphics, including bar charts and box plots, were used to demonstrate menstrual phases, intake of calories and macronutrients, and type of intake, including fat, protein, and carbohydrates. A final table showed the relationship between each type of intake and the menstrual phases, along with associated frequencies and p values. The authors noted which relationships were statistically significant throughout the tables and figures.

These data confirm that appetite for some types of foods is associated with the menstrual cycle. This information can help the nurse counsel women about their nutrition in order to minimize the potential for obesity and weight gain during menstruation.

Source: Chung, S., Bond, E., & Jarrett, M. (2010). Food intake changes across the menstrual cycle in Taiwanese women. *Biological Research for Nursing, 12*(1), 37–46.

Introduction

If descriptive analysis answers the question, "What is going on?" then inferential analysis answers the question, "Are you sure?" The word *inferential* means that the reader can infer something about a population's response to an intervention based on the responses of a carefully selected sample. Inference requires the calculation of numerical values to enhance confidence that the intervention resulted in the outcome and to rule out the possibility that something else did. In quantitative inferential analysis, that "something else" is error in all its forms—sampling error, measurement error, standard error, even random error—and inferential analysis allows the researcher to quantify its effect.

Inferential statistics are those that enable the researcher to draw conclusions about a population given a sample. Because these are calculations, they are by necessity focused on numerical representations of reality. Inferential analysis, then, is based on evaluation of numbers using quantifiable variables. Inferential analysis is the most common type of quantitative analysis used in research for evidence.

When reading quantitative analysis, it is important to focus on both the probability of error and the certainty of the estimates. When quantitative analysis is used as evidence for nursing practice, the nurse should also consider the size of the effect and whether it attains both statistical and clinical significance. When creating quantitative analysis, the focus is on choosing the correct test and making appropriate decisions about its application. All are critical for ensuring that the relationship between intervention and outcome is one that is defined with certainty so the results can be expected to be replicated in different settings among different people.

Some General Rules of Quantitative Analysis

Quantitative analysis is a highly systematic and organized process. Data for quantitative analysis are represented numerically, and so reliability of data collection, accuracy of data entry, and appropriateness of analytic processes are critical for drawing the correct conclusions. These types of analyses can be complex, and so a plan for analysis and reporting is determined when the methods and procedures are designed. A wide variety of statistical tests is available, and each has specific requirements for data preparation and analysis. There are, however, some general guidelines for the way quantitative analyses are conducted:

- *Select tests a priori:* The specific statistical tests that will be used for quantitative analysis are selected before the experiment begins. The selection of specific tests is based on the research question to be answered, the level of measurement, the number of groups, and the nature of the data.
- *Run all the tests identified:* The researcher must run all tests that were identified *a priori.* Looking at the data and then deciding which tests to run can create bias. Although the specific version of a test may be dictated by the nature of the data (for example, using a test for nonnormal data), the researcher should not pick and choose tests after reviewing the data.
- *Report all the tests that were run:* The researcher must report the results from each test that was run. Selectively reporting or retaining data to support a personal viewpoint is a form of researcher bias that is unethical.

Types of Quantitative Analysis

Quantitative analysis refers to the analysis of numbers. Quantifying the values of variables involves counting and measuring them; these counts and measures result in numbers that can be mathematically manipulated to reveal information. The researcher can think of quantitative analysis as an interpreter that takes raw data and turns it into something understandable.

There are many types of quantitative analyses. The types of quantitative analyses available to the researcher can be categorized in several ways: by the goals of the analysis, the assumptions made about the data, and the number of variables involved.

Goals of the Analysis

Quantitative analyses are useful for many research goals. In particular, research questions that focus on evaluating differences between groups (for example, between an experimental and a control group) are amenable to quantitative analysis. Quantitative tests are also appropriate to assess the nature and direction of relationships between subjects or variables, including the capacity to predict an outcome given a set of characteristics or events. Researchers also use quantitative methods to sort data (for example, a clinician may identify characteristics that enable him or her to differentiate people at risk for falls from those who are not at risk). Quantitative analyses are helpful in data reduction by grouping variables into overall classifications. This approach is helpful in determining clusters of symptoms that may predict complications.

Quantitative analyses are also classified as descriptive or inferential based on the aims of the study. Descriptive studies are concerned with accurately describing the characteristics of a sample or population, and were addressed in detail in Chapter 13. Inferential analyses are used to determine if results found in a sample can be applied to a population. The latter is a condition for confidently generalizing research as a basis for evidence for nursing practice (Machin & Fayers, 2010).

Assumptions of the Data

Quantitative analyses are generally grouped into two large categories based on assumptions about the data: parametric and nonparametric. These two groups of tests have one large differentiating factor: the assumptions about the distribution, or shape, of the data. Parametric tests are based on the assumption that the data fall into a specified distribution—usually the normal (bell-shaped) distribution. This can be assumed only when interval- or ratio-level measures are collected or when samples are large enough to achieve normality. In reported healthcare research, parametric tests are the most common, even when it is questionable whether the basic assumptions have been met. However, there is a group of tests that is specific to data that are not normally distributed. If a normal distribution cannot be assumed, then nonparametric tests are needed. This group of tests is "distribution-free," meaning the tests do not rely on a specific distribution to generate accurate results. Nonparametric tests are becoming more common, particularly in health care, where many variables are not normally distributed.

Parametric tests: Statistical tests that are appropriate for data that are normally distributed (fall in a bell curve).
Nonparametric tests: Statistical tests that have no assumptions about the distribution of the data.
Robust tests: Statistical tests that are able to yield reliable results even if underlying assumptions are violated.

Parametric tests are usually desirable because they are sensitive to relatively small differences, they are commonly available in most software packages, and they are readily recognizable by the reader. However, it is not uncommon for them to be applied in data sets where the distribution of the data has not been shown to be normal, and in this case, they may result in misleading conclusions. Small deviations from normality may be acceptable with these tests because most parametric tests are described as robust, or capable of yielding reliable results even when underlying assumptions have been violated. But some data are so nonnormal as to require a test that makes no such assumptions.

Nonparametric tests are not as commonly applied, are less recognizable, and are not always available in analytic packages. These tests are also relatively insensitive and require large samples to run effectively. When possible, researchers should strive to collect data in a form that can be expected to be normally distributed and to create sample sizes that allow them to use parametric tests. However, the researcher should use the appropriate category of test for the data, meaning he or she should specifically evaluate the results for distribution prior to final test selection. Most parametric tests have a nonparametric counterpart, enabling the researcher to apply the correct class of test to the data.

Number of Variables in the Analysis

Quantitative analyses can be classified in terms of the number of variables that are to be considered. These tests are classified by both the number and type of variables involved. Univariate analysis involves a single variable. Univariate analyses are the primary focus of descriptive and summary statistics. This term is also applied when the study involves a single dependent variable or when only one group is included. For example, differentiating whether blood pressure is affected more by exercise in the morning or the evening is a univariate analysis. Even though there are two groups (morning and evening), the analysis focuses on a single dependent variable: blood pressure. Bivariate analysis is the analysis of the relationship between two variables. The most common bivariate analysis is the correlation. Bivariate analysis is also used to determine if a single variable can predict a specified outcome. For example, determining if blood pressure is associated with sodium intake is a bivariate analysis. Two variables—blood pressure and sodium—are analyzed to determine any relationship between them. Multivariate analysis is the simultaneous analysis of multiple variables. This may reflect the analysis of multiple predictors on a single outcome, the differences between groups on several effects, or the analysis of the relationships between multiple factors on multiple outcomes. For example, determining if blood pressure is different in the morning or evening, and is associated with sodium intake, weight, and stress level, is an example of a multivariate analysis.

> **Univariate analysis:** Analysis of a single variable in descriptive statistics or a single dependent variable in inferential analysis.
> **Bivariate analysis:** Analysis of two variables at a time, as in correlation studies.

> **Multivariate analysis:** Analysis of the effects of an independent variable on two or more dependent variables simultaneously.

These analyses become more sophisticated and complex as more variables are added to either side of the equation. A research study may require a simple univariate analysis to achieve a descriptive goal. On the other hand, an experiment may require the complexities of a full factorial multivariate analysis of variance—a calculation of the effect of multiple factors on multiple outcomes, taking into account both their main effects and the effects of the interaction of factors. Quantitative analyses can accommodate the complexity of human responses to interventions and illness by reflecting the multivariate nature of health and illness.

An Overview of Inferential Statistics

Inferential statistics are used to determine if a specific result can be expected to occur in a population, given it was observed in a sample. In statistics, a sample (part of the population) is used to obtain results that represent a target population (all of the population). Quantitative research as evidence for practice is only useful when it can be generalized to larger groups of patients than those directly studied in the experiment. Inferential analysis allows the researcher to recommend that an intervention be used and to do so with an identified level of confidence.

Inferential analysis is fundamentally an analysis of differences that occur between samples and populations, between groups, or over time because something changed. In experimental research, the change is an intervention. In case–control studies, the "change" is a risk factor; in causal–comparative studies, it is a characteristic or an event. Inference is used to determine if an outcome was affected by the change.

It is not enough, however, to see a difference between two samples and assume that the difference is the same as would be expected in a population. Samples, by nature, are different than the populations from which they were drawn. Samples are made up of individuals and, particularly in small samples, we cannot be sure the sample exactly matches the population characteristics. These differences—the ones that are due to the sampling process—are quantified as standard error. One might view standard error as the differences between samples and populations that are expected simply due to the nature of sampling.

Any differences between groups are compared to their standard error to determine if the differences are real or if they are due simply to the differences that exist between the sample and the population. This comparison of observed differences to standard error forms the basis for most inferential tests. The certainty with which a researcher can say "these effects are not due to standard error" is subjected to rules of probability. The calculations produce a *p value*, or the probability the results were due to standard error. If the p value is very small, then the probability that results were due to error is very small, and the researcher can be very confident that the effects of the intervention are real. If the p value is very large, then the probability that results were due to error is very large, and the researcher cannot draw a conclusion that the intervention had an effect greater than would be expected from random variations.

It is the comparison of differences to standard error and the calculation of the probability of error that gives inferential analysis its strength. This set of statistical tests enables the researcher to do two very important things: calculate whether an intervention has an effect that is real, and quantify if the difference is important. Inferential analysis enhances the researcher's capacity to draw conclusions about whether a similar result can be expected for all members of the population. This type of analysis forms the basis of some of the strongest scientific evidence for effective nursing practices.

Sampling Distributions and Standard Error

To determine the probability that a result is due to standard error, the researcher needs an understanding of sampling distributions. A sampling distribution is extremely useful because it allows the researcher to make statements about the probability that a specific observation will occur (Dawson, 2008). A sampling distribution is defined by the specific statistic of interest. For example, sampling distributions can be developed for the mean, a proportion, the standard deviation, or the variance. These distributions can be used to determine how likely it is that any specific measurement in the sample also appears in the population with the same relative frequency. Understanding sampling distributions is central to understanding how inferential results are calculated and reported. Applying probabilities from sampling distributions enables the analyst to calculate estimates and test hypotheses.

A sampling distribution is different from a simple distribution of values from individual observations. If a researcher wished to estimate the birth weight of babies in a population of women from a developing nation, a single sample of babies would provide a basis for calculating a sample mean. On the other hand, it is unlikely that this number would exactly represent the mean value for the entire population, no matter how carefully the sample was drawn. The estimate would likely get more accurate if a second sample was drawn and the mean calculated again. Theoretically, as more samples are drawn, the estimate of the mean for the population becomes more and more accurate as the total number of observations increases. If all these mean values were aggregated into a single distribution, this distribution of mean values from the samples would form a sampling distribution. The mean of this sampling distribution, then, would have the greatest likelihood of accurately reflecting the actual mean value from the population (Motulsky, 2010).

However, generating the sampling distribution each time an investigator wants to ask a statistical question would be extraordinarily time-consuming and it is unlikely a researcher would convince a huge proportion of the population to participate. Instead, a statistical theory called the central limit theorem provides a basis for drawing conclusions about populations from smaller samples. Basically, this theorem supports the following ideas:

> **Central limit theorem:** A mathematical theorem that is the basis for the conclusion that larger samples will represent a population more accurately than small ones.

- The mean of the sampling distribution equals the mean of the population.
- If the population distribution is normal, then the sampling distribution will also be normal.
- The standard deviation of the sampling distribution is equal to standard error.

Standard error is a statistic that is calculated to reflect the effects of normal variability, taking into account sample size. FIGURE 15.1 represents the calculation of standard error. Standard error can be thought of as "random variability," or variability that is due to the way samples are drawn. The central limit theorem helps the researcher understand how to manage standard error. As samples get larger, standard error will by necessity get smaller. This is particularly relevant in cases of samples with a great deal of variability among subjects. Table 15.1 depicts the effects of sample size and variability on the magnitude of standard error. In this case, standard error is the standard against which real changes are compared. When interventions produce effects that are greater than standard error, then the results are said to be statistically significant. Sampling distributions enable the

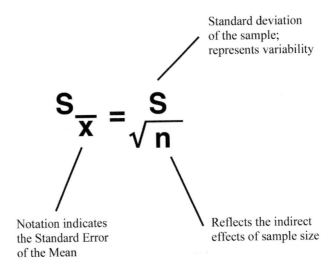

$$S_{\overline{X}} = \frac{S}{\sqrt{n}}$$

Standard deviation of the sample; represents variability

Notation indicates the Standard Error of the Mean

Reflects the indirect effects of sample size

Standard error is calculated by creating a ratio of standard deviation (a measure of variability), compared to the square root of sample size. The calculation is expressed as a decimal.

FIGURE 15.1 What Makes Up Standard Error?

Table 15.1

The Role of Variability and Sample Size in Standard Error

Variable: Length of Stay for Community-Acquired Pneumonia	Mean	Standard Deviation	Sample Size	Standard Error
Group 1: Age group 5 years through 12 years	2.2 days	0.62 days	100	0.06
Group 2: Age group 13 years through 19 years	2.2 days	0.64 days	418	0.03
Group 3: Age group 20 years through 65 years	2.2 days	1.22 days	32	0.22
Group 4: Age group 66 years and older	2.2 days	2.02 days	1060	0.06

Interpretation of standard error: Note that all four groups have the same mean length of stay but that standard error is dramatically different for the groups.

- *The effects of variability:* Group 3 has nearly twice as much variability (reflected in the standard deviation) when compared to group 1. Although the means are similar, group 3 has a much larger standard error. This is directly due to the differences in variability between the two groups, but also partially due to the smaller sample size in group 3.
- *The effects of sample size:* Group 3 has less variability than group 4 (as reflected in standard deviation) but more standard error. This is because group 3 has a much smaller sample size than group 4. The large sample size for group 4 decreases standard error, even with a large amount of variability. In particular, note the differences between the standard errors of groups 1 and 2. Although these two groups have identical mean values and nearly identical standard deviation values, group 2 has half the standard error due to the increased sample size over group 1.

researcher to reach a conclusion by using established probabilities so conclusions can be drawn using much smaller (and achievable) sample sizes.

Goals of Inference

The central limit theorem and sampling distributions enable the researcher to draw conclusions about the data using probability. For example, a unit manager may want to determine the average length of stay on the unit. The manager can collect data from a sample of months and estimate a mean range of values. A sampling distribution can be used to determine a level of confidence that the actual population value is reflected by the sample mean. This use of inference is to estimate a population value and is the basis for the calculation of confidence intervals.

Inference also can be used to determine the probability that an outcome was due to error. For example, the researcher may want to calculate the probability that a mean value in a sample is the same as that of a population; a hospital may want to determine if its mean length of stay is longer than the national average. A sampling distribution would enable the researcher to determine if the differences between the hospital's length of stay and the national average are due to standard error by calculating the difference, expressing it as a ratio to standard error, and consulting a sampling distribution to identify the probability this difference is due to chance.

Both of these applications of inferential analysis are common in quantitative analysis. Confidence intervals are used to represent population estimates, estimate the differences between groups, or estimate the possibility that error affected an outcome. As such, generating confidence intervals also helps the reader judge the clinical importance of outcomes.

Estimation and Confidence Intervals

Estimates of population values can be expressed as **point estimates** or interval estimates. A point estimate represents a single number. In other words, a researcher measures a value in a sample, calculates a statistic, and then concludes that the population value must be exactly that number. In reality, however, samples rarely produce statistics that exactly mimic the population value (called a parameter). In this respect, a point estimate is less accurate than an estimate that includes a range of numbers. The likelihood that a single point represents a population value is quite small; the likelihood that the actual value could be captured in a range of numbers is considerably better. This range of numbers represents a **confidence interval** and is used to estimate population parameters.

Point estimate: A statistic derived from a sample that is used to represent a population parameter.
Confidence interval: A range of values that includes, with a specified level of confidence, the actual population parameter.

A confidence interval enables the researcher to estimate a specific value, but it also provides an idea of the range within which the value occurs by chance. It is defined as a range of values that the researcher believes, with a specified level of confidence, contains the actual population parameter. Although it sounds counterintuitive, confidence intervals are more accurate in representing population parameters than are point estimates because of the increased likelihood that an interval will contain the actual value.

Confidence intervals are helpful in quantitative analysis in a variety of ways. Because a point estimate is expressed as a single number, it gives the researcher no idea of the effects of standard error on the estimate. The calculation of a confidence interval takes into account the effects of standard error, and so the probability that the interval actually contains the population value can be determined. Confidence intervals allow the measurement of the effect of sampling error on an outcome and express it in numeric terms. Confidence intervals also are useful in interpreting the results of hypothesis tests. They provide more information than p values do; they enable the evaluation of magnitude of effect so the nurse can determine whether results are large enough to be of clinical importance. Confidence intervals are constructed using several pieces of information about the data, combined with a decision made by the researcher regarding how much confidence is necessary. Confidence intervals may be constructed around any statistic, but the most common is the mean. Confidence intervals for mean estimates and for estimates of the mean differences between groups are common ways to measure experimental differences. This requires that the researcher calculate the mean value and then determine the range around the mean that is due to standard error. This range is affected by how much confidence the researcher must have (usually 95 or 99 percent), the amount of variability among subjects, and the size of the sample. **FIGURE 15.2** represents how a confidence interval of the mean is constructed.

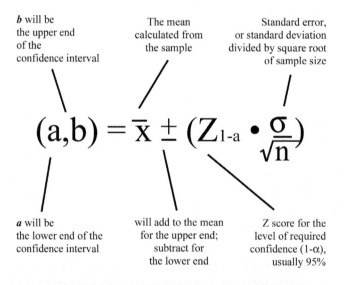

b will be the upper end of the confidence interval

The mean calculated from the sample

Standard error, or standard deviation divided by square root of sample size

$$(a,b) = \bar{x} \pm \left(Z_{1-a} \cdot \frac{\sigma}{\sqrt{n}}\right)$$

a will be the lower end of the confidence interval

will add to the mean for the upper end; subtract for the lower end

Z score for the level of required confidence (1-α), usually 95%

The confidence interval is calculated by taking into account the amount of error in the sample and the level of confidence required. This creates a range above and below the sample mean that we are confident contains the population mean.

FIGURE 15.2 What Makes Up a Confidence Interval?

Table 15.2

Confidence Intervals Interpreted: An Example

Statistic	Confidence Interval	What It Means
Mean number of distressful symptoms reported by terminal cancer patients	3.5 to 4.1 symptoms	Terminal cancer patients have, on average, between 3.5 and 4.1 distressful symptoms, inclusive.
Proportion of terminal cancer patients who report distressful symptoms	79.2 percent to 88.7 percent	Between 79.2 percent and 88.7 percent of terminal cancer patients report distressful symptoms, inclusive.
Mean difference between number of symptoms experienced by men and women as distressful	–0.24 to 1.4 symptoms	The average difference between the number of symptoms reported as distressful by men and women could be nothing (zero, which appears in this interval). There are no statistical differences between these groups.
Mean difference between number of symptoms experienced by those in a treatment group and those in a control group	–1.2 to –0.3 symptoms	A nursing intervention had the effect of reducing the number of symptoms perceived as distressful. The decrease could be as little as 0.3 of a symptom or as much as 1.2 symptoms. There is a significant effect, but it is very small.
Mean difference between number of symptoms experienced by those early in the disease and those late in the disease	2.1 to 4.3 symptoms	People late in the terminal stages of cancer experience more distressful symptoms than those in early stages. They could experience as few as 2.1 or as many as 4.3 symptoms, which demonstrates a significant effect of considerable magnitude. This is a clinically meaningful finding.

Confidence intervals may be quite precise and narrow or very broad and general. A very small estimate is quite precise; a large interval indicates a lack of precision. For example, estimating weight within 4 ounces may be quite acceptable for an adult male; it is not at all acceptable for a preterm infant. Table 15.2 illustrates how confidence intervals are interpreted. The width of a confidence interval reflects its precision; clearly, a researcher desires the most precise estimates possible. The precision of estimates is affected by some factors that are under the control of the researcher and some that are not:

- *Sample size:* The most direct impact on precision is the size of the sample. Because sample size improves the accuracy of estimates (via the central limit theorem) and reduces standard error, larger samples will yield more precise confidence intervals.
- *Variability of the sample:* Samples that have a great deal of diversity will have less precise estimates unless very large samples are used. Variability is represented by standard deviation, a direct element in the calculation of standard error. Increasing variability results in a larger standard error, making precise estimates more difficult.
- *Confidence level:* High levels of confidence require less precise intervals. For example, if a researcher needs 95 percent confidence that an interval contains a population parameter, then a narrower interval will suffice. However, if the

researcher needs to ensure that the interval contains the parameter 99 percent of the time, the interval will have to get broader to ensure it is "hit" more frequently. A 95 percent confidence interval will actually contain the mean fewer times, but it will represent a narrower interval.

The researcher can maximize the confidence in an estimate by representing it as an interval with an appropriate level of confidence. Requiring a confidence level in excess of what the research question demands may seem to be a way to enhance quality, except it will necessarily require that estimates are less precise. Ensuring an appropriate sample size (increasing even more when a great deal of variability is present) can ensure that confidence intervals are useful in application to practice.

Hypothesis Testing

Hypothesis testing is a central feature of quantitative analysis, particularly in evidence-based practice. Hypothesis testing is the process that enables the nurse to draw conclusions about the relationship between an intervention and its effect; it is the predominant method for analyzing the results of experimental designs. As such, it is a critical element of the research process that generates evidence for nursing practice.

On the other hand, hypothesis testing is difficult and counterintuitive to understand. The way hypotheses are written and tested are logical—when viewed as a mathematician or statistician would view them. The process is less clear to the average clinician who simply wants to know if an intervention works.

Hypothesis testing begins with the construction of an actual hypothesis. This is not a simple statement about what the researcher expects to find. Indeed, many hypotheses are written to reflect the exact opposite of what the researcher expects to find. This is referred to as a null hypothesis, or a hypothesis written to reflect that no relationship is expected. This seemingly counterproductive approach is actually logical when one understands that hypotheses are tested not to determine if a relationship exists, but to calculate the probability that it does not.

Null hypothesis: A translation of the research question into a testable statement that reflects the notion that no differences exist between groups.

Why Test Hypotheses Instead of Research Questions?

Why such a circuitous approach to testing a research question? There are several reasons, and each affects the way a hypothesis is constructed and the rules for testing it. Hypothesis testing is needed to answer quantitative research questions because

- A research question is not directly testable.
- A hypothesis enables calculation of the probability of alternative explanations.
- Testing a hypothesis allows the researcher to report results with a specified level of certainty.

A Research Question Is Not Directly Testable

Research questions specify the variables to be tested, the population of interest, and the outcome expected. However, these questions are not constructed in a way that is amenable to mathematical testing. The question "What are the effects of caffeine on test scores of undergraduate nursing students compared to nursing students who do not ingest caffeine?" is not directly tested with calculations. However, the hypothesis "There will be no difference between the test scores of nursing students who drink caffeine and those who do not" can be tested. It is even easier to see the way to test this textual hypothesis when it is translated into a statistical hypothesis. For example, H_0: The mean score of group 1 (with caffeine) will equal the mean score of group 2 (without caffeine). Represented mathematically, this hypothesis is $H_0: \mu_1 = \mu_2$. It is easier to see how this final hypothesis is tested than the original question. Hypotheses, then, give the researcher a way to express research questions in a manner that directs and guides the statistical tests required to answer them.

A Hypothesis Enables Calculation of the Probability of Alternative Explanations

Even if a statistical test shows that an intervention was associated with a change in an outcome, the researcher can never be sure the intervention was the only possible explanation for the outcome. Suppose a nurse decided to try a new pressure ulcer treatment on patients in a nursing home who are at risk for skin breakdown. The nurse randomly selects half of her high-risk patients, obtains adequate informed consent, and uses the new treatment. The patients that are not selected get the traditional treatment. After 2 weeks, the nurse measures skin breakdown and determines that the group with the new treatment had fewer pressure ulcers than the group without. Can the nurse researcher draw a definitive conclusion that the treatment caused the outcome?

There are many other possible explanations for this outcome. The patients in the experimental group may have been more active. They may have had more family members to help monitor their skin condition. They may have had a better nutritional status. So even though the statistics showed a difference, the researcher cannot be certain there was no other possible explanation for the outcome.

This is where hypothesis testing is helpful. A hypothesis test yields a calculation of the probability that something else—in this case, standard error—was responsible for the outcome. Hypothesis testing, in essence, allows the researcher to decide if something other than the intervention may have been responsible for the outcome and to judge the probability of these rival explanations in relation to a preset criterion called alpha.

Alpha: The risk of erroneous conclusions that the researcher is willing to accept; the standard for statistical significance.

Testing a Hypothesis Allows the Researcher to Report Results with a Specified Level of Certainty

Hypothesis testing allows the researcher to calculate the probability that an outcome is due to something other than the intervention. It also enables the researcher to document the amount of confidence the reader can have in the findings. For example, if a researcher calculates the differences in mean scores between nursing students who ingest caffeine and those who do not, the researcher can express that mean difference with an identified level of confidence, usually 95 or 99 percent.

Although it may appear to be a circuitous way to test a research question, hypothesis testing is actually a more accurate way of representing the effects of interventions on outcomes. This process enables the researcher to both reassure the reader that the chances are quite low that other explanations are possible and report findings with a documented level of confidence.

Types of Hypotheses

One kind of hypothesis, the null hypothesis, has already been introduced. The null hypothesis states the research question in a way that suggests there will be no difference between groups, no relationship among variables, or no effect generated from an intervention. It is stated this way so that it is directly testable, can quantify the probability of error, and generate a level of confidence in the outcomes. Table 15.3 demonstrates the translation of research questions into text and mathematical hypotheses.

To make a decision about a hypothesis, researchers usually construct a null hypothesis and an alternative hypothesis. The alternative hypothesis is sometimes referred to as a research hypothesis. The alternative hypothesis states the expected relationship, and it is usually the opposite of the null hypothesis. For example:

The null hypothesis is H_0: The mean score of group 1 (with caffeine) will equal the mean score of group 2 (without caffeine).
The alternative hypothesis is H_A: The mean score of group 1 (with caffeine) will be different from the mean score of group 2 (without caffeine).
The statistical hypothesis for this example is a null of $H_0: \mu_1 = \mu_2$ and an alternative of $H_a: \mu_1 \neq \mu_2$

In this example, the alternative hypothesis is stated as a nondirectional hypothesis. In other words, although the alternative hypothesis expresses an expected relationship,

Table 15.3			
Translating Research Questions into Hypotheses			
Research Question	Null Hypothesis (Text and Statistical)	Alternative, Nondirectional Hypothesis	Alternative, Directional Hypothesis
Are symptoms of myocardial infarction recognized in a shorter period of time in men than they are in women who present to an emergency department?	H_a: There will be no difference in mean time to diagnosis of myocardial infarction between men and women. $H_a: \mu_1 \neq \mu_2$	H_a: There will be a difference in mean time to diagnosis of myocardial infarction between men and women. $H_a: \mu_1 = \mu_2$	H_a: Men will have a shorter mean time to diagnosis of myocardial infarction than women. $H_a: \mu_1 < \mu_2$
Does the introduction of bar coding on a patient care unit result in lower medication error rates when compared to patient care units without bar coding?	H_a: There will be no difference in the medication error rate between units that do and do not have bar coding. $H_a: \pi_1 \neq \pi_2$	H_a: There will be a difference in the medication error rate between units that do and do not have bar coding. $H_a: \pi_1 = \pi_2$	H_a: Units with bar coding will have a lower medication error rate than units without bar coding. $H_a: \pi_1 < \pi_2$

it does not designate a particular direction for the relationship; it simply states the means will be "different." Nondirectional hypotheses are most common for exploratory studies or studies in which little literature exists that forms a basis for believing a particular relationship will emerge. On the other hand, if a strong theoretical or literature basis exists for a particular direction of effect, then a hypothesis will be written that reflects this expectation. These are called directional hypotheses. For example, a directional alternative for the previous example is $H_a: B_1 > B_2$ or $H_a: B_1 < B_2$.

The directionality of a hypothesis is important from a theoretical and a practical standpoint. A directional hypothesis only makes sense when there is a strong theoretical reason to believe a direction of effect will be revealed. From a practical standpoint, a directional hypothesis is more liberal than a nondirectional one because all of the error is in one tail, moving the cut point for a hypothesis decision toward the mean. Directional hypotheses will be supported more often than nondirectional ones for this mathematical reason alone, resulting in a less conservative result. Directional hypotheses are supported more often than their nondirectional counterparts, and this characteristic should be considered when the researcher contemplates the role of error in the experiment and the stakes of being wrong.

The Hypothesis Testing Procedure

Hypothesis testing is used when the analysis is focused on whether an intervention had an effect. It is used to determine if results that are observed are greater than those that would be expected based on standard error alone. The steps of the hypothesis-testing procedure appear in **Table 15.4**.

Several choices must be considered and decisions made as part of the hypothesis-testing procedures. Each of these is made based on the specifics of the research question, the resources available to the researcher, and the stakes of being wrong. The probability of error is a major consideration in determining the specifics of the analytic process, as is a consideration of the size of effect that is clinically meaningful.

Hypothesis testing requires that the researcher determine an acceptable risk level for error. This is called alpha, and it represents the probability of an error that the researcher is willing to risk. This decision is based on the nature of the research question and the stakes of being wrong. Alpha is set by the researcher; it is compared to the actual amount of error in the experiment to determine the level of significance of the result. The researcher calculates a **test statistic**, which in most cases is a calculation of differences compared to an expected amount of error. When a result has an identified level of error that is lower than that which was set before the experiment began (as alpha), then the results are called **statistically significant**, and it is assumed the intervention had an effect.

> **Test statistic:** A calculation of differences in group values compared to standard error.
> **Statistically significant:** Differences between groups exceed standard error; the probability that differences are due to chance is less than 5 percent.

If the calculated amount of error is lower than the preestablished standard, then the null hypothesis can be rejected and the alternative accepted. Rejecting a null hypothesis—in other words, saying that "no difference" is wrong—means that a difference was measured and the difference was greater than chance. Accepting an alternative

Table 15.4

Steps in Hypothesis Testing

1. State the research question as a mathematically testable statement.
   a. Translate the variables into statistics (mean, proportion, variance).
   b. State the expected relationship between the statistics (alternative hypothesis).
   c. Restate the relationship as a null hypothesis.
2. Decide on the appropriate test statistic.
   a. For tests of two means, use z or t statistic.
   b. For tests of proportions or rates, use chi square statistic.
   c. For tests of variance, use f statistic.
3. Select the level of error that is acceptable (alpha; usually 0.05 or 0.01).
   a. Determine the value the test statistic must achieve to be declared significant.
   b. Determine the critical value of the test statistic.
   c. Determine what divides the "error" section from the "real effect" section of the distribution.
   d. Determine the cut point at which a result is statistically significant.
4. Compute the test statistic from the raw data using one of the following:
   a. Compare the test statistic to a tabled value to determine significance.
   b. Compare the calculated p value to the *a priori* alpha.
5. Make a decision about the hypothesis and draw a conclusion.
   a. Rejecting a null hypothesis (if p is less than 0.05) means the difference is statistically significant.
   b. Accepting an alternative hypothesis (if p is less than 0.05) means the difference is statistically significant.

(whether directional or nondirectional) indicates that the preconceived difference actually occurred.

The accuracy of hypothesis tests, like any other statistic, is affected by a multitude of factors. One of the greatest impacts is sample size, but other aspects of the experiment, such as random selection, variability, and reliability, may also affect the outcome. These errors can be classified according to their type, interpretation, and impact.

Errors in Hypothesis Tests

Type I error: Concluding that a null hypothesis is false when in fact it is true; claiming a treatment has an effect when it does not.

Two errors can be made in drawing conclusions about a hypothesis test. A **Type I error** occurs when the null hypothesis is true and the researcher rejects it. In other words, there is no relationship among variables or differences between group responses to the intervention, but the researcher claims there is. This is the most serious type of error in health care because it means we impart false hope to patients. We believe that a treatment or intervention will be effective, when in fact it is not. In truth, Type I error is usually a design problem; rival explanations for the outcome are responsible for the results, or a threat to internal validity presents itself. But Type I errors have a tremendous impact on interpreting the results of quantitative studies because they often do not reveal themselves through the analytic process.

Type II errors are also serious, but they represent errors of missed opportunity. A Type II error occurs when the intervention is effective, or there is a relationship among variables, and the researcher concludes there is not. In other words, the intervention works but the researcher claims it does not. Type II errors are common in healthcare studies, unfortunately, because they are almost always a result of inadequate sample size. A Type II error most likely occurs in a study that finds no significant results and was based on a small sample. Type II error is not a concern if differences were detected, no matter how small the sample was. If a difference was found, then the sample was obviously large enough to detect it, and Type II error did not occur.

> **Type II error:** Concluding that a null hypothesis is true when in fact it is false; claiming a treatment does not have an effect when it does.

Type I and II errors always involve balancing tradeoffs between competing demands. One might consider using a highly restrictive alpha—99 percent, for example—to limit the potential for a Type I error. However, this would increase the possibility that a significant finding existed but was overlooked because of the stringent standard for significance that was imposed. The best approach is to set alpha appropriately to avoid reasonable concerns about Type I error and use an adequate sample size to avoid Type II error. Table 15.5 depicts the two types of errors and common means to control them.

A Contrast of Statistical and Clinical Significance

Statistical significance means that the results of a test are greater than would be expected from standard error alone. This means the results are real and not attributable to the ways samples are drawn and variables are measured. On the other hand, because the standard for statistical significance (standard error) is greatly affected by sample size, a very large sample will have an extremely small standard error, making the standard for statistical

Table 15.5

Type I and Type II Errors and Their Control

Condition	Decision	Error	Means of Control
The null hypothesis is true; there is no difference between groups.	Reject the null and accept the alternative; draw the conclusion there is an effect when in fact there is none.	Type I error	Set alpha at the appropriate level; if too liberal, may reject when there is no difference. Design studies that have strong internal validity to minimize effects of rival explanations.
The null hypothesis is not true; there is a difference between groups.	Accept the null and reject the alternative; draw the conclusion there is no effect when in fact there is one.	Type II error	Recruit adequate sample sizes to achieve sufficient power.

significance an easy one to meet. In this case, differences of inconsequential size may be statistically significant when they are of no real importance.

The researcher is wise to include in hypothesis tests a discussion of both statistical significance and clinical importance. Clinical importance is usually represented by **effect size** or the size of the differences between experimental and control groups. Effect size can provide the nurse with a yardstick to represent how much of an effect can be expected, and, therefore, it provides more information than statistical significance alone.

Effect size: The size of the difference between experimental and control groups compared to variability; an indication of the clinical importance of a finding.

Effect size is calculated in many different ways, but all have in common a formula that takes into account the size of differences and the effects of variability. Interpreting effect size is relatively easy; larger numbers represent a stronger effect, and smaller numbers represent a weak one. Effect size can also be discerned from a confidence interval. If the confidence interval for a mean difference includes zero, or nears zero on one end, then it can be concluded that the difference could be nothing. In this case, clinical significance becomes a critical consideration.

Both statistical significance and clinical significance are needed to ensure that a change in practice is warranted. A change in practice should not be recommended if the researcher cannot demonstrate that the results are real; in other words, the results are not due to sampling error. Change also is not warranted if the results are not big enough to warrant the effort involved in changing a practice. Effect size is needed to draw this conclusion.

Designs that Lend Themselves to Hypothesis Testing

Some research questions naturally lend themselves to hypothesis testing. Experimental, quasi-experimental, causal–comparative, and case–control designs are all studies that are particularly suited to hypothesis testing. A research question must lend itself to numerical identification to be appropriate for hypothesis testing, and a relationship, difference, or effect must be the focus of the study. Qualitative studies, then, do not lend themselves to hypothesis testing because they do not involve analysis of numbers.

Predictive and correlation studies also yield a hypothesis test, but these are not necessarily about differences in groups. A correlation coefficient yields a p value that represents the probability that the relationship that is observed is not due to standard error. That relationship, however, may be a weak one, and so the hypothesis test is less important for a correlation study than interpretation of the size and direction of the coefficient. Predictive studies involving regression also yield hypothesis tests, but in this case, the hypothesis is that the regression line is a straight one with no slope. The regression itself is compared to the mean to determine the value of the prediction. So a p value in a regression simply indicates that the values are related in a linear way, and that the regression line is a better predictor than the mean.

The primary consideration in hypothesis testing, however, is appropriate interpretation. A hypothesis decision must be framed in the terms used for the original hypothesis, and interpretation should not exceed what the data will support. Appropriately reporting hypothesis tests and associated effect sizes, along with confidence intervals, is a complete and accurate way to draw conclusions about evidence for nursing practice. All three should be incorporated into the quantitative research report.

Selecting the Appropriate Quantitative Test

Conducting an appropriate quantitative analysis is dependent on the ability of the researcher to select the appropriate statistical test for the hypothesis. This is often the most daunting part of the analysis process because many statistical tests are available to the nurse researcher. Each has specific requirements and is appropriate to yield particular information. The researcher must make decisions about the appropriateness of a statistical test based on the following factors:

- The requirements of the research question
- The number of groups to be tested
- The level of measurement of the independent and dependent variables
- The statistical and mathematical assumptions of the test

Each of these elements is considered in determining which group of tests is selected and, from that group, which particular version will best answer the question without misleading results. Questions about differences between two groups will be answered with different tests than would be used with three or four groups. Interval data, which are assumed to be normally distributed, are tested differently than nominal data, which must be represented as proportions or rates. All statistical tests have assumptions; the data have to meet the assumptions for the results to be interpreted correctly.

The most common tests used in intervention research are tests of means and proportions. When dependent variables are measured as interval numbers (for example, heart rate, length of stay, and cost), then the mean value can be calculated and compared. When dependent variables are nominal or ordinal, then frequencies, rates, or proportions are tested. In each case, tests may be conducted to determine if differences exist between two, three, or more groups.

Tests of Differences Between Two Group Means

Frequently, the research question of interest is whether an intervention, risk factor, or condition made a difference in a specific outcome between two groups. The typical experiment, in which the outcomes from a treatment group are compared to a control or comparison group, falls into this category. If the outcome can be expressed as a mean, then a z or t test is appropriate to use for these differences. The z or t test is a hypothesis test to determine whether the differences in mean values between two groups are statistically significant and clinically important. FIGURE 15.3 depicts the decision process that results in a z or t test for a quantitative analysis.

The two tests essentially accomplish the same end: They generate a test statistic that reflects the differences between the groups compared to standard error—a p value that quantifies the probability that standard error is responsible for the outcome and a confidence interval for mean differences that enables the quantification of effect size. The z

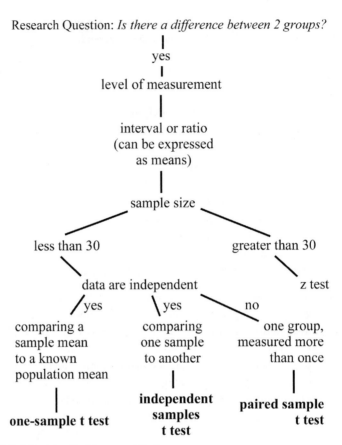

Research Question: *Is there a difference between 2 groups?*

yes

level of measurement

interval or ratio
(can be expressed
as means)

sample size

less than 30   greater than 30

data are independent   z test

yes   yes   no

comparing a   comparing   one group,
sample mean   one sample   measured more
to a known   to another   than once
population mean

one-sample t test   **independent samples t test**   **paired sample t test**

FIGURE 15.3 A Decision Tool for a z or t Test

test is appropriate for large samples or when testing an entire population. The t test is for smaller samples, generally with fewer than 30 subjects (Motulsky, 2010). **FIGURE 15.4** shows how the t test is calculated and the calculations that are represented by each part of the formula.

Because most experiments involve samples, the remainder of this discussion will focus on the t test. There are essentially three versions of the t test that can be applied to determine differences in mean values:

- The one-sample t test quantifies the difference between a mean value in a sample and a population. For example, a one-sample t test could test the difference between a hospital's mean length of stay and the national average.
- The independent-samples t test quantifies the difference between the mean in one group and the mean of another group. An example would be a test to determine if mean length of stay were different for rural and urban hospitals. This could also be a test of effectiveness by comparing the mean in an experimental group to a control group value. For example, an independent-samples t test would be

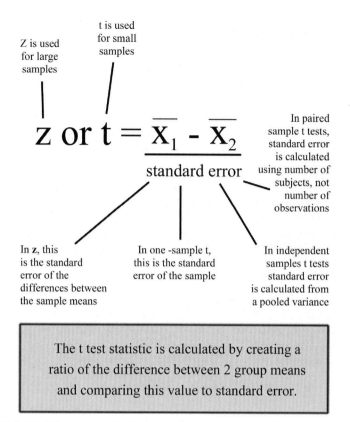

FIGURE 15.4 What Makes Up a t Test?

appropriate to determine if units that used standard order sets had a shorter length of stay than units that did not.

- The paired-samples t test quantifies the difference between a mean value measured in the same group over time. A paired-sample t test could be used to answer questions about average length of stay before and after a change in Medicare reimbursement.

Table 15.6 shows research questions that are addressed by each type of t test. In general, t tests are appropriate when two groups or time periods are compared against some value that is well represented by a mean. Data must be normally distributed to lend themselves to a t test; therefore, interval or ratio data (or ordinal data from large samples) are the only appropriate variables evaluated with a t test.

The results of a t test are used to determine if an intervention is effective in achieving an outcome that can be measured with an interval-level number. Appropriately reported results include the test statistic (t or z), the p value, the mean difference between groups, and a confidence interval for the mean difference.

If the results of a t test are statistically significant, then the differences observed between the groups are real and are not due to standard error. If the results are not

Table 15.6

Research Questions Answered by the t Test

Question	Characteristics	t Test
Is there a difference between mean costs per patient day in an urban-based rehabilitation hospital and the national average for rehabilitation hospitals?	Comparing a sample mean to a known population value	One-sample t test
Is there a difference in mean costs per patient day in urban-based rehabilitation hospitals and rural rehabilitation hospitals?	Comparing the mean value in one group to the mean value in another group; the groups have no influence on each other	Independent-samples t test
Is there a difference in mean costs per patient day for patients in rehabilitation hospitals who are managed with a pharmacist/nurse/physician team and patients who are managed with a traditional model?	Comparing the mean value in one group to the mean value in another group; the groups have no influence on each other	Independent-samples t test
Is there a difference in mean costs per patient day before and after Magnet designation of a rehabilitation hospital?	Comparing the mean value in a group measured over time; a value in the first sample can be "paired up" with a value in the second sample	Paired-samples t test

statistically significant—in other words, if the p value exceeds 0.05—then the remaining numbers in the output need not be interpreted. If, on the other hand, the results are statistically significant, then the size of the test statistic and the specifics of the confidence interval give clues as to the size of the difference. A relatively large test statistic means that a greater effect was achieved relative to standard error; the reverse is also true. A confidence interval that has one end near zero means the difference could be near nothing, and so a smaller effect is expected. Conversely, if the ends of the confidence interval are some distance from zero, then the effect is likely quite large. More detailed statistical texts, specifically Portney and Watkins (2008) and Dawson (2008), can provide formulas for calculating effect size.

The t test is widely used in health care, is relatively simple to calculate, and is easily interpreted. It is included in most introductory statistics classes, so it is meaningful to a wide range of readers. The test is robust, meaning it may still be effective even if data are not normally distributed, and it will work well even with small samples. It is a relatively simple test, however, and it cannot accommodate multiple independent or dependent variables, so it is used primarily for univariate analysis.

Researchers are commonly interested in outcomes that are summarized as average scores, although by no means does this cover all the range of tests that nurse researchers may wish to use. Often, variables in health care are expressed as rates, frequencies, proportions, or probabilities, and these do not lend themselves to analysis with a t test. If a dependent variable must be expressed as a nominal or ordinal number (for example, gender, satisfaction, or presence of a risk factor), then a t test is not appropriate. In these cases, the nonparametric chi square test is appropriate (Norman & Streiner, 2008).

Tests of Differences in Rates and Proportions

Healthcare variables are often expressed as rates or proportions. Events that either occur or do not (e.g., a medication error), characteristics that are either present or not (e.g., risk factor or no risk factor), or variables that describe characteristics in a categorical way (e.g., ethnicity or gender) cannot be expressed as intervals. These variables are not expressed as means, so they are inappropriate for tests using the z or t distribution. FIGURE 15.5 depicts the decision process leading to a chi square test. In this case, tests that are based on a chi square distribution are appropriate.

Three kinds of chi square tests are commonly used in hypothesis testing:

- The chi square test of model fit is used to determine if a sample proportion is independent of a population; it is analogous to the one-sample t test and is used for the same purposes. A chi square test of model fit could be used to determine if a hospital's infection rate were the same as the national rate.
- The chi square test of independence is used to determine if two samples are independent of each other. It is analogous to the independent-samples t test and is used for the same reasons. An example of an appropriate application of the chi square

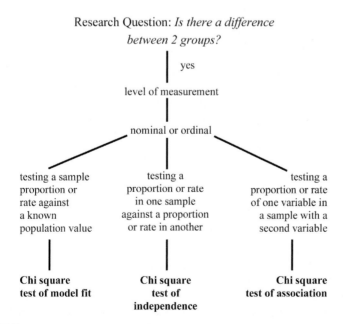

FIGURE 15.5 A Decision Tool for the Chi Square Test

test of independence would be to determine if the infection rate in one nursing home is the same as the infection rate in another nursing home.

- The chi square test of association is used to determine if there is an association between the presence or absence of a characteristic and the occurrence of an event. It is analogous to the paired-samples t test. A chi square test of association could be used to determine if there is an association between the infection rate on a unit and attendance at a unit-based educational event.

Table 15.7 shows research questions that are addressed by each type of test. The chi square test essentially determines an occurrence rate that is expected, based on prior probabilities, or alternatively by assuming equal distribution across all groups. These expected rates are then compared to the rates observed in the experiment. A probability is calculated for the differences between observed and expected values, which yields a p value. This p value is interpreted identically to the way it is used in z tests, t tests, or other hypothesis tests. If the p value is less than the preset alpha, then the fit, association, or independence is considered statistically significant and the differences are real. FIGURE 15.6 demonstrates the calculation and meaning of a chi square statistic.

The chi square test is based on the assumption that the data are not normally distributed and that variables are measured in a categorical manner. Therefore, only nominal or ordinal data (or interval data that have been turned into categories) are appropriate for this test. There are several different versions of the actual chi square statistic. The version used and a rationale for its selection should be provided. The test statistic (the chi square) should be reported, as well as the p value for the test. Confidence intervals are not generally reported for chi square tests, but proportions in each group should be specified.

Table 15.7

Research Questions Answered by the Chi Square

Question	Characteristics	Chi Square
Is the proportion of patients who fall the same on a rehabilitation unit as it is for the rest of the hospital?	Comparing a sample proportion to a known population value	Chi square test of model fit
Is the proportion of patients who fall the same on the day shift as it is on the night shift?	Comparing a sample proportion to another sample's proportion	Chi square test of independence
Is the proportion of patients who fall the same on a shift that received Internet-based training and a shift that received coaching-based training?	Comparing a sample proportion in an experimental group (coaching-based training) to a comparison group (Internet-based training)	Chi square test of independence
Is there an association between falls and the use of diuretics?	Comparing two characteristics of a single sample	Chi square test of association

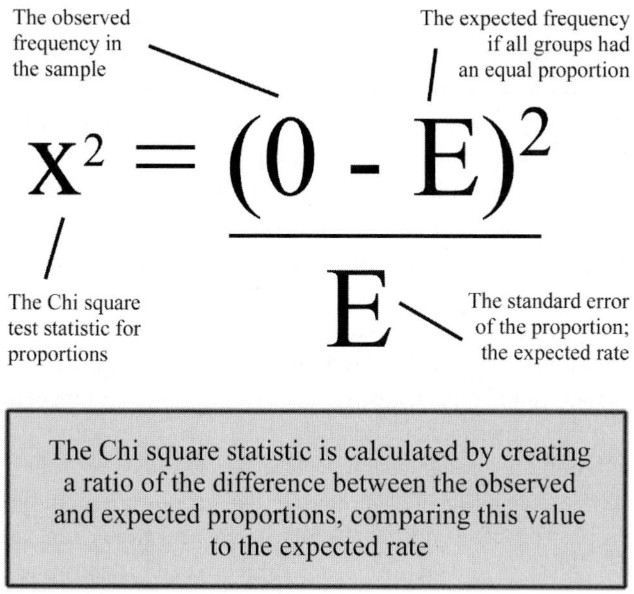

The observed frequency in the sample

The expected frequency if all groups had an equal proportion

$$X^2 = \frac{(0 - E)^2}{E}$$

The Chi square test statistic for proportions

The standard error of the proportion; the expected rate

The Chi square statistic is calculated by creating a ratio of the difference between the observed and expected proportions, comparing this value to the expected rate

FIGURE 15.6 What Makes Up a Chi Square?

Chi square is a common and simple test to run. It is available in nearly all statistical analysis software, and it is a readily recognizable test. It is easy to run and to interpret. However, it is a relatively insensitive test due to its nonparametric nature. Large samples are needed to ensure avoidance of Type II error, and results provide very little information. Aside from the proportion of a variable and a p value, little else is generated from these tests. Still, the chi square is widely used for assessment of research involving everything from risk prediction to model testing; therefore, it is a versatile test for the healthcare researcher.

Tests of Differences in Means with Many Groups

Although tests for differences in means and proportions will answer many evidence-based research questions, all these tests assume that only two groups will be compared. In some cases, more than two groups are involved in an experiment. For example, a researcher may control for the placebo effect by introducing an intervention to one group, withholding the intervention from the control group, and delivering a "sham" intervention to a third comparison group. In this case, the researcher is interested in comparing the intervention group to each comparison group, and then comparing the two controls to each other. Differences between the intervention groups and the nontherapeutic groups will support a treatment effect; differences between the control and comparison groups supports a placebo effect. If treatment effects are identified without placebo effects, the results of the study are particularly strong.

The analysis of more than two groups creates a problem, however. Each statistical test is based on the idea that there is less than a 5 percent chance that the results are due to standard error. The key word here is *each*. When three groups are involved, three actual comparisons are needed: group 1 compared to group 2, group 2 compared to group 3, and group 1 compared to group 3. Each of these tests carries with it a 5 percent error rate. By making three comparisons instead of a single comparison (as we would do with two groups), the error rate has tripled from 5 percent to 15 percent. This **error of multiple comparisons** affects statistical tests in which multiple tests are carried out within the same analysis. Analysis of variance, or its acronym ANOVA, avoids this problem when an interval outcome is compared in more than two groups (Motulsky, 2010).

Error of multiple comparisons: The increased error associated with conducting multiple comparisons in the same analysis; the 5 percent allowable error for each test is multiplied by the number of comparisons, resulting in an inflated error rate.

ANOVA is one of the most frequently used statistical tests in evidence-based research studies. It is a staple for testing the effectiveness of interventions because of its versatility and capacity to produce a tremendous amount of information. It is effective for experimental and quasi-experimental designs, particularly those such as the Solomon four group design, which, as it sounds, tests four groups simultaneously. ANOVA is helpful when more than two groups are required. Studies that compensate for placebo effects or that test for extraneous variables are also suitable for ANOVA. ANOVA and its variants may also be used to determine if factors have interaction effects. **Factors** in ANOVA are the broad categories by which subjects are categorized into levels (for example, gender is a factor in which there are two levels, male and female). Research questions that search for the interactions between characteristics, events, and responses are well addressed with the full factorial versions of ANOVA. A full factorial ANOVA can be used to test all the main effects and interactions involved in an experiment with multiple groups. FIGURE 15.7 depicts a decision tool for the application of ANOVA.

Factors: Independent variables in an ANOVA that are measured as categories.

For example, a researcher may be interested in determining if guided imagery can reduce preoperative anxiety. In this case, the researcher can randomly assign preoperative

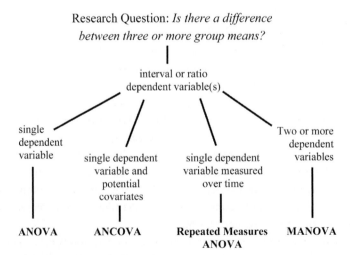

FIGURE 15.7 A Decision Tool for Applying ANOVA

patients to three groups: One group receives formal training in guided imagery, one group receives nonspecific guidance in relaxation, and one group receives no formal intervention. The differences among the three groups would be classified as a main effect. Finding a difference between the guided imagery group and the two comparison groups would provide evidence that the imagery worked. Finding a difference between the control group and the group receiving nonspecific relaxation guidance would provide evidence of a placebo effect. If the researcher were concerned that gender might have an effect on acceptability of guided imagery, the researcher could test for an interaction effect between gender and group membership. Testing both main effects and interaction effects makes up a full factorial ANOVA and enables the researcher to appraise both the effects of the intervention and its interaction with other variables.

ANOVA is used for data that meet some fundamental assumptions. Although ANOVA is focused on the analysis of variance, it is actually a test of means. Therefore, the dependent variable must be numerical and one that is approximately normally distributed. ANOVA possesses a considerable amount of robustness and can still generate good conclusions even if this assumption is somewhat violated. ANOVA also depends on a random sample for generalizability. Unless a special version of the test is used, ANOVA data must be independent, meaning the score at each level has no effect on other scores. In other words, the data must not be repeated measures.

ANOVA is used to determine if the differences between multiple groups are greater than standard error. The test accomplishes this by comparing the variance between treatment groups to the variance within each group. The variance between treatment groups is assumed to be attributable to the different applications of the intervention, called levels. Levels of an intervention might be an experimental treatment, no treatment, and a sham treatment. The variance within each group is assumed to be attributable to standard error. For example, if one subject getting the treatment is different from another subject getting the treatment, these differences are assumed to be attributable to the way the samples were drawn. If this description sounds familiar, it is because within-groups variation is considered and used in ANOVA in the same way standard error is used in a t test—as a surrogate for random chance. If the variance between groups exceeds the variance within groups, then it is assumed that differences between groups are real and are attributable to the intervention.

Levels: The categories that make up factors in an ANOVA.

Four basic kinds of ANOVA are useful for evaluating experiments:

- Univariate ANOVA is applied to determine if there is a difference among groups on a single numerical outcome. Groups may be formed in multiple ways (for example, by treatment condition, demographic characteristics, or other classifications). Multiple groupings with a single dependent variable are called univariate because only a single outcome is measured. Main effects and interaction effects are measured. An example of a univariate ANOVA would be an experiment with treatment, sham, and control conditions measured with respect to gender on an outcome such as time to treatment for chest pain.

- Repeated measures ANOVA is used to determine if time is a factor in treatment conditions. Because these data are not independent, a different version of ANOVA must be applied. For example, a study of the differences in functionality between a treatment group and a control group at four different time periods of recovery would be analyzed with repeated measures ANOVA.

- Analysis of covariance or ANCOVA is used to determine if a covariate—commonly an extraneous variable—has an impact on the experiment. For example, one might want to determine if socioeconomic status was a reason for a poor outcome in a treatment group as opposed to treatment conditions.
- MANOVA, the multivariate version of ANOVA, is the most complex version of the test. MANOVA can accommodate multiple groups and multiple dependent variables, and it is particularly useful when the researcher believes that multiple dependent variables are related to one another. For example, a researcher could use MANOVA to determine if a combination of music therapy and relaxation techniques affected anxiety and panic attacks during painful procedures.

Table 15.8 provides examples of research questions answered by ANOVA. ANOVA and its variants are powerful tools for quantitative analysis. It is a robust test with broad applicability, and it is familiar to the reader of research. It enables the researcher to determine the effects of multiple variables on multiple outcomes, and to do so in a way

Table 15.8

Research Questions Answered by Analysis of Variance (ANOVA)

Question	Characteristics	ANOVA
Is mean length of stay in a rehabilitation facility different for children who have constant parental presence, periodic but daily parental presence, or periodic but not daily parental presence?	Comparing a mean value among three groups	Analysis of variance (ANOVA)
Is mean length of stay in a rehabilitation facility different for children who have constant parental presence, periodic but daily parental presence, or periodic but not daily parental presence? Is this relationship mediated by socioeconomic group?	Comparing a mean value among three groups while controlling the effects of a potential extraneous variable	Analysis of covariance (ANCOVA)
Are mean length of stay and mean functional status on discharge different for children who have constant parental presence, periodic but daily parental presence, or periodic but not daily parental presence?	Comparing mean values on two outcome variables among three groups	Multivariate analysis of variance (MANOVA)
Does functional status after discharge from a pediatric rehabilitation facility change the most in the first month, between 1 and 3 months, between 3 and 6 months, or after 6 months?	Comparing a mean value over time periods	Repeated measures analysis of variance

that minimizes error associated with multiple comparisons. However, it can be a complex test to carry out. As more variables and interactions are considered, the size of the required sample increases. Beyond a fundamental univariate ANOVA, it requires specialized software and training to run and interpret. It remains, however, one of the most widely used tests in healthcare research and yields high-quality evidence for practice.

The results of an ANOVA test are reported similarly to other tests of group differences. The p value indicates if the overall model is statistically significant; in other words, are the differences between groups greater than one would expect from standard error alone? If the p value for the ANOVA is less than 5 percent, however, it only indicates that some group mean is different. If this is the case, then post hoc tests, or tests that look for specific group means, are appropriate. Post hoc tests allow for all groups to be freely compared to all other groups, and all interactions to be tested, while overall error is controlled. If no statistical significance is determined for the overall ANOVA, however, then any group differences are due to standard error, and no additional testing is required.

Tests for Non-normal Data

Although most data questions can be addressed with statistical tests intended for normally distributed data, some data do not conform to this standard. A moderate violation of the assumptions of a statistical test may still yield accurate results; many tests that depend on normal distributions are "robust" in this way. However, some data are so skewed as to be inappropriate for tests intended for normally distributed data. If there are no "tails" in the distribution, then finding statistical significance is a more challenging proposition.

For these data—data that are ranked, ordinal data, or data that are skewed—nonparametric tests are available. These tests are "distribution-free," meaning the test relies on no underlying assumptions about the way the variable is distributed. As such, they can be useful in cases of non-normality. However, these tests are also less sensitive, leading to more Type II error. Avoiding error requires large samples. Further, little information is yielded by these tests (for example, they do not yield confidence intervals), so application of these tests is limited.

This group of tests depends on the ability to rank data, and so are suited for ordinal data. Examples of these tests are the Mann Whitney U, the Wilcoxon Signed Rank test, and the Kruskal Wallis test. The choice of specific tests depends on whether the data are independent or paired sample data.

Reading the Analysis Section of the Research Report

The statistical analysis of a research study provides the tools to determine if interventions do, indeed, make a difference. Without statistical analysis, a researcher cannot quantify if results are attributable to the experiment or to some random effect. Yet the statistical section of a research article is the one area that is often a mystery, a collection of daunting tables, figures, and numbers that seem to confuse more than they clarify. It is a common approach for clinicians to focus on the methods and then flip the pages to the discussion and conclusion section, taking on faith that the statistics are appropriately reported.

This is insufficient, however, to judge the value of a research study as evidence for practice. Studies do get into print with faulty statistical conclusions; errors (both Type I and II) are made; authors go beyond what the statistics will support in interpreting output (Girden & Kabacoff, 2010). The nurse must be able to review the statistical section of a research report both to judge the quality of the article and to decide if the findings should be applied to practice.

There is little reason to be intimidated by the statistical section of a research article. Numbers in research are just tools that are used to convert raw data into information. Statistical numbers are used in research to measure the effects of sampling, to quantify the amount of error in measurement, and to put a value on the effects of chance. These numbers in a research study can help determine if the findings are clinically relevant. Whether a finding is of practical use depends on the magnitude of the effect, and statistics help to evaluate effect size. These are numbers that provide a yardstick to assess whether estimates are precise and useful. Fundamentally, the numbers in a research study help determine if the results are credible, and ultimately if they should be applied to practice.

That is not to say that the nurse must understand every variant of every statistical test. Understanding the ways numbers are used, combined with a focus on some of the

Where to Look

Where to look for quantitative results:

- The text of the section labeled "Methods and Procedures" should include a description of each test that was planned and run. If plans were modified, this should be clearly identified with the reasoning for changing the *a priori* plan.
- The report of quantitative analysis will be clearly identified as a separate section of the report, typically called "Results" or "Findings."
- The text of the "Results" section should include a description of the most important results, along with numbers that are critical for understanding the nature of the findings. For each test, this should include at least the test statistic and the p value. Many authors also report degrees of freedom (a number reflecting the effects of sample size) and confidence intervals for the results.
- Look for confidence intervals to help determine how "close" the results were and to estimate the

magnitude of effect. The inclusion of confidence intervals is becoming more common—and, in fact, is required by some journals—and indicates a thorough report on the part of the authors.

- The "Results" section will often include detailed tables, graphs, and figures to support the text, which generally includes only the most important results.
- The p values may be reported as the actual, calculated probability of error, or they may be identified as "$p < 0.05$" or "$p < 0.01$," which is acceptable. The latter forms are more common when a single table reports multiple test results, or when there are a large number of insignificant results mixed with significant ones. Authors may also simply note nonsignificant results as "NS."

most important numbers, can help determine whether the results can be trusted. A quality evaluation of a research study should focus on the appropriateness of tests and on numbers that provide critical information. The following are the most common types of numbers reported in the quantitative results section:

- Descriptive statistics about the sample and variables
- Analysis of sample subgroups for group equivalency
- Statistics to evaluate the role of error in measures and results
- Statistics to evaluate the magnitude of effect (if there is one)
- Statistics to determine the level of confidence in the findings

Descriptive Statistics About the Sample and Variables

Quantifying characteristics of the sample is important for many reasons. Numbers provide information about the size of samples and the way adequacy of sample size was determined. Descriptive and summary statistics provide the reader with an overall familiarity with the characteristics of the subjects, their baseline conditions, and their responses to treatments. The initial part of the results section should provide sufficient descriptive statistics about the sample and each variable so the reader has a good sense of the characteristics of this sample in this study. This provides a basis for understanding how these subjects responded to treatment and supports generalization to other groups.

Analysis of Sample Subgroups for Group Equivalency

Numbers related to the sample can tell us whether the experimental and control groups are similar enough that extraneous variables are controlled. Deciding whether results are due to a treatment requires that other potential explanations for a result can be eliminated. Differences in key characteristics of subjects (for example, age, severity of illness, activity level, or ethnicity) may compromise internal validity.

Many researchers provide statistics to document the similarity of the treatment groups on key characteristics that might affect the outcome. The effects of these extraneous variables can be minimized if they are distributed equally between the experimental and control groups, and so documenting this equivalence statistically enhances confidence in the results. When groups have been evaluated for comparability, the researcher should provide the results of inferential tests to determine if the groups are the same on key characteristics. In this case, the statistical tests should *not* be statistically significant, meaning that any differences between groups are due to chance. When tests of group comparability are provided in a research study, look for a p value that is greater than 0.05, meaning the groups are statistically identical.

Statistics to Evaluate the Role of Error in Measures and Results

If a researcher could include every member of a population in a study, then sampling error would be nonexistent. That is rarely possible, however, so it is inevitable that there will be some differences between the characteristics of a population and the characteristics of the sample, no matter how carefully the sample is drawn. These differences are

---

SKILL Builder | Reading Statistical Tables and Graphs in
                    Research Reports

Details of quantitative analyses are often displayed in tables and graphs to present them more efficiently and so the text can focus on the most important findings. Although this is an effective way to present a large volume of results, it can be difficult to sort through and evaluate. Tables may be filled with numbers that are confusing, and it is common that the results have to be read and reread to determine their importance. The wide array of graphical presentations that is available means that the reader may have to figure out exactly what the graph itself represents before determining the implications of the results. A challenge for the reader is the fact that no universal method for reporting data in tabular or graphical form is available, either through style manuals or in authors' guidelines. As a result, authors generally provide the numbers in a way that makes sense to them—which does not always translate into an interpretable approach from a reader's perspective.

A systematic approach to evaluating tables and figures can help the nurse reader determine if the results are represented accurately in the discussion and conclusions; this is essential to the critical evaluation of a research report. Do not expect that every research report will have every statistic reported in the same way. It takes some persistence on the part of the reader to track down the numbers that are important for his or her evaluation of the study as effective evidence for practice.

Although tables present numbers efficiently, the reader should begin his or her evaluation by looking at the words in the text. When reading the results that are reported in the text, refer to the tables at the same time to determine the meaning of the findings. For example, if the authors note that a finding was "statistically significant at 0.01," then expect to find more detailed data in the table that matches with the text report. Use the text to guide reading of the data in the table, and refer back to the table to expand understanding of the information provided in the text.

Do not rely solely on the numbers in the table to draw conclusions. The titles of tables and footnotes that accompany them often illuminate the most critical information from the table. Footnotes often contain information about statistical significance, particularly if they are reported in aggregate form. Check each column and row heading to determine the information that is being reported and match it with the text description.

Information in tables and graphs should always be consistent with the textual report; discrepancies between the numbers that are in a table and those reported in the text are causes for grave concern about the accuracy of the researcher's conclusions. It can be helpful to write in the article margin what each test means so that an aggregate of all the findings can be reviewed prior to reading the author's conclusions.

---

quantified as standard error and are directly affected by variability and indirectly affected by sample size. As samples get larger, standard error gets smaller.

How big is an unacceptable standard error? There is no easy answer for that question; standard error is a relative number, specific to the measures that are used and their scale. However, when a standard error is very large relative to the mean value, you can draw the conclusion that a lot of sampling error is present in the experiment. Standard error is, in general, the comparison value to determine statistical significance, so it may be difficult to find statistically significant results when standard error is large. The researcher can reduce standard error by using a sound sampling strategy and drawing a sample that is as large as is practical.

Even when sampling error is small and the sample size is large, however, misleading results may be caused by error associated with the measurement itself. Measurement error can be directly evaluated if the authors provide numbers that reflect the reliability and validity of the measures that are used. Measurement error can be directly evaluated by scrutinizing the reliability of the measures; subtracting the reliability coefficient alpha from 1 results in an approximation of the amount of error contributed by the measure. For example, a measure with a coefficient alpha of 0.72 is contributing 28 percent measurement error to the experiment.

Random events can also create error. All of these taken together provide a rough estimate of the chance of concluding an intervention caused an effect when it did not. The probability of a Type I error is reflected in the p value that is reported with test statistics. When the p value is very small, then the role of error is also very small. Likewise, a large p value indicates a large probability that error is responsible for the result. The p value is not the sole number of interest in a statistical report, but it should be one of the first that is appraised when reading research.

The p value in actuality tells very little about the effectiveness of an experiment, but it does reflect whether any effects that were demonstrated were due to chance. If the probability that error is responsible for the outcome is very large, then any other calculations are irrelevant and should be dismissed. On the other hand, if the probability of error is very low, then the chances that results are real is very high and the reader should move on to look for signs of effect size and clinical importance.

Statistics to Evaluate the Magnitude of Effect

Studies that include inferential tests report several numbers. One of these, the test statistic, enables the reader to judge the magnitude of effect, or the size of the differences between groups. This allows the nurse to conclude whether the difference is large enough to be of practical use. The magnitude of effect helps the nurse make the critical decision of whether to use the results with specific patients. Magnitude of effect can be calculated, but often it is just "eyeballed" by appraising the relative size of the test statistic. Keep in mind that the test statistic is generally a ratio of the effect of treatments to error. As such, this number can provide a rough idea of the importance of any differences that were identified.

> **Magnitude of effect:** The size of the differences between experimental and control groups; supports clinical significance of the findings.

How do you know when a test statistic is large? Again, this is a relative number; in general, the larger the test statistic, the greater the effect. Test statistics that are decimals or low single digits may have very little practical effect, even if the p value shows statistical significance. Test statistics that are in the tens or hundreds usually indicate a good deal of effect. When test statistics show a great deal of effect, then the final consideration is how much confidence the nurse has that this statistic can estimate the effect on another population with accuracy. It may be difficult to judge magnitude of effect from the test statistic, however. In particular, chi square yields a test statistic that is difficult to interpret directly. On the other hand, it is becoming more common to report confidence intervals for mean differences, and these provide a great deal of information about the size of an effect as well as its direction.

Numbers that Reflect Confidence in Estimates

When a test statistic is reported, the researcher should report confidence intervals for the results. Confidence intervals indicate the precision with which the researcher has been able to estimate various characteristics or differences between groups. Confidence intervals get larger as they get more precise; they get smaller as they get more accurate.

Looking at a confidence interval with the test statistics can give the reader an idea whether the results were close or whether the results are precise enough for generalization. For example, if the confidence interval for a mean difference is "0.01 to 6.5," it means the average difference could be as little as a hundredth of a unit or as big as six and a half units. In other words, the difference could be next to nothing. On the other hand, if a confidence interval for a mean difference indicated "12.6 to 12.8," there were quite a few units of average difference between groups and the estimation of the difference is very precise.

Although quantitative results can appear daunting, a systematic appraisal of the most important numbers can provide the nurse with enough information to determine if the findings should be applied in practice. The usefulness of clinical research depends on clinical importance more than statistical significance. Once it has been determined that effects are statistically significant, then the focus of evaluation should be on the size of effects, confidence in the results, and descriptions that enable appropriate generalization of findings.

Using Quantitative Results as Evidence for Practice

Statistical significance is a requirement for using evidence in practice; if results are due to error, then their application is irrelevant. On the other hand, statistical significance tells the nurse little about whether the results will have a real impact in patient care. For this, the nurse must focus on measures of magnitude of effect and clinical significance.

Even with that caveat, inferential results are some of the strongest evidence for practice. Considered the "top of the heap" in most evidence hierarchies, experimental designs provide evidence about the effectiveness of interventions that can be used with a great deal of confidence.

When considering the application of inferential results, nurses should evaluate whether the effects make sense in light of the kinds of patients and outcomes that are found in their specific practice. In other words, can the results be generalized to the setting in which the reader is practicing? All the numbers in the study, taken together, help to answer that question. It requires a systematic appraisal of quantitative information about the sample, the role of error, and the size of effects to draw a conclusion about using quantitative research as evidence.

Checklist for Evaluating Quantitative Results

✔ The statistical tests are appropriate for the research question and the goals of the analysis.

✔ The statistical tests are appropriate for the level of measurement of the variables.

✔ Assumptions of the data were tested and meet the requirements of the tests used.

✔ If groups were compared, inferential analyses were used.

✔ Hypotheses decisions were reported for each hypothesis test and appropriate supporting statistics are provided (test statistic, p value, and confidence interval).

✔ If more than two groups were compared, the researcher compensated for the error of multiple comparisons by modifying alpha or running a test such as ANOVA.

✔ Tables and graphs are clear and labeled correctly.

✔ Results reported in tables and graphs are consistent with the summary report in the text.

✔ The researcher reports findings objectively and accurately.

Creating a Quantitative Analysis

Creating a quantitative analysis requires selecting the right test, using software correctly, interpreting the output, and reporting the results appropriately and completely. Decision trees in this chapter have provided guidance in choosing the correct test. In general, selection of a test is based on the research question, the level of measurement, the specific statistics used to represent the variables, and the number of groups to be compared.

The Research Question

Specific research questions dictate specific methods of analysis. If the words *relationship* or *association* appear in the research question, then correlation or chi square statistics should be used. If the words *differences* or *cause and effect* are inferred by the research question, then inferential tests of group differences are required, such as t tests, ANOVA, or Mann-Whitney U. If the words *explanation* or *prediction* appear in the research question, then regression tests should be used. The research question will also drive the choice of variables and the level at which they are measured.

The Level of Measurement

Not all numbers are created the same, and not all numbers in a research study can be treated the same way mathematically. Whether data are nominal, ordinal, interval, or ratio will drive the specific test that can be applied. For example, nominal data can only be expressed as frequencies, proportions, or rates, and so require tests that accommodate these numbers. Interval and ratio data can be analyzed using a wide range of tests, but they are not appropriate for tests of frequency. An early step for the researcher is to identify the unit of analysis and level of measurement of each variable so the correct statistical tests can be selected.

The Statistics Used to Represent the Variables

The selection of a specific test depends on the statistics used to represent the variables. For example, when testing interval-level data, means are often used to represent a typical response. Tests of means include several varieties of the t test or ANOVA. Frequencies, proportions, and rates are tested with chi square. The choice should also consider the relationship that is expected between variables. Associations and relationships are tested with different statistics than are the effects of treatments. Sample size will also support or limit the selection of a specific test.

The Number of Groups to Be Compared

When only two groups are compared, the role of error is not an issue. When more than two groups are compared, however, the error of multiple comparisons should be controlled. This can be done by restricting the alpha level considered statistically significant. More commonly, tests are applied that are intended to be used as omnibus tests that avoid the multiple comparisons error. It is important, then, that one of these two approaches be applied when more than two group comparisons will be carried out.

Availability of Statistical Software

From a practical standpoint, the final selection of a statistical test is based on access to software that supports the particular analysis chosen. Statistical analysis is much less burdensome with adequate statistical software. Many packages are available for inferential analysis (indeed, even Excel will conduct most common statistical tests), and so there is little motivation for doing manual calculations. The selection of a specific software

---

 CRITICAL APPRAISAL **EXERCISE**

Retrieve the following full text article from the Cumulative Index to Nursing and Allied Health Literature or similar search database:

Baba, L., McGrath, J., & Liu, J. (2010). The efficacy of mechanical vibration analgesia for relief of heel stick pain in neonates. *Journal of Perinatal and Neonatal Nursing, 24*(5), 274–283.

Review the article, focusing on the sections that report the results of the quantitative analyses. Think about the following appraisal questions in your critical review of this research article:

1. Identify the hypothesis. Is it directional or nondirectional? Is it stated as a null?
2. How did the authors ensure that measurement error was minimized? How did blinding strengthen the internal validity of the study?
3. What inferential tests were used in the analyses of data in this study? How are they appropriate for the research questions?
4. Discuss whether the authors use tables and graphs appropriately to represent the data. How could results reported in the tables be clearer?
5. Is sufficient numerical data provided to determine if the results are accurately reported in the text? Are the tables and text reports consistent?
6. Do the authors draw appropriate conclusions? Are the data overinterpreted, underinterpreted, or appropriately reported in the discussion and conclusion sections?

package depends on many factors, including the user's skill and knowledge, financial resources, and statistical acumen. Some software, such as AnalyzeIt and StatsDirect, are simple to run and inexpensive; these packages enable analysis of the most common types of questions. More sophisticated software such as SPSS and SAS require substantial training and investment to maximize usefulness. Regardless of the complexity of the analysis programs, statistical software is simply a tool; without making the appropriate decisions and interpretations, software is of little assistance.

Summary of Key Concepts

- Inferential analysis is the most common analytic tool used in quantitative studies; it enables a researcher to draw a conclusion about a population given the results from a sample.
- Quantitative tests should be selected *a priori*; all identified tests should be run and reported.
- Parametric tests are appropriate for normally distributed data; otherwise, non-parametric tests should be used.
- Statistical analyses can be univariate, bivariate, or multivariate depending on the nature and number of variables involved.
- Statistical significance indicates that a result is not due to standard error; therefore, the effect can be assumed to be real.
- Standard error is the amount of variability in the sample that is due to the sampling procedures; it is directly affected by variability and indirectly affected by sample size.
- A confidence interval is a way of reporting results so the precision and accuracy of the estimates can be evaluated.
- Hypothesis testing is the appropriate way to translate research questions into testable statements. Null hypotheses are used to enable mathematical testing and determination of the probability that results were due to chance.
- Directional hypotheses are more liberal than nondirectional ones; therefore, they will produce statistically significant findings more often.
- Type I error is drawing an erroneous conclusion that a treatment works when it does not; Type II error erroneously concludes a treatment does not work when it does.
- Effect size is a better basis for clinical importance than statistical significance. Effect size indicates the relative size of differences that can be expected under similar circumstances.
- The appropriate statistical test is selected based on the requirements of the research question, the number of groups to be tested, the level of measurement of variables, and the assumptions of the statistical test.
- The z or t test is appropriate for testing differences between means; therefore, these tests are useful when differences in interval-level variables are contrasted in two groups.

- The chi square is appropriate for testing differences between proportions; therefore, it is useful when differences in a nominal- or ordinal-level variable are contrasted between two groups.
- The ANOVA is appropriate for testing differences among three or more group means and is applied to avoid the error of multiple comparisons.
- Some data are so non-normal that they require tests that do not rely on a specific distribution. These tests are described as nonparametric, require large samples, and are not as sensitive as other tests.
- When reading the quantitative analysis section of a research report the nurse should focus on the appropriateness of the statistical selection and key numbers that reflect the role of error and the amount of certainty that exist in the estimates.

For a full suite of assignments and additional learning activities, use the access code located in the front of your book to visit this exclusive website: http://go.jblearning .com/houser. If you do not have an access code, you can obtain one at the site.

References

Chung, S., Bond, E., & Jarrett, M. (2010). Food intake changes across the menstrual cycle in Taiwanese women. *Biological Research for Nursing, 12*(1), 37–46.

Dawson, G. (2008). *Easy interpretation of biostatistics: The vital link to applying evidence in medical decisions.* Philadelphia: W.B. Saunders.

Girden, E., & Kabacoff, R. (2010). *Evaluating research articles from start to finish.* Thousand Oaks, CA: Sage.

Machin, D., & Fayers, P. (2010). *Randomized clinical trials: Design, practice and reporting.* Hoboken, NJ: Wiley Blackwell.

Motulsky, H. (2010). *Intuitive biostatistics: A nonmathematical guide to statistical thinking.* Oxford University Press.

Norman, G., & Streiner, D. (2008). *Biostatistics: The bare essentials* (3rd ed.). Hamilton, Ontario, Canada: B.C. Decker.

Portney, L., & Watkins, M. (2008). *Foundations of clinical research: Applications to practice* (3rd ed.). Upper Saddle River, NJ: Prentice Hall.

part VI

Research that Describes the Meaning of an Experience

chapter 16

Qualitative Research Questions and Procedures

 ## CHAPTER OBJECTIVES

The study of this chapter will help the learner to

- Discuss the purpose of qualitative research as evidence for nursing practice.
- Define characteristics of the qualitative research question.
- Relate sampling strategies and data collection procedures to qualitative design.
- Determine the ways in which credibility, confirmability, dependability, and transferability are demonstrated in qualitative design.
- Review the classifications of common qualitative traditions, including appropriate questions, methods, strengths, and limitations of each.

 ## KEY TERMS

Audit trail	Habituation	Qualitative meta-synthesis
Bracketing	Integrative review	Reflexivity
Case research methods	Investigator triangulation	Saturation
Constant comparison	Member checking	Snowball sampling
Constructivist research	Method triangulation	Stratified purposive sampling
Data source triangulation	Participant observation	
Ethnography	Phenomenology	Theory triangulation
Extreme case sampling	Prolonged engagement	Traditions
Field notes	Purposeful sampling	Transferability
Grounded theory		Triangulation

An Introduction to Qualitative Research

Research that focuses on the effectiveness of interventions is critical evidence for nursing practice, but it is not the only evidence that is important. The definition of evidence-based practice has equal focus on scientific studies, clinical experience, and the preferences of patients. It is these last two—clinical experience and patient preferences—that are commonly answered with qualitative study. Qualitative research is grounded in the belief that reality can never be completely known because it is constructed by each individual (Nicholls, 2009a). Attempts to *measure* reality are limited to methods that are focused on defining variables and finding manifestations of them. But there is much of the human experience that is not easily defined, and outward expressions may be difficult, if not impossible, to detect. Although blood pressure and circulating blood volume are relatively easy to define and measure, experiences such as grief and quality of life are much more difficult to assess.

There are fundamental reasons why qualitative research is important in nursing practice. Nursing is a humanistic, holistic approach to promoting health and minimizing the effects of disease. These are fundamental elements of care on which the profession of nursing is based. Understanding the human experience of health and disease is central to appreciating how to help patients manage them.

The impetus behind qualitative research is to discover the meaning of the phenomenon under study; in quantitative research, determining cause and effect is the main goal. Qualitative research integrates the use of language, concepts, and words rather than numbers to produce evidence. Qualitative research can be either descriptive or interpretive (Munhall, 2010). Descriptive qualitative research is used in a preliminary way to establish basic knowledge about a group or individual's response to health and illness. Interpretive qualitative research is a more complex form of analysis that involves extracting meaning from data in a way that requires inductive thought on the part of the researcher. Interpretive research emphasizes understanding the meaning individuals ascribe to their actions and to the reactions of others (Streubert & Carpenter, 2010). This type of research also emphasizes process and context in understanding the meaning of an experience (Nicholls, 2009c). The point of qualitative research is to elicit a description of a social experience that is so detailed and insightful that one who has not experienced it can understand and appreciate its nuances. The researcher accomplishes the research goals by establishing a relationship with informants and by considering the contextual issues that may shape inquiry.

In many ways, qualitative research is the polar opposite of quantitative research. Designs are not preplanned; the details of a particular study are "emergent," meaning the specifics of the study adapt to the emerging characteristics of the data. Qualitative research is focused on understanding the meaning of an event, rather than measuring effects, and so issues of internal validity, control, and avoidance of bias are not central concerns. Instead, trustworthiness is the guide for appraising the validity of a qualitative study (Ryan-Nicholls & Will, 2009). Sampling strategies, analysis procedures, and reporting of results are all considerably different for qualitative studies than quantitative ones.

Scenes from the Field

Nurses were first deployed to war zones in the Middle East in 2003. Assigned to forward surgical teams and mobile hospitals, U.S. military nurses cared for more than 35,000 injured U.S. soldiers and tended to the more than 5000 Americans who perished there. Although caring for the wounded has required both the resolve and competence of U.S. nurses, very little has been written about the U.S. military nurse experience in the Iraq and Afghanistan wars. Scannell-Desch and Doherty (2010) used a phenomenological approach to study the experiences of these nurses after their return to the United States.

The population for this study consisted of male and female military registered nurses who served in Iraq or Afghanistan during the war years 2003 to 2009. Very few criteria were set for participation—informants had to be a registered nurse, able to speak English, current or former military service, and willing and able to discuss their war experiences. Active duty, reserve, and National Guard nurses were included. The authors used snowball sampling to get an adequate response. They began by contacting two women who had served in the military, and through their contacts, a final sample of 37 nurses was recruited. Individual interviews were used to collect recollections from these nurses.

These authors put in place rigorous guidelines to ensure trustworthiness. Comprehensive field notes—including an audit trail—were kept. Triangulation was sought through inter-coder agreement and member checking. Transferability was enhanced by using multiple sources to recruit participants from all U.S. military branches. Thick description and verbatim quotes were incorporated into the study findings to augment dependability.

Seven themes emerged about the experience of war. The theme of "deployment to war" included description of living conditions, working conditions, and the nurses' attempts to find diversion from the war. A second theme, "most chaotic scene," involved descriptions of soldier patients, children caught in the crossfire, and the difficulty of caring for the injured enemy. Other themes included feelings that the war experience was "more than I bargained for," experiences of bonding with military "family," a sense of being changed by the war, the difficulty adjusting to homecoming, professional growth, and advice for deploying nurses. In particular, these nurses struggle with posttraumatic stress disorder and finding normalcy in their postmilitary lives.

This study provides a clear look at the challenges faced by military nurses in the Middle East and their difficulties reclaiming their lives in the United States. Research such as this study can help develop strategies for preventing postmilitary problems and enhancing the quality of life of those who serve.

Source: Scannell-Desch, E., & Doherty, M. (2010). Experiences of U.S. military nurses in the Iraq and Afghanistan wars, 2003–2009. *Journal of Nursing Scholarship, 21*(1), 3–12.

On the other hand, qualitative and quantitative researchers have many characteristics in common—both are focused on a rigorous approach to eliciting the best possible answer to a research question, and both are a disciplined inquiry aimed at finding the truth.

The Purpose of Qualitative Research

The intent of qualitative research is to gather data that illuminate the meaning of an event or phenomenon. The main purpose is to develop an understanding of meaning from the point of view of the informants. Data are gathered directly from informants or through the investigator's observations. Qualitative research has been called constructivist research because it is grounded in the assumption that individuals construct reality in the form of meaning and interpretation (Holloway & Wheeler, 2010). It is defined as research that is applied to discover the meaning and interpretations of events, phenomena, or experiences by studying cases intensively in natural settings and by subjecting the resulting data to analytic interpretation. Qualitative designs answer questions about the human experience by exploring motives, attitudes, reactions, and perceptions.

Constructivist research: Research that is applied to discover the meaning and interpretations of events, phenomena, or experiences by studying cases intensively in natural settings and by subjecting data to analytic interpretation.

Qualitative designs are particularly useful in evidence-based practice for determining patient needs, preferences, and motives. Although quantitative studies are useful in determining the *effectiveness* of an intervention, qualitative studies are helpful in describing the *acceptability* of an intervention. Interventions that require lifestyle adjustment, attitude changes, or behavioral alterations are particularly suited to qualitative study. Nursing practices that support adaptations on the part of the patient are well addressed by qualitative study, as are counseling and therapeutic communication. Qualitative study is appropriate for addressing a wide variety of research questions that focus on the needs, responses, and experiences of patients.

The Uniqueness of Qualitative Study

Qualitative inquiry is unique in terms of the researcher's beliefs about the nature of reality and in the methods and procedures used to describe the informant's worldview. Although quantitative researchers focus on a single, objective reality, the lens of a qualitative researcher is based on a social construction of reality in which multiple realities are acceptable. In the world of the qualitative researcher, all variables are dependent on each other, and the context of the study is naturalistic. Control and validity are not issues so much as credibility and trustworthiness.

Integration of Qualitative Research into Evidence-Based Practice

In the past, evidence-based practice focused on the medical model, with an overall emphasis on experimental designs that yielded an evaluation of the effectiveness of an intervention. Discovery of this evidence was through systematic reviews of quantitative studies or meta-analysis of aggregate effect size. Nursing practice is a profession focused on the human experience, however, and a reliance solely on experimental designs produces evidence that lacks dimension. As a result, evidence of nursing practice has expanded to include qualitative studies that illuminate the nature of the patient's experience.

In current practice, researchers now realize that, to gain a full understanding of the needs of a patient, an integration of quantitative and qualitative research is needed. Quantitative evidence is widely incorporated into practice, but qualitative evidence is not as commonly used. However, both types of inquiry are helpful in determining best practices. The nurse must examine scientific evidence of best nursing interventions, but he or she must also understand a social or human problem through the eyes of the patient (Streubert & Carpenter, 2010). Qualitative research provides a depth of understanding and adds another dimension to quantitative evidence: one based on the human experience.

Evidence of nursing practice is often discovered through methods that integrate both quantitative and qualitative studies in what is referred to as qualitative meta-synthesis and integrative review. A qualitative meta-synthesis is analogous to a systematic review; it is based on a pre-established set of selection criteria and a systematic appraisal of study quality. An integrative review is one that encompasses both quantitative and qualitative studies, resulting in a practice guideline that incorporates elements of both types of research. This integrative view focuses both on the effectiveness of an intervention and how the treatment affects a patient's life; both are required to assess efficacy (Pearson, 2011).

> **Qualitative meta-synthesis:** A review of qualitative studies that combines a number of studies based on pre-established selection criteria and systematic appraisal of study quality.
> **Integrative review:** A review of both qualitative and quantitative studies that results in a practice guideline incorporating elements of both types of research and focusing on how a treatment affects a patient's life.

Attaining health involves health-promoting behaviors, lifestyle adaptations, knowledge, and an attitude that supports these efforts. Qualitative study is used to discover how the nurse can support the patient's health-promoting actions. These studies are helpful in addressing complex problems, such as perception of care or quality of life. Qualitative research helps to explain the experiential and behavioral components of illness and health care.

The Qualitative Research Question

The fundamental characteristics of the research question will determine if it is best answered with a qualitative approach. Questions that reflect exploration of feelings, perceptions, attitudes, motives, quality of life, and other subjective experiences are well addressed with qualitative inquiry. Table 16.1 provides examples of research questions that are suited to qualitative study and the specific designs that are appropriate to answer them.

In qualitative designs, researchers specifically state questions, not objectives, aims, or hypotheses. There is often a central, broad question and several subquestions. The central question is written in such a way that it accommodates the emerging design that is characteristic of qualitative inquiry. It is often written in broad terms and is open-ended. These questions commonly begin with the words *what* or *how* to convey an open mind and lack of preconceived notions. The verbs in the research question are exploratory and do not reflect directionality; there is no expectation of demonstrating cause and effect. Qualitative research questions often include words such as *discover* and *explore*.

Table 16.1	

Examples of Qualitative Research Questions

Research Question	Design Used to Answer It
What are the responses of a patient with chronic pulmonary hypertension to a lung transplant?	Case research methods
What are the responses of the nurses on a neonatal unit to a medication error causing a death?	Case research methods
How are nurses portrayed in the media?	Content analysis
What are the perceived barriers for ethnically diverse students in nursing programs?	Content analysis
What is the nature of moral distress in nurses related to witnessing futile care in the critical care unit?	Phenomenology
What are the long-term implications for intimacy of couples in which the husband has been treated for prostate cancer?	Phenomenology
What are the cultural issues that emerge during a merger between a for-profit and a not-for-profit hospital?	Ethnography
What is the culture of the waiting room for the open-heart surgery unit?	Ethnography
What are the relationships and interactions that affect intimate partner violence?	Grounded theory
What are the relationships and reactions that lead to teen pregnancy?	Grounded theory

This broad, general approach to the topic conveys the expectation that specifics of the study will emerge. It is also likely that the question itself may evolve and change as the study progresses. The continual review and reformulation of the research question are characteristic of qualitative inquiry. The question should, however, focus on a single phenomenon or concept; a lack of specificity should not be construed as a lack of focus. The researcher should be clear about the fundamental purpose of the study. These studies frequently have more specific subquestions that address particular areas of interest. These subquestions narrow the focus and become the explicit topics that are explored through interviews, focus groups, observations, and other sources (Creswell, 2008).

Although the qualitative research question may evolve as the study progresses, the researcher must still start with a general approach that is consistent throughout the study. The specifics of the research question guide the selection of a particular design that is best used to address it. Qualitative research designs are sometimes called "traditions" when they refer to qualitative approaches. Each tradition is intended to answer a particular kind of question.

Traditions: Particular designs or approaches in qualitative research used to answer specific types of study questions.

The way a question is worded determines the specific tradition the researcher will select to fully answer it. For example, phenomenology is focused on determining the essence of a lived experience. The following are two examples of questions that might be answered with phenomenology: "What is it like to be wheelchair-bound?" "What is it like to be a freshman student in an inner city university?" Ethnography is used by nurse researchers to examine the interrelationship among people, environment, culture, and health: "What is the culture of the department of nursing and how does it affect the university as a whole?" "How do the health beliefs and practices of Asian Americans integrate with Western medicine?" Another question that lends itself to qualitative research is steeped in examining processes, interactions, and interrelationships through grounded theory: "What are the social processes that nursing students must attend to in order to be successful in the nursing program?" There should be an identifiable link between the research question and the specific question used to answer it, even though the details of the design may take some time to emerge.

Characteristics of Qualitative Research Methods

Qualitative research is a systematic approach to understanding the experiences of others. This research is characterized by sampling procedures, data collection processes, and analytical processes that are aimed at achieving this understanding. Although internal validity and external validity are not paramount for qualitative researchers, there is concern for trustworthiness (Ryan-Nicholls & Will, 2009). Strong qualitative research studies include attention to actions that can support confidence in the results. Table 16.2 contrasts the characteristics of quantitative and qualitative research processes.

Table 16.2

Comparison of Quantitative and Qualitative Characteristics

Element	Quantitative Version	Qualitative Version
Research question	Specific; includes identification of population, variables, and outcome	General and broad; may be stated as a purpose instead of a question
Design	Preplanned and specific	Emergent in response to data collection and ongoing analysis
Sample selection	Random selection to achieve maximum representation of identified population	Purposeful selection to achieve maximum information about the topic of interest
Inclusion/exclusion criteria	Strictly adhered to; based on demographic or other characteristics	Loosely applied; based on shared experience or group membership
Sample size	Based on power calculation	Based on achievement of saturation
Data collection	Achieved through measurement of a quantifiable characteristic	Achieved through observation, interaction, or document review
Instrumentation	Measurement instruments are calibrated or otherwise determined to be reliable and valid	The researcher is the measurement instrument
Analysis of data	Preplanned; does not begin until all data have been collected	Emergent; data are analyzed as they are collected and compared to previous results

Sampling Strategies

In qualitative research, subjects are referred to as "informants," "respondents," or "participants." As in other types of research, the qualitative sampling strategy is concerned with how participants are selected and how many are enough. The way these two elements of the strategy are addressed is unique for qualitative research.

The first element of the qualitative sampling strategy is the selection procedure. Qualitative samples are most commonly selected using a purposeful sampling method. Purposeful sampling is a characteristic of qualitative research in which the researcher identifies criteria for the type of informant most likely to illuminate the research question, actively seeks out these individuals, and personally invites their participation. These criteria often involve a shared experience, a specific demographic group, or simply the willingness to share information with the researcher. The researcher is usually the person who approaches the accessible informants, informs them about the study, and obtains their consent to participate. Informed consent is as important in qualitative research as in quantitative; concerns for confidentiality, anonymity, and protection of privacy also are important in these studies. These issues may be of particular concern because of the often sensitive nature of the subject matter.

The researcher is involved in each step of the sampling process. Selection bias is not a concern if clear criteria are used and the researcher is aware of his or her biases. Qualitative researchers acknowledge the potential for bias and make an assumption that it is inherent in any study of an interpretive nature. This active process of identifying biases and making them explicit is a control for validity called bracketing (Creswell, 2008).

Most qualitative samples are purposeful, but there are several other types of sampling strategies. Stratified purposive sampling involves sampling participants who meet certain inclusion criteria and then stratifying them according to age, gender, ethnicity, and other criteria. For example, the researcher may be interested in how older women react to an unplanned pregnancy, and so might stratify the sample by age. Snowball sampling is useful when one cannot locate a list of individuals who share a particular characteristic. As participants are identified, they in turn are asked to identify others who meet the inclusion criteria, thus the sample snowballs. This is a common approach for working with sensitive populations such as drug addicts or pregnant teens. Extreme case sampling focuses on cases that are unusual or special. These individuals exhibit the phenomenon of interest in its extremes. These may be useful for studying the characteristics of individuals who exhibit superior abilities or those who are considered worst cases. An example of the former might be studies of the characteristics of nurses who have zero errors; the latter might be exhibited in a study of nurses who made a serious error resulting in patient death.

A second consideration is sample size. Qualitative studies are not intended to be generalized to populations, and they are not tests of cause and effect. Issues such as power and Type I and II errors are not applicable. And so the question arises: When is the sample big enough? Saturation is the key consideration for the sample

---

Purposeful sampling: A technique used in qualitative research in which the subjects are selected because they possess certain characteristics that will enhance the credibility of the study and because they can reliably inform the research question.

Stratified purposive sampling: Sampling of participants who meet certain inclusion criteria and then stratifying them according to other criteria (for example, age, gender, and ethnicity).

Snowball sampling: A nonprobability sampling method that relies on referrals from the initial subjects to recruit additional subjects. This method is best used for studies involving subjects who possess sensitive characteristics or who are hard to find.

Extreme case sampling: Sampling of unusual or special participants who exhibit the phenomenon of interest in its extremes.

Saturation: The point at which no new information is being generated and the sample size is determined to be adequate.

size in a qualitative study (Creswell, 2008). Saturation is reached when themes become repetitive, suggesting no new input is needed. The sample size is not predetermined, although the researcher may consider a general sample size as a goal at the beginning of data collection. Once the study has been initiated, recruitment of informants and data collection continue until the researcher finds that no new information has been elicited. This is referred to as the point of saturation, and it is the standard for adequacy of the sample size. Saturation may be achieved with as few as five or six informants, or it may take a considerably larger number of participants in studies of complex or sensitive topics. Determination of saturation is up to the researcher, but it should be reported that it was reached.

Data Collection Methods and Procedures

Data may be collected through a variety of methods. Qualitative data are usually collected through a combination of methods, including observation, interaction, or document review. Interaction data may be collected via essay questions, interviews, focus groups, or conversation. These data are often recorded on audiotape and transcribed for analysis of the data. Some researchers are turning to photographic methods to capture observations, document interactions, and even stimulate discussion (Hansen-Ketchum & Myrick, 2008). Video may also be used with individuals or focus groups to capture both verbal and nonverbal responses to questions.

With most qualitative research traditions, analysis occurs simultaneously with data collection—another significant departure from quantitative research. This method of analysis is called constant comparison, a common approach in the qualitative traditions. Data are reviewed and analyzed as they are gathered, and new data are compared to what has been interpreted to support or disprove earlier conclusions. This process results in an emergent analytic process that evolves and focuses as more data are gathered. The analytic process involves coding units of meaning into themes; these processes will be covered in-depth in the next chapter.

Observations of body language, the surroundings, and other factors are also an important part of the data collection. These are often referred to as field notes, and they enrich the data interpretation process with detailed descriptions of the context, environment, and nonverbal communications. These observations are generally inserted into the transcripts as soon as possible to ensure they are recollected correctly and completely. It is not uncommon for the researcher to maintain a personal journal as well to capture his or her individual responses and reactions to the research process.

The researcher must be attentive to how the data are collected. For example, when there are sensitive issues under study, the researcher needs to create an environment of safety and trust for the participants. Conducting interviews in natural settings (for example, observing and speaking with nurses in the unit conference room or meeting with an informant in the informant's home) are appropriate for qualitative studies and elicit the most natural responses. It is important to anticipate the concerns participants may have regarding the phenomenon under discussion (Nicholls, 2009b). The researcher

Constant comparison: A method of analysis in qualitative research that involves a review of data as they are gathered and comparison to data that have been interpreted to support or reject earlier conclusions.

Field notes: Detailed descriptions of the context, environment, and nonverbal communications observed during data collection and inserted by the researcher into the transcripts to enrich the data interpretation process.

must maintain an approach based on engendering mutual respect and maintaining confidentiality throughout the data collection process.

Enhancing the Trustworthiness of Qualitative Study

Qualitative study is not subject to concerns about internal or external validity because these studies do not focus on cause and effect, and they are not intended to be generalized to larger populations. However, rigor and truth are still concerns; no researcher wants his or her findings to be misleading or in error. But the rigor of qualitative research is judged differently. The seminal works of Guba (1981) and Guba and Lincoln (1989) advance the notion that qualitative research is based on trustworthiness rather than reliability and validity. Trustworthiness includes the following specific characteristics:

- *Credibility:* The results of the study represent the realities of the participants as much as possible.
- *Confirmability:* The researcher attempts to enhance objectivity by reducing bias in methods and procedures.
- *Dependability:* Repetition of the study with similar subjects in similar circumstances results in consistent findings.
- *Transferability:* Results can be transferred to situations with similar subjects and settings.

Methods to support these characteristics should be built into the study methods and procedures. One of the most common threats to credibility of a study is bias. Drawing premature conclusions, basing themes on isolated responses, and incorrect interpretations can all influence the strength of a qualitative study. The nurse researcher can limit the effects of bias through bracketing, prolonged engagement, triangulation, member checking, and audit trails. Some of these processes are built into the design of a qualitative study; others are initiated during analysis of results. **Table 16.3** depicts the methods used to achieve trustworthiness in qualitative inquiry. It is difficult, however, to separate the specific strategies that are used in each phase of a qualitative study because emergent design and data analysis often overlap. These controls will be discussed in this chapter as they relate to design and in Chapter 17 as they relate to analysis.

Bracketing, one method of limiting the effects of researcher bias, is a means of demonstrating an awareness of the potential assumptions and preconceived notions of the researcher. Bracketing includes three phases:

1. The researcher examines and reflects on his or her own standpoint regarding the topic.
2. The researcher identifies his or her own assumptions, based on theory or experience.
3. The researcher explicitly identifies the process for setting aside, suspending, or holding at bay personal biases (Creswell, 2008).

---

gray matter

Threats to the credibility of qualitative research may include the following errors:
- Drawing premature conclusions
- Basing themes on isolated responses
- Incorrectly interpreting data

Bracketing: A method of limiting the effects of researcher bias and setting them aside by demonstrating awareness of potential suppositions of the researcher.

Methods Used to Achieve Trustworthiness in Qualitative Inquiry

Consideration	Qualitative Version	Methods to Achieve
Internal validity	Credibility: Can the results be believed?	■ Prolonged engagement ■ Researcher reflexivity ■ Bracketing of researcher bias ■ Member checking ■ Triangulation
External validity	Transferability: Can the results be transferred to other people and situations?	■ Purposeful sampling ■ Inclusion/exclusion criteria ■ Thick description of the setting ■ In-depth description of informants
Reliability	Dependability: Would the results be similar if the study was repeated with similar subjects in similar circumstances?	■ Audit trail ■ Researcher journal ■ Detailed descriptions of research methods ■ Triangulation ■ Peer examination of procedures and results ■ Measures of interrater reliability
Objectivity	Confirmability: Was objectivity enhanced by reducing bias?	■ Bracketing of researcher bias ■ Researcher reflexivity ■ Triangulation

Qualitative researchers have to be sensitive to the ways in which the researcher and the research process have shaped the data (Munhall, 2010). This is referred to as reflexivity and is based on introspection and acknowledgment of biases, values, and interests. Reflexive introspection is a key component of bracketing and requires maturity and honesty on the part of the researcher.

Prolonged engagement with the participants involved in the study supports the credibility of conclusions. Extended contact with informants and the setting is a means of controlling the biases that result in premature conclusions. Included in this process is the investment of sufficient time in the data collection process that the researcher gains an in-depth understanding of the culture, language, or views of the group under study. Sustained involvement also helps build the trusting relationships and rapport that are necessary to elicit accurate and thorough responses.

Triangulation is a useful strategy for the enhancement of credibility. A qualitative researcher employs triangulation when at least three sources of information are used to support each major conclusion. The researcher uses a variety of methods or informants to capture a more complete and insightful portrait of the phenomena that are being studied. Four types of triangulation have been described by Farmer et al. (2006):

- Data source triangulation involves the use of multiple data sources in a study (for example, interviewing diverse key informants to give credence to the findings).

Reflexivity: A sensitivity to the ways in which the researcher and the research process have shaped the data; based on introspection and acknowledgment of bias.

Prolonged engagement: Investment of sufficient time in the data collection process so that the researcher gains an in-depth understanding of the culture, language, or views of the group under study.

Triangulation: Enhancing credibility by cross-checking information and conclusions, using multiple data sources, using multiple research methods or researchers to study the phenomenon, or using multiple theories and perspectives to help interpret the data.

Data source triangulation: A type of triangulation in which multiple data sources are used in a study.

Investigator triangulation: A type of triangulation in which more than one person is used to collect, analyze, or interpret a set of data.

Theory triangulation: A type of triangulation in which multiple perspectives are obtained and used from other researchers or published literature.

Method triangulation: A type of triangulation in which multiple data collection methods are used, such as interviews, observation, and document review.

Member checking: A method of ensuring validity by having participants review and comment on the accuracy of transcripts, interpretations, or conclusions.

Audit trail: A thorough and conscientious reflection and recording of the decisions that were made, procedures that were designed, and questions that were raised during analysis of data.

- Another method is investigator triangulation, which involves more than one person to collect, analyze, or interpret a set of data.
- Gaining and using multiple perspectives from other researchers or published literature accomplishes theory triangulation.
- The use of multiple data collection methods (for example, interviews, observation, and document review) results in method triangulation.

Performing external checks on the data and their interpretation is a common method of ensuring validity via member checking. Researchers use member checking when they ask participants to review and comment on the accuracy of transcripts, interpretations, or conclusions. Member checking requires that contact be made with each informant twice: once to collect data and a second time to review their accuracy and completeness.

An audit trail supports the dependability of a study and its analysis. An audit trail is a thorough, conscientious reflection on and documentation of the decisions that were made, the procedures that were designed, and the questions that were addressed during analysis. A thorough record of the emerging design decisions helps other researchers confirm the findings.

Qualitative research has a subjective focus, but it is not without rigor. Methods of ensuring trustworthiness enable the researcher to support the validity and usefulness of his or her conclusions. These strategies should be evident throughout the research process and documented in the research report.

Classifications of Qualitative Traditions

Multiple strategies are available to the qualitative researcher. The selection of a particular tradition depends on the purpose of the research and the nature of the research question. Some traditions are more common in nursing and health care in general. These designs, which include those in the following list, are regularly used because they answer questions about human reactions and interactions.

- *Case research methods:* Intense study of a single subject or small group of subjects
    - *Content analysis:* Interpretation of the meaning in verbal responses or in documents
    - *Phenomenology:* Investigation of the meaning of a phenomenon among a group that have experienced it
    - *Ethnography:* Study of the features and interactions of a given culture
    - *Grounded theory:* Research aimed at developing a theory of process, action, and interaction

gray matter

The following traditions are commonly used in qualitative studies by nurses:

- Case study
- Content analysis
- Phenomenology
- Ethnography
- Grounded theory

Although these are the most common qualitative methodologies, often no specific tradition is identified. Rather, a researcher refers to the study as "qualitative research" without discriminating a specific approach. Shin et al. (2010) reviewed more than 500 articles in two qualitative nursing research journals to determine the most common methods identified. In nearly 30 percent of the articles, no specific method was identified. So it is common that qualitative design principles are applied with no specific methodology identified. Still, there are guidelines for specific methodologies that should be matched appropriately to research questions when possible.

Case Research Methods

Research is often aimed at understanding entire populations, but nursing practice is concerned with the health of individuals. Case research methods involve the in-depth study of a single participant or a single group over an extended period of time so the impact of health and illness on an individual can be described. Multiple data collection methods are used, including observation, interviewing, and/or instrumentation (Anthony & Jack, 2009). Mixed methods, which combine qualitative and quantitative data collection, are also common. This is an appropriate method for studying the responses of individuals and small groups related to interventions, health behaviors, and perceptions of illness. It may be the only way to study individuals with rare conditions.

Case research methods: The meticulous descriptive exploration of a single unit of study such as a person, family group, community, or other entity.

Case research methods are often the basis for teaching strategies. "Grand rounds" had its roots in the medical model, but it has become a valuable teaching tool in all health professions. Using in-depth analyses of individuals and groups helps bring the human dimension to the healthcare experience and enables a rich, multidimensional picture of the subjects to emerge.

Questions that Are Addressed with Case Research

Research questions that focus on the effects of treatments or conditions for individuals are appropriately answered with case study. The case research method is valuable because it can be used to generate evidence about the impact of health and illness for an individual who presents as a unique or interesting subject. Often these cases are ones that present challenges for nursing care. Exploratory questions and questions that are intended to produce potential interventions for later testing are also well addressed with case research methods. Because case research allows for a thorough analysis of a rare or uncommon situation, it often leads to the discovery of relationships that were not obvious or observed prior to the experiment (Payne et al., 2007).

Methods and Procedures for Case Research

Case research is an intensive investigation designed to analyze and understand factors that are important to the cause of health problems, care of patients, and outcome of interventions (Anthony & Jack, 2009). An individual is identified who meets the criteria or (more often) presents him- or herself as a patient with a challenging or unusual condition. Data are collected over an extended period of time using multiple data collection methods. A case analysis begins with a description of the patient's history and demographic, social, and environmental factors that are relevant to the subject's health care. Data collected via observation and interactions are usually qualitative, but quantitative data may also be collected to augment the subjective responses.

Case in Point: A Case Research Method Example

Nearly one in three young people in the United States and Canada report drug use before the age of 15. Illegal drug use presents direct health risks, and in this age group, is associated with self-harm, suicide, risky sexual behavior, and youth offending. Understanding the ways that this use might be influenced by the school context is important in determining how to stop it.

Fletcher et al. (2009) used a case study approach to explore young people's experiences of school influences on drug use. The authors used semi-structured interviews with 30 students and 10 teachers in two case-study schools to gather data. The students were purposively sampled to achieve broad demographic representation. Content analysis was used to arrive at the potential pathways through which school affects drug use.

One strong pathway was through the peer group as a source of identity among students who feel disconnected from the mainstream. A second pathway was the students' desire to "fit in" at schools that were believed to be unsafe. A third source was drug use as a strategy to manage anxiety about school, particularly when the teen had few effective social support systems. These findings support the notion of "whole school" interventions to reduce drug use through promoting a sense of belonging, reducing bullying and aggression, and providing additional social supports.

This study was typical of case research in that a limited number of "cases" were studied in depth, specifically two schools. Both teachers and students were interviewed to achieve triangulation, supporting credibility. Verbatim quotes were used to demonstrate the themes, which were described in sufficient detail that the reader could understand the experiences of these young people. The researcher spent prolonged time in the schools, gaining the trust of the students and establishing a rapport that led to in-depth interviews.

Source: Fletcher, A., Bonell, C., Sorhaindo, A., & Strainge, V. (2009). How might schools influence young people's drug use? Development of theory from qualitative case study research. *Journal of Adolescent Health, 45*, 126–132.

Strengths of Case Research

Case research methods have some clear strengths in generating evidence for nursing practice:

- Case research is a practical method for studying individuals or small groups.
- Case research has direct applicability to patient care.
- Case research demonstrates the impact of health and illness on individuals.

Limitations of Case Research

Case research methods have some inherent limitations:

- In-depth analysis requires extended contact and involvement in the research; attrition of the subjects limits the usefulness of the entire study.
- Studies apply only to individuals and are not applicable to other groups or people.
- These studies have an inherent lack of control over extraneous variables, so conclusions about the effects of treatments cannot be drawn.

Case research is a useful methodology for determining how individuals in unique circumstances respond to their health and disease conditions. It is also an effective way to communicate with colleagues and teach others about challenging cases.

Content Analysis

Content analysis is technically not a specific qualitative research design; it is more accurately described as a data analysis method. The term, however, is commonly used to describe designs that rely on data collected via interviews or document analysis and that use interpretive coding to arrive at themes and patterns. These designs are sometimes referred to as descriptive qualitative designs, but even that term is misleading because these studies may be interpretive as well. In reality, content analysis is often used when no other classification "fits."

The purpose of content analysis is to discover and interpret the meaning in the words of respondents or in historical or written documents. Content analysis as an analytic method may be used in any of the other traditions, but when a qualitative study does not neatly fit into one of the more formal classifications, it is often referred to simply as a content analysis study.

Questions that Are Addressed with Content Analysis

The primary usefulness of content analysis is to answer a research question that explores feelings, perceptions, thoughts, attitudes, or motives related to a concept of interest to the researcher. Content analysis can be used for either descriptive or interpretive studies.

Methods and Procedures for Content Analysis

Content analysis requires the researcher to gather in-depth data in word form. Purposeful sampling is used to identify and recruit appropriate informants who can best

---

Case in Point: A Content Analysis Example

A focus on healthcare quality has intensified in the past two decades. Documentation of the number of deaths that are caused by healthcare providers' errors sent shockwaves through the profession of nursing. Although the quality of nursing care is clearly vital to achieving optimal patient outcomes and ensuring the safety of patients, improvements have been slow. This may be in part because practicing nurses are rarely involved in developing or defining improvement programs for quality nursing care. These authors propose that quality nursing care must be meaningful and relevant to nurses, and uncovering the meaning of quality for nurses could facilitate more effective improvement approaches.

Burhans and Alligood (2010) used a content analysis approach to determine the meaning of quality nursing care for practicing nurses. Twelve nurses from medical-surgical units were interviewed, and emerging themes were discovered through reflective analysis of verbatim transcripts. The themes that described quality included meeting human needs through caring, empathetic interactions; responsible, intentional advocacy for patients; and accountability for achieving quality outcomes.

This study was typical of content analysis in that no specific analytic method was identified. One could assume that content analysis was used from the description of the analytic processes of the authors, but it was not explicitly identified. Because content analysis is a tool—not a design—this is typical of many qualitative studies that use a general approach to exploring a topic of interest.

Source: Burhans, L., & Alligood, M. (2010). Quality nursing care in the words of nurses. *Journal of Advanced Nursing, 66*(8), 1689–1697.

help the researcher answer the specific research question. General interview questions are designed and/or document retrieval guidelines are developed. Interviews and focus groups are the most common ways to gather data for content analysis, but document review may be the focus of the study. It is not uncommon for researchers to use all three as a method of triangulation of the data. Interviews and focus groups are more common for phenomenological study or research focused on subjective aspects of a concept. Document review is more common in studies that involve historical reviews, biographies, or secondary data analysis.

Data are collected and transcribed in their entirety, and thematic coding is applied to draw meaning from the content. Thematic coding will be described in-depth in Chapter 17. Procedures for data management and maintenance of confidentiality are critical in the design of content analysis studies.

Strengths of Content Analysis

Content analysis is a common method applied to answer qualitative research questions. It has some definite advantages as an approach to qualitative inquiry:

- Content analysis is relatively uncomplicated to carry out.
- Extended time periods of observation are generally not needed; saturation may be achieved with relatively few interviews or focus groups.
- Content analysis results in identification of general themes that allow the researcher to report and answer the question in a straightforward, concise way.

Limitations of Content Analysis

Content analysis is not appropriate for all studies because it has the following limitations:

- Content analysis relies on the informant's recall, ability to report, and willingness to talk.
- Selection effects may be in play because those who agree to respond to interviews may not be representative of all of those who are affected.
- The researcher's bias may affect the interpretation and coding of themes in the data.

Content analysis is common in nursing and healthcare research, and it is considered one of the less-complex qualitative methods. It is useful in identifying themes, patterns, and common experiences among individuals related to their health and disease.

Phenomenology

Phenomenology is concerned with the lived experiences of humans in relation to a shared phenomenon. Researchers use this tradition to describe how unique individuals respond to the circumstances of their health and illness. Phenomenology may be either descriptive or interpretive. It is based on a philosophical premise that it is possible to capture and articulate the "essence" of an experience that can be explored and understood (Flood, 2010). Phenomenology is defined as a research methodology that is rigorous, critical, and systematic in its investigation of a human experience in context (Fain, 2009). Phenomenology is useful for understanding the way in which patients react and respond to both everyday experiences and unique events.

Phenomenology: Investigation of the meaning of an experience among a group that has lived through it.

It is useful for evidence of nursing practices that support and enhance the ways patients respond to the challenges in their health care.

Questions that Are Addressed with Phenomenology

Phenomenological research always focuses on a variation of the following question: "What is this experience like?" The goal of this research is to develop rich, detailed, insightful descriptions of the way individuals react to the experiences in their lives. It is particularly helpful when an experience of interest has been poorly defined or explored. It can be helpful in determining interventions that support or enhance the experiences of patients who are facing healthcare decisions or conditions.

Methods and Procedures for Phenomenology

Phenomenological study begins with the articulation of an experience of interest. This becomes the focus of the research question, sample selection, and data collection. In this sense, phenomenological research questions are specific to a single experience. Although the exact nature of the study and data collection may evolve and change, the focus on the experience of interest does not.

Case in Point: A Phenomenology Example

One of the most disturbing errors in an operative unit is the unintended retention of foreign bodies from surgery. Ensuring correct pre- and postsurgical counts is a primary responsibility of perioperative nurses and surgical technicians. However, these incidents continue to occur. To determine how incorrect surgical counts occur, Rowlands and Steeves (2010) conducted a qualitative analysis of the tasks and challenges faced by perioperative nurses and surgical technologists in a busy surgical suite.

Informants for the study were recruited from two hospitals, one an academic medical center with a high volume of surgical procedures, and one a smaller community hospital with general surgical services. Subjects were recruited if they were the nurse responsible for providing direct patient care at a time when an incorrect surgical count occurred. Individual face-to-face interviews were conducted by the researcher and transcribed verbatim for coding. A constant-comparison approach was used to generate three overarching themes.

A theme of "bad behavior" was reported by several of the nurses. Examples include poor decision making, lack of respect for others, nonadherence to standards and policies, and "sloppiness" in meth-

ods. A second theme was "general chaos," blamed on the fast pace of a surgical suite, lack of educational preparation, quickly changing assignments, and loud noise levels. A final theme was "communication difficulties," which involved difficulty working together, overuse of idle chatter, lack of sharing of information, and lack of proper equipment. These themes can be used to design organizational strategies to reduce these serious errors.

This phenomenological study was typical in that subjects were selected because they had a shared experience (incorrect surgical counts) and were willing to discuss the experience. This study is a good example of the use of phenomenology to build evidence for leadership practices. The authors arrive at recommendations for organizational actions based on the perceptions of the informants who have experienced this phenomenon. This study provides an excellent description of the way inclusion criteria are used to guide selection of a purposive sample and of the unique way phenomenological data are analyzed.

Source: Rowlands, A., & Steeves, R. (2010). Incorrect surgical counts: A qualitative analysis. *AORN Journal, 92*(4), 410–419.

Once a question has been articulated, the researcher must identify informants who have experienced the phenomenon. Subjects are purposefully selected based on this central characteristic, but other criteria may also be included, such as demographic, social, or relationship roles. It is not uncommon for samples to be small, although data collection should continue until saturation is achieved (Connelly, 2010).

In phenomenology, the researcher is the primary data collection instrument. It is important, then, for the researcher to conduct a reflective self-assessment for the purposes of bracketing prior to initiation of data collection. Phenomenological study requires that an individual be able to reflect on and report reactions to a specific phenomenon in his or her life. Data collection is generally through interview or focus group. There is less concern for the facts of an experience than for the meaning these facts hold for the people experiencing them. A general interview guide may be developed for data collection, but the interviewing process is guided by the respondent as the interviewer follows the thoughts and ideas of those who have experienced the phenomenon. Data are transcribed and analyzed using coding and content analysis.

Phenomenology generates large amounts of data, and so a method for filing, coding, and retrieving data should be planned into the research procedures. Analysis is through constant comparison, and so continuous reflection on the meaning in the data, use of analytic memos, and comparison of emerging data with existing data are essential in determining the essence of the experience for informants.

Strengths of Phenomenology

Phenomenology has several advantages as an approach to generating evidence for nursing practice:

- The phenomenological tradition can be used to study a wide range of phenomena, including both common and uncommon experiences.
- The interviewing process that is characteristic of phenomenology enables exploration of a wide range of responses.
- Phenomenology lends itself well to focus groups and as such may be more transferable than other types of qualitative study.
- The procedures for phenomenological research are relatively straightforward, and questions are usually more focused than for other types of qualitative study (Flood, 2010).

Limitations of Phenomenology

Phenomenology is a valuable source of evidence for nursing practice, but it also has some limitations:

- Phenomenology generates large amounts of data that must be carefully managed. Because the reports of experiences may be sensitive, protection of confidentiality is paramount.
- Bias is a potential problem in drawing conclusions and exploring experiences. Bracketing of researcher bias may be difficult to accomplish if the researcher is inexperienced or feels strongly about the subject of interest.

- The interview process in phenomenology requires a high level of skill in eliciting clear and accurate responses from informants.
- Respondents must be able to reflect on their experience and report their responses, and so recall and willingness to share sometimes painful events may be stressful for participants.

In general, phenomenology requires a skilled researcher who is capable of identifying and setting aside his or her bias about an experience. The analysis of the essence of an experience requires reflection and careful interviewing techniques. The outcome can provide a valuable addition to evidence about the way individuals respond to events and the meaning of their lived experiences.

Ethnography

Ethnographic studies focus on the culture of a group of people. The assumption underlying this tradition is that every group of individuals evolves a culture that guides the way members structure their experiences and view the world (Creswell, 2008). This qualitative approach to inquiry gives the researcher an opportunity to conduct studies that attend to the needs and relationships of members of a culture. In ethnography, participant observation is the norm; the researcher is more than an observer. He or she becomes an active participant in the culture under study to more thoroughly understand its experiences and worldview. As such, the aim of the ethnographic researcher is to learn from, rather than study, the members of a culture (Roberts, 2009). This does not mean the researcher attempts to have an effect on the members of the culture. Rooted in anthropology, the ethnographic researcher attempts to understand a culture without changing it.

> **Ethnography:** A study of the features and interactions of a given culture.
> **Participant observation:** Involvement of the researcher as an active participant in the culture under study to more thoroughly understand the culture without changing it.

Questions that Are Addressed with Ethnography

Ethnographic research questions are unique in that they focus exclusively on understanding the culture of a group of individuals (Nicholls, 2009b). Many ethnographic questions focus on large-scale studies (e.g., What is the culture of a Samoan village?). Nursing research usually focuses on smaller, more narrowly focused cultural studies (e.g., What is the culture of a critical care waiting room?).

Methods and Procedures for Ethnographic Study

Ethnographers use extensive fieldwork to learn about the culture under study. It is a time-consuming and labor-intensive type of research. One of the goals of ethnography is to reveal information that is so embedded in a culture that it may not be discussed. In fact, members may not even be aware of the cultural implications of their lived experiences. This level of understanding of a group requires an extended period of participant observation, multiple methods for collecting data, and rigorous data analysis procedures.

Gaining entry into the cultural setting may be one of the greatest challenges in an ethnographic study. There are no strict rules about how to enter a field setting to make observations; the procedures for gathering data will be based on the characteristics of the field setting, its members, and where the researcher intends to situate him- or herself on the continuum from complete participant to participant-observer (Clarke, 2009).

Much as in phenomenology, the concept of researcher as instrument is inherent in ethnography. The study of a culture requires rapport, trust, and, ultimately, intimacy with the members of the culture. The researcher plays a significant role in generating relationships that will result in reflection on the part of members of the culture and a willingness to share thoughts, feelings, and perceptions.

Ethnographers begin with general questions about the nature of reality for a given culture. Three types of information are usually collected for analysis:

- *Cultural behavior:* Collected via extended observation, this information is used to describe what members of a culture do, the ways they interact, and the outcomes that are achieved.
- *Cultural artifacts:* These are objects and materials that the members of the culture make, use, and consider valuable. Information about cultural artifacts is also collected by observing, but historical artifacts may be described by informants.
- *Cultural speech:* As the title implies, cultural speech is gathered verbally through interaction with members of the culture (Roberts, 2009).

It is clear that the ethnographer relies on multiple sources of information and a variety of data collection methods. Although some of these may be preplanned, most are discovered during extended observational periods. Data are collected as detailed field notes, and they may include words as well as drawings. Some ethnographers use audio or video recordings of activity as well. Observers should strive to collect field notes that are detailed and concrete rather than vague and overgeneralized. This supports credibility and reduces bias in reporting. Ethnographers analyze data through rich and detailed descriptions and interpretations of the culture. These interpretations may include descriptions of normative behaviors, reactions and interactions among members, and observable social patterns.

Strengths of Ethnography

Ethnographic studies provide rich information about a culture and insight into its reactions and interactions. The following are some of the strengths of this design:

- These studies provide insight about the way unique groups will react to health and illness and give the nurse information to design effective interventions that will support health.
- Ethnography is a naturalistic inquiry that enables the nurse to draw conclusions about how health and illness are addressed in "real life."
- Many different kinds of cultures can be defined for the purposes of ethnography. It lends itself to groups as small as "children in a third-grade health class" or on a grand scale such as "members of an ethnic subgroup."

Limitations of Ethnography

Ethnography can help nurses understand how cultural groups respond to health and illness, but these studies have some limitations as well:

- These studies are labor-intensive and time-consuming. Achieving the rapport and intimacy necessary for honest sharing of the lived experience may require years

Case in Point: An Ethnography Example

Deitrick et al. (2006) used ethnographic methods as a means to examine problems related to answering patient call lights on one medical-surgical inpatient unit. This methodology was chosen so the authors could get deeper insights into patient and provider perspectives directly at the point of care. The data were collected simultaneously from multiple sources:

- Mapping was used to depict the clinical unit, particularly the nurses' station and room layout.
- Photographs were taken at intervals to capture workflow and status of the call bell console.
- An ethnographer observed for 60 hours over 3 months on all shifts to gain detailed descriptions of workflow and to measure the time it took to answer a call light.
- Interviews were conducted with staff, patients, family members, and one physician.

The data were analyzed using a coding scheme to identify themes that were triangulated to multiple sources. The authors concluded there was a disconnect regarding perceptions of the call bells, the patients who used them, and whose job it was to answer them. Three interrelated components of call bells were identified; all had an impact on the efficiency of communication between unit staff and patients.

1. The most problematic aspect was the actual answering of the call (that is, who answers the light and how long it takes to answer a light). The ethnographer noted that many patient care-givers viewed the lights as an interruption of their work.
2. Transmitting the information to the patient's nurse accurately was sometimes problematic.
3. Follow-through on patient requests was not always consistent or timely.

These authors determined that the patient's perception about staff response to his or her call bell is a key component of patient satisfaction, and the use of an ethnographic study helped the staff identify changes in responses that were needed. The authors updated this study in 2010 and found that staff behaviors regarding call lights could be enhanced with upgraded technology, a relationship-centered leadership style, and a culture of service.

This research is a good example of an ethnographic study with immediate application to practice. This study was used to improve care on a single unit, and its findings could be translated to similar units. As is common with ethnography, multiple data collection methods were employed, and analysis involved triangulation as a basis for ensuring credibility of the findings.

Source: Deitrick, L., Bokovoy, J., Stern, G., & Panik. A. (2006). Dance of the call bells: Using ethnography to evaluate patient satisfaction with quality of care. *Journal of Nursing Care Quality, 21*(4), 316–324; Deitrick, L., Bokovoy, J., & Panik, A. (2010). The "dance" continues: Evaluating differences in call bell use between patients in private rooms and patients in double rooms using ethnography. *Journal of Nursing Care Quality, 25*(4), 279–287.

of involvement on the part of the researcher. Some researchers spend their entire professional lives studying a particular culture.

- The researcher must take extreme care not to overinterpret his or her observations but rather to report them objectively; otherwise, biased, incorrect conclusions may result.
- Members of the culture may react to the observer's presence, inhibiting accurate conclusions about natural behavior. Extended contact enables habituation, or a reverting to natural behaviors, as members of the culture come to disregard the observer's presence.

Habituation: A process that occurs when an observer has extended contact with the subjects of a study. The subjects revert to natural behaviors and come to disregard the observer's presence.

- Observers may become so immersed in the culture that they become involved in a way that changes the cultural behaviors of the members. This is a particular concern in the study of developing groups or groups that have not had contact with outsiders.

Grounded Theory

**Grounded theory: ** Aimed at discovering and developing a theory based on systematically collected data about a phenomenon. The intent is to discover a pattern of reactions, interactions, and relationships among people and their concerns.

Grounded theory is the discovery of theory from systematically obtained data through qualitative means. It does not begin with theory but leads to a theory to explain the phenomenon. The intent of grounded theory is to discover a pattern of reactions, interactions, and relationships among people and their concerns (Moore, 2010). It is a complex type of qualitative research and requires a high level of skill and the capacity to suspend bias related to the topic of interest.

Questions that Are Addressed with Grounded Theory

Grounded theory rarely has a central research question. Instead, the research problem is discovered, as is the process that resolves the problem (Fain, 2009). The purpose is to develop theory, and so the grounded theory study begins with a general area of interest and proceeds to explore how individuals frame the problem, variations that arise as a result, and how people deal with it. Grounded theory provides evidence about the ways people react and interact with each other and with their own health and illness (Hernandez, 2010). The basic elements of grounded theory include answering the following questions: "What is the chief concern of people regarding this area of interest?" "What accounts for the way people deal with this concern or problem?"

Methods and Procedures for Grounded Theory

Grounded theory studies are the least preplanned of any of the qualitative methods. The researcher begins with a general research problem, selects individuals who are most likely to illuminate the initial understanding of the question, and collects data using a variety of methods. Interviewing, observation, and document review may all be used in establishing grounded theory.

The researcher interprets and codes data constantly and at each stage decides what data to collect to continue developing the theory. After initial identification of a purposeful sample, data collection, and analysis, the emerging theory drives subsequent decisions about continuing data collection and analytic processes. Additional sampling may be undertaken based on this preliminary analysis of results. These subsequent samples may have relaxed inclusion criteria to gather data that possess more variability and expose relationships. This use of a theoretical sample is characteristic of this tradition.

The sample size, data collection, and analytic processes are not planned and finite but rather emerge throughout the study. Rather than making the study easier to conduct, this lack of guidelines for implementation calls for a highly skilled and competent researcher to accomplish well.

Strengths of Grounded Theory

Grounded theory is a method for developing the very basis of nursing practice via the proposition of theories for subsequent testing. The following list includes some of the strengths of grounded theory:

- Grounded theory provides the basis for testing theories about reactions and interactions.
- Grounded theory enables the exploration of human action and interaction related to subjects in which very little knowledge is available.
- Grounded theory allows researchers to determine what is rather than suggesting what should be.
- These studies help build models that can be used to assess human reactions to nursing interventions.

Limitations of Grounded Theory

Grounded theory is essential for the development of nursing theory, but it has significant limitations, particularly for a novice researcher:

- Grounded theory is difficult to conduct well and requires a high level of competence on the part of the researcher.
- Theoretical development is a complex process that has many points at which the investigator's bias may interfere with accurate theory development.
- Grounded theory studies are lengthy, time-intensive, and require a great deal of effort and skill on the part of the researcher (Elliott & Jordan, 2010).

Reading Qualitative Research Studies

Qualitative research as evidence for nursing practice is appraised for its trustworthiness, just as quantitative research is evaluated for reliability, validity, and generalizability. However, considerable controversy exists regarding the standards that are used to evaluate qualitative research. Some researchers argue that the same standards that are applied to quantitative research should be used to appraise qualitative studies. It is likely, however, that the nurse reader will become frustrated (and seriously limit the number of qualitative studies included in a review) if this approach is used. Others question whether any predetermined criteria are appropriate to judge these primarily emergent designs. This conclusion is based on the belief that there is no unified qualitative research paradigm, and so there is little impetus to define predetermined criteria with which to evaluate it (Rolfe, 2006).

However, when qualitative research is used in supporting evidence-based practice, it is most common to approach the evaluation with criteria that are specific to qualitative inquiry rather than quantitative study. To effectively determine if the results of a qualitative study apply in a specific patient care situation, the standards for design, implementation, and analysis of qualitative inquiry must be used as a basis for appraisal.

Because qualitative research is not aimed at testing hypotheses about cause and effect, issues of internal validity, measurement reliability, hypothesis testing, and statistical analysis are not of concern. There is no attempt to evaluate effect size, and so power is not of concern. Generalizability is not a goal; qualitative research is either descriptive or interpretive, and so it is not intended to generate conclusions that can be generalized to entire populations. As a result, random sampling is unnecessary and generation of confidence intervals, probability of error, and p values is not of concern.

Instead, the methodological rigor of the sampling strategy is assessed by evaluating how well the researcher used purposeful sampling to select participants who could best inform the question. Appropriate selection criteria should be reported, and methods of recruiting and informing subjects of their rights should be described. Although power is not the primary issue in evaluating sample size, saturation of data should be achieved to indicate that an adequate sample was accessed. The researcher should report both the way saturation was evaluated and how many subjects were required to reach it.

Although internal validity is not a concern, credibility and trustworthiness of the conclusions are. The researcher should report the ways in which credibility and reliability were maintained. A report of how bracketing was accomplished and the use of triangulation, extended contact, and member checking enhance reliability of the conclusions. An audit trail gives the reader an indication that decisions and design processes were systematically recorded and supports the confirmability of the study.

Three tools have been developed to appraise the validity of qualitative research studies. The primary focus of these tools has been to translate qualitative research into evidence for nursing practice, specifically to the development of practice guidelines. Hannes, Lockwood, and Pearson (2010) compared three online appraisal instruments, the Joanna Briggs Institute tool (JBI), the Critical Appraisal Skills Program (CASP), and the Evaluation Tool for Qualitative Studies (ETQS). All three instruments were comprehensive and rigorous in their respective standards. The JBI tool requires completing a series of statements about the research; the CASP and ETQS rely on questions to guide an appraisal. Table 16.4 depicts the type of validity tested by each instrument, and the criteria that make up the evaluation.

Transferability: The ability of qualitative research findings to apply in other settings or situations.

The reader of qualitative research should not broadly generalize the results to his or her population. However, qualitative research is transferable. Transferability refers to the ability of the nurse to transfer the findings to patients who are in similar situations and who have similar characteristics (Tan, Stokes, & Shaw, 2009). Describing the sample carefully enables more confidence in transfer of the findings to other practice settings or patients. The thick description that is characteristic of qualitative research reporting gives the reader sufficient information to be able to judge the applicability of the findings to other settings and people.

Using Qualitative Research Studies as Evidence

The integration of qualitative research findings into nursing practice is a strategy receiving increasing attention (Ryan-Nicholls & Wills, 2009). Qualitative research can help the nurse better understand the nature of the effectiveness of interventions. In other words, what about the intervention was helpful to the patient? What was clear? What was unclear? How did the patient respond to the treatment? Conversely, qualitative research can be invaluable in determining why an intervention did not work. What about the treatment was unacceptable to the patient? What affected his or her life in an adverse way? What caused complexity or confusion or was not sustainable? A treatment may be shown to be effective in a controlled setting, such as that of a randomized controlled trial, but it

Table 16.4

Types of Validity Addressed in the Critical Appraisal Instruments

Types of Validity	Description	Criteria	Appraisal Instruments
Descriptive validity	The degree to which descriptive information such as events, subjects, setting, time, and places are accurately reported.	Impact of investigator Context	Evaluated in JBI, CASP, & ETQS JBI & ETQS
Interpretive validity	The degree to which participants' viewpoints, thoughts, intentions, and experiences are accurately understood and reported by the qualitative researcher.	Believability	Evaluated in JBI & ETQS
Theoretical validity	The degree to which a theory or theoretical explanation informing or developed from a research study fits the data and is, therefore, credible and defensible.	Theoretical framework	Evaluated in JBI & ETQS
Generalizability	The degree to which findings can be extended to other persons, times, or settings than those directly studied.	Value and implications of research	Evaluated in CASP & ETQS
Evaluative validity	The degree to which an evaluative framework or critique is applied to the object of study.	Evaluation/ outcome	Evaluated in JBI & ETQS

Note: JBI = Joanna Briggs Institute; CASP = Critical Appraisal Skills Program; ETQS = Evaluation Tool for Qualitative Studies

Reprinted with permission, Sage Publications, Hannes, K., Lockwood, C., and Pearson, A. (2010). A comparative analysis of three online appraisal instruments' ability to assess validity in qualitative research. *Qualitative Health Research, 20*(12), page 1740.

is not sustainable in a natural setting. Interventions may produce side effects that are not tolerated or that are undesirable. Quality of life may be affected in a way that is not acceptable to the patient or that is difficult to manage on an everyday basis. Qualitative research is helpful in discovering the ways that nursing interventions affect the everyday life experience of an individual, in both positive and negative ways. As such, these studies provide the evidence that is needed to help patients sustain their treatments and get the most benefit from them.

Qualitative research adds a dimension to interventional study that is not obtained through the measurement of variables alone. Much of the human experience—particularly with health and illness—is affected by motivation and perception as much as by therapies. These aspects are some of the qualities most suited to qualitative inquiry.

Schumacher et al. (2005) identified some of the ways in which qualitative research can be linked to interventional analysis. They note that qualitative study can help nurse researchers

- Identify the needs of a target population.
- Design interventions that are most likely to be acceptable to patients.
- Address the process and implementation issues associated with an intervention.
- Improve the understanding of the impact of an intervention in a natural setting.

Where to Look for Information About Qualitative Methods

- Some qualitative research reports do not explicitly report the classification of the research design. It may be up to the reader to infer the specific type of design that was used. The study may simply be described as "qualitative" or "content analysis." The types of research questions that were asked, the informants selected, and the methods used to collect and analyze data may provide hints to the categorization of the study.

- The conversational style of qualitative writing, which is often reported in first person, and the liberal use of quotations from informants make the report an interesting one to evaluate. This is not a weakness, but rather a characteristic of qualitative reports. The insights provided by qualitative research are engaging and can provide the reader with personal insights as well, increasing the value of the reading experience.

- Conversely, the lack of consistent criteria for evaluating these studies and the controversy surrounding the use of standards for evaluating reliability and validity frequently make them more difficult to evaluate. The use of criteria specific to qualitative study reduces frustration and enhances the ability of the reader to have confidence in the findings.

- The sequence of information in a qualitative report may be quite different from that of a quantitative report. This is not a drawback, but an inherent characteristic of these studies. The literature review may be at the beginning or provided during interpretation. The methods and procedures are often clearly described, but they may not be labeled as such. The reader must thoroughly review the entire study before determining that a particular aspect has been omitted.

- Whether labeled as such or not, a qualitative study should outline the sampling procedure, any inclusion criteria, how the data were collected, and an overview of analysis. These may not be standard, but they should be recognizable.

- Information about efforts to establish credibility, trustworthiness, dependability, and confirmability may appear nearly anywhere in the article, but in general:

- Bracketing is described near the beginning of a research study.

- Purposive sampling, inclusion criteria, and saturation will likely be described in the sampling strategy.

- Triangulation, member checking, and peer debriefing are usually described with the data analysis procedure.

- Documentation of an audit trail may appear anywhere in the report, although it is frequently mentioned near the end of the procedures section.

- Understand the reasons for attrition, cessation of treatment, or lack of adherence to a treatment protocol.

These are all ways that the nurse can integrate qualitative research into the evaluation of interventions and the design of evidence-based practices. It is particularly important to recognize the humanistic, holistic nature of nursing practice, and qualitative research is invaluable in adding this facet to the evidence that is the basis for nursing knowledge.

How does one determine whether to use a qualitative research study as sound evidence for practice? Henderson and Rheault (2004) recommend four rules for determining whether to include qualitative research studies in evidence-based practice.

- *The study must satisfy the general assumptions for the development of a practice guideline.* The study must support the topic under study and meet the inclusion criteria, and it must be retrieved from a peer-reviewed journal.

Checklist for Critically Reading a Qualitative Research Study

✔ The central phenomenon, event, experience, or conceptual basis of the study is clearly stated in the research question.

✔ The research tradition that is chosen is linked to the research question and the nature of the information that is sought.

✔ The study participants are chosen using a purposeful method based on established criteria.

✔ Evidence of saturation is provided to justify sample size.

✔ The researcher provides evidence of bracketing of personal preconceptions and biases to mitigate their effects.

✔ The study includes description of methods to enhance trustworthiness. For example:

- Prolonged engagement
- Triangulation
- Member checking

✔ The author mentions the documentation of an audit trail to support dependability.

✔ Sufficient description is provided of the context and informants to determine transferability of the findings to other settings or people.

- *The study must meet the qualitative screening criteria.* The study involves observation of social or human problems in a natural setting, and observations are interpreted by the researcher. The study is conducted in conformance with ethical principles for research.

- *The study exhibits the criteria for trustworthy qualitative evidence.* The study is designed and carried out in a way that supports credibility, transferability, dependability, and confirmability.

- *The strength of recommendations is based on the quality of the evidence.* Qualitative studies are graded according to their strength, and subsequent recommendations are consistent with the level of the evidence.

Qualitative studies are valuable additions to the evidence that supports nursing practice. These studies are subjected to the same appraisal process as quantitative studies, albeit one that is based on characteristics that are specific to qualitative research.

Creating Qualitative Evidence

The creation of qualitative research requires patience, persistence, and a passion for the subject under study. Although qualitative studies are emergent designs, they are no less rigorous because of it. The lack of preconceived design elements does not mean the study is unfocused. It does mean, however, that extended contact is required, meaning the nurse researcher must devote substantial time and effort to carrying out the study effectively. Analysis can be a complex process, and the

gray matter

The following key steps help create a strong qualitative study:

- Determine a broad research question.
- Select a research tradition.
- Determine criteria for selection of participants that can best inform the question.
- Locate a source of participants and invite participation through informed consent.
- Design general data collection procedures.
- Transcribe data in their entirety and add field notes.
- Analyze data as they are collected.
- Develop a codebook of themes and code units of meaning.
- Check the conclusions with participants.
- Report the themes with supporting examples from informants.

software that supports statistical analysis has no use in qualitative coding. Software is available for qualitative analysis (and will be discussed in more detail in the chapter that follows), but it does not analyze the data for the researcher; these processes still require substantial time and skill.

With that said, qualitative research enables the nurse researcher to identify rich, interesting, and insightful information about the experiences of patients. Health and illness are humanistic considerations, and qualitative inquiry is well suited to help the nurse understand them.

The approach to a qualitative study is not preconceived, but it is systematic. The following key steps can help the nurse researcher create a qualitative study that meets standards for trustworthiness and makes a strong addition to the evidence for nursing practice:

- *Determine a broad research question.* The central question is broad and general, but it should focus on a single phenomenon or concept. Sub-questions can add detail to the central question, but these may evolve and change as the study emerges. Sub-questions often provide guidance for the development of specific interview guides, procedures, or sampling considerations.
- *Select a broad research tradition.* A specific classification of qualitative research is selected next based on a match between the research question and the characteristics of the tradition. This classification generally does not change and evolve with the study.
- *Determine criteria for selection of participants that can best inform the question.* These criteria may be characteristics (for example, gender or age), experiences (for example, recent diagnosis of breast cancer), or membership in a particular group (for example, drug addicts). Criteria may also be developed that support the methodology and conduct of the study. For example, in a study of teen attitudes toward drug rehabilitation, the willingness of the teen to talk with an adult about his or her experience is paramount.
- *Locate a source of informants and invite participation through informed consent.* The researcher must find an accessible group of informants that meets the criteria. An invitation is issued, and participants are thoroughly informed about the nature of the study, associated risks, and benefits.
- *Design general data collection procedures.* If interviews are the data collection process, then a general interview guide should be designed. No more than a handful of questions should be determined. The interviewer should, in essence, "go where the informant goes." Having too many questions may lead the informant to the researcher's preconceived conclusions. Open-ended questions that enable exploratory interviewing are best for beginning interviews. Focus group and observation guides should similarly be broad and enable exploration on the part of the researcher. Table 16.5 depicts an example of an interview guide for a qualitative study.
- *Transcribe data in their entirety and add field notes.* Data of any type—interviews, focus group recordings, or observational records—should be transcribed in their

Table 16.5

Example of a Qualitative Interview Guide

Purpose of the Study

Determine the aspects of nursing work that are considered "caring."

Interview guide

What are the kinds of things that you do for patients that you consider "caring," that is, not tasks or procedures?

What are the characteristics of patients that you have found mean they will require more caring?

What are the characteristics of patients that you have found mean they will not require as much caring?

What are the kinds of responses you get from patients when you have exhibited caring behaviors?

What are the kinds of responses you find in yourself when you have exhibited caring behaviors?

entirety. This requires a high level of organization and data management because a large volume of data will be generated. The researcher should add field notes to the transcribed data as soon as possible after the experience to capture contextual issues and nonverbal responses while they are still fresh in his or her mind.

- *Analyze data as they are collected.* Analytic memos, or short notes indicating the potential for emerging themes or exemplar quotations, should be added to the data as they are collected and reviewed. As new data are collected, they should be compared to the existing data to determine the themes that are supported or not supported by the emerging information. This constant comparison also enables the identification of saturation when it occurs.

- *Develop a codebook of themes and code units of meaning.* The development of a codebook supports reliable coding of units of meaning—whether they are words, phrases, or observations—into overall themes that make up the key components of the conclusions. Because qualitative analysis is a complex undertaking, a detailed description of analytic processes appears in the next chapter.

- *Check the conclusions with participants.* Member checking is a method to ensure that the interpretations of the researcher are valid and that their assumptions and preconceived ideas have not affected the analysis of the data.

- *Report the themes with supporting exemplars from informants.* Reporting themes and using the words of informants to support these conclusions is the accepted way to report qualitative studies. The use of direct quotations enables the reader to judge the credibility of the interpretations of the researcher.

Qualitative studies are invaluable tools for adding to the body of evidence that supports nursing practice. A systematic approach and attention to methodological rigor are not unique to quantitative research, but serve the qualitative researcher equally well.

Qualitative research provides a rich dimension to the design of nursing interventions and gives voice to patients' needs, preferences, and concerns.

Summary of Key Concepts

- The impetus behind qualitative research is to identify the meaning of a phenomenon, event, or experience for an individual.
- Evidence of clinical experiences and patient preferences is often discovered through qualitative research.
- Qualitative research is grounded in the belief that reality can never be completely known because it is constructed by each individual, and so discovery of meaning must be collected using methods that do not rely on measurement.
- Qualitative research is important in nursing because it is a humanistic, holistic profession and knowledge of human reactions to illness and health is important.
- Qualitative research may be descriptive or interpretive; it does not result in conclusions about cause and effect but about meaning.
- The point of qualitative research is to elicit a description of a social experience that is so detailed and insightful that one who has not experienced it can understand and appreciate its nuances.
- Qualitative research involves an emergent design in which details of the research unfold as the study progresses. It is based on rigorous principles focused on credibility, trustworthiness, and confirmability.
- Data are gathered directly from informants via interview or focus groups, through researcher observation, or through review of documents and artifacts.
- Interventions that require lifestyle adjustment, attitude changes, or behavioral alterations are particularly suitable for qualitative study.
- Questions that reflect exploration of feelings, perceptions, attitudes, motivation, quality of life, and other subjective experiences are well addressed with qualitative inquiry. The central question is written in such a way that it accommodates the emerging design that is characteristic of qualitative inquiry.
- Qualitative research designs are sometimes referred to as "traditions." Each tradition is intended to answer a particular kind of question.
- Qualitative samples are most commonly selected using a purposeful sampling method.
- Saturation, or the point at which no new information is being generated, is the standard for sample size in a qualitative study.
- Data are analyzed using a constant-comparison method in which data are reviewed and analyzed continuously as new data are compared to existing data to confirm or disprove emerging themes.
- Qualitative researchers are concerned with credibility and trustworthiness, which are supported by the following methods:
  - Bracketing of the researcher's biases to "set them aside"

CRITICAL APPRAISAL EXERCISE

Retrieve the following full text article from the Cumulative Index to Nursing and Allied Health Literature or similar search database:

 Nolbris, M., Abrahamsson, J., Hellstrom, A., Olofsson, L., & Enskar, K. (2010). The experience of therapeutic support groups by siblings of children with cancer. *Pediatric Nursing, 36*(6), 298–304.

 Review the article, focusing on the sections that report the question, tradition, methods, and procedures. Consider the following appraisal questions in your critical review of this research article:

1. What is the purpose of this research?
2. What is the methodology selected to answer the question? What makes this tradition appropriate for this purpose?
3. Describe the data collection methodology. Why was it appropriate for this study? Why might focus group interviews yield better information than individual interviews for this subject?
4. How was the sample selected? What are the strengths and weaknesses of this sampling strategy? Is evidence provided that saturation was achieved?
5. What analytic process was used? Is the report of the process complete enough to judge the validity of the conclusions? Did the tables help illuminate the analytic process?
6. How did the authors support their report of the final themes? Are sufficient data provided to confirm the author's conclusions?
7. What evidence is provided for the trustworthiness of the methods and procedures applied in the study?

- Triangulation of conclusions based on at least three separate data sources
- Prolonged engagement with participants
- Member checking to ensure that conclusions accurately represent the thoughts of informants
- An audit trail to enable confirmability of the study

■ Qualitative research is not intended to be generalized but transferred to similar situations and individuals.

■ The traditions that are commonly used as evidence for nursing practice are case study, content analysis, phenomenology, ethnography, and grounded theory. It is common, though, that no specific tradition is identified in qualitative study.

For a full suite of assignments and additional learning activities, use the access code located in the front of your book to visit this exclusive website: http://go.jblearning.com/houser. If you do not have an access code, you can obtain one at the site.

References

Anthony, S., & Jack, S. (2009). Qualitative case study methodology in nursing research: An integrative review. *Journal of Advanced Nursing, 65*(6), 1171–1181.

Clarke, D. (2009). Using qualitative observational methods in rehabilitation research: Part two. *International Journal of Therapy and Rehabilitation, 16*(8), 413–419.

Connelly, L. (2010). What is phenomenology? *MedSurg Nursing, 19*(2), 127–128.

Creswell, J. (2008). *Research design: Qualitative, quantitative, and mixed methods approaches* (3rd ed.). Thousand Oaks, CA: Sage.

Elliott, N., & Jordan, J. (2010). Practical strategies to avoid the pitfalls in grounded theory research. *Nurse Researcher, 17*(4), 29–40.

Fain, J. (2009). *Reading, understanding, and applying nursing research* (3rd ed.). Philadelphia: F. A. Davis.

Farmer, T., Robinson, K., Elliott, S., & Eyles, J. (2006). Developing and implementing a triangulation protocol for qualitative health research. *Qualitative Health Research, 16*(3), 377–394.

Flood, A. (2010). Understanding phenomenology. *Nurse Researcher, 17*(2), 7–15.

Guba, E. (1981). Criteria for assessing the trustworthiness of naturalistic inquiries. *Educational Communication and Technology Journal, 29*(2), 75–92.

Guba, E., & Lincoln, Y. (1989). *Fourth generation evaluation.* Newbury Park, CA: Sage.

Hannes, K., Lockwood, C., & Pearson. A. (2010) A comparative analysis of three online appraisal instruments' ability to assess validity in qualitative research. *Qualitative Health Research, 20*(12), 1736–1743.

Hansen-Ketchum, P., & Myrick, F. (2008). Photo methods for qualitative research in nursing: An ontological and epistemological perspective. *Nursing Philosophy, 9*, 205–213.

Henderson, R., & Rheault, W. Q. (2004). Appraising and incorporating qualitative research into evidence-based practice. *Journal of Physical Therapy Education, 17*(3), 35–40.

Hernandez, C. (2010). Getting grounded: Using Glaserian grounded theory to conduct nursing research. *Canadian Journal of Nursing Research, 42*(1), 150–163.

Holloway, I., & Wheeler, S. (2009). *Qualitative research in nursing and healthcare.* San Francisco: Wiley Blackwell.

Moore, J. (2010). Classic grounded theory: A framework for contemporary application. *Nurse Researcher, 17*(4), 41–48.

Munhall, P. (2010). *Nursing research: A qualitative perspective* (5th ed.). Sudbury, MA: Jones & Bartlett.

Nicholls, D. (2009a). Qualitative research: Part one—philosophies. *International Journal of Therapy and Rehabilitation, 16*(10), 526–533.

Nicholls, D. (2009b). Qualitative research: Part two—methodologies. *International Journal of Therapy and Rehabilitation, 16*(11), 586–592.

Nicholls, D. (2009c). Qualitative research: Part three—methods. *International Journal of Therapy and Rehabilitation, 16*(12), 638–647.

Payne, S., Field, D., Rolls, L., Hawker, S., & Kerr, C. (2007). Case study research methods in end of life care: Reflections on three studies. *Journal of Advanced Nursing, 58*(3), 236–245.

Pearson, A. (2011). Evidence-based healthcare and qualitative research. *Journal of Research in Nursing, 15*(6), 489–493.

Roberts, T. (2009). Understanding ethnography. *British Journal of Midwifery, 17*(5), 291–294.

Rolfe, G. (2006). Validity, trustworthiness and rigour: Quality and the idea of qualitative research. *Journal of Advanced Nursing, 53*(3), 204–210.

Ryan-Nicholls, D., & Will, C. (2009). Rigour in qualitative research: Mechanisms for control. *Nurse Researcher, 16*(3), 70–85.

Schumacher, K., Koresawa, S., West, C., Dodd, M., Paul, S., Tripathy, D., et al. (2005). Qualitative research contribution to a randomized control trial. *Research in Nursing and Health, 28*, 268–280.

Shin, K., Kim, M., & Chung, S. (2010). Methods and strategies utilized in published qualitative research. *Qualitative Health Research, 19*(6), 850–858.

Streubert, H., & Carpenter, D. (2010). *Qualitative research in nursing: Advancing the humanistic imperative.* Philadelphia, PA: Lippincott Williams & Wilkins.

Tan, T., Stokes, T., & Shaw, E. (2009). Use of qualitative research as evidence in the clinical guideline program of the National Institute for Health and Clinical Excellence. *International Journal of Evidence Based Healthcare, 7*, 169–172.

chapter *17*

Analyzing and Reporting Qualitative Results

CHAPTER OBJECTIVES

The study of this chapter will help the learner to

- Describe the challenges facing the qualitative research analyst.
- Discuss the importance of developing an organized approach to managing qualitative data.
- Summarize the steps that make up an overall approach to qualitative analysis.
- Explain the purpose and process of constant comparison as an analytic technique.
- Express the process for coding data and development of a codebook.
- Review methods for establishing the trustworthiness of qualitative conclusions.
- Describe how qualitative data are reported and presented for publication.

KEY TERMS

Codebook	Immersion/crystallization analysis	Recontextualizing
Codes		Schematic
Cohen's kappa	Inquiry audit	Template analysis
Constant comparison	Margin notes	Themes
Decision trail	Parsimonious	Theoretical sampling
Dictionary	Peer debriefing	Unit of analysis
Editing analysis		

Introduction to Qualitative Analysis

The qualitative analyst is much like the leader of a jazz band. Although he or she may start out with a general idea of what is to be accomplished, the leader follows each musician as he or she improvises on a basic theme. It is not so much that the music is composed as that

❝ *Scenes from the Field* ❞

Hope is a necessity for humans; it is the belief in a future that holds the promise of a better life. When one gives up hope, however, reversing this state is necessary to restore or preserve one's well-being. Through the transformation of despair into hope, people can transcend their current difficulties and improve quality of life.

For most societies, becoming a parent is one source of hope. Children enable people to envision a future filled with potential. Parenting is a social norm; most couples hope to become parents and may lose hope when they are persistently unable to do so. For these couples, achieving parenthood is fraught with frustration and anguish. Many infertile couples feel compelled to pursue all possible avenues to achieve their goal of parenthood. The development of reproductive technology has provided infertile women with the hope of a pregnancy, but it is not always successful. At present, the pregnancy rate of in vitro fertilization is between 20 percent and 50 percent; this obviously means that half or more of women who try it will fail. Those women who fail typically describe the experience as an emotional roller coaster.

The factors that influence the success of in vitro fertilization are complex. Although scientists can identify predictors of success, women who are in the midst of treatment often do not know whether the treatment should be terminated or not. Su and Chen (2006) set out to explore this phenomenon and sought to understand the lived experiences of infertile women who decided to terminate treatment after in vitro fertilization.

The informants in this study were infertile women who experienced in vitro fertilization failure and decided to terminate treatment. Twenty-four women eventually participated in the study via telephone interviews. The subjects were asked to talk about their experiences of discontinuing treatment and were encouraged to express their feelings, perceptions, and thinking. The interview began by addressing several general questions regarding health conditions, the process of discontinuing treatment, the reasons for it, their feelings, their life at the present, and reflections on the previous year. The data were analyzed using a constant-comparison approach, coded into categories of meaning, and summarized as themes.

The essence of the experience of infertile women who discontinued treatment after in vitro fertilization failure is embedded into the main theme of transforming hope. They felt the impossibility of accomplishing the goal of pregnancy and transformed their hope of doing so. These women found realistic ways of perceiving an entirely new set of possibilities; this was described as changing from "hope of pregnancy" to "acceptance of reality." This process included three stages.

- *Accepting the reality of infertility:* This stage involved being convinced that they had done everything possible to become pregnant, accepting that pregnancy was not going to happen, and reducing the pressure to become a biological mother.
- *Acknowledging the restrictions of treatment, including the limitations on technology:* This stage involved accepting that technology and in vitro fertilization could not solve all reproductive problems.

- *Re-identifying their future, reestablishing the importance of personal well-being, and reject-ing obsessiveness about infertility:* This last stage enabled the couples to begin making new plans for the future and considering alternatives, such as other methods of building a family or considering a life without children.

The stress experienced by these women began to decrease as they accepted the fact of infer-tility. Support from family and spouse helped ease the process of transforming hope. Although the authors note that these lived experiences were as complex, rich, and varied as the women involved, they theorize that a common understanding can help the nurse provide therapeutic support to help infertile women begin the process of identifying meaningful ways of life without biological motherhood.

Source: Su, T., & Chen, Y. (2006). Transforming hope: The lived experience of infertile women who terminated treatment after in vitro fertilization failure. *Journal of Nursing Research, 14*(1), 46–54.

it emerges. It is similar with qualitative analysis: The final product of the analysis emerges as the researcher follows the informants as they illuminate the question more and more.

Jazz compositions are often longer than traditional compositions. Chasing interpreta-tions of themes takes time and effort, and so a lot of music is generated. Qualitative study also results in volumes of information. The thick description and prolonged engagement that produce credible, trustworthy results also generate a tremendous number of words. The sheer volume of data that is characteristic of qualitative inquiry produces challenges in both data management and drawing sensible conclusions. This is why qualitative data analysis is sometimes referred to as data reduction. The goal is to reduce the data to meaningful units that can be described, interpreted, and reported in an understandable way. The analysis of numerical data is relatively straightforward: The correct statistical test is selected and applied, and results are interpreted. Qualitative analysis, on the other hand, requires a different skill set—even a different state of mind—and the methods that are used are not standard, even within a single tradition.

The intent of data analysis, regardless of the approach, is to organize, provide struc-ture to, and draw out meaning from the data collected. The challenges the qualitative researcher faces in the analysis process are threefold.

First, qualitative analysis offers no single standard for the analytic process. On its surface, this might seem to simplify the analytic process, but in execution, the lack of clearly defined steps often results in false starts, backtracking, and an enormous use of time. Even within traditions, recommendations may vary widely as to the appropriate steps to take. Some authors argue that having steps at all means that preconceptions exist, and the avoidance of a systematic process enables more creative and insightful conclusions. Regardless, the qualitative researcher is faced with a perplexing array of possibilities for approaching the analytic process.

The work of the qualitative researcher is further complicated by a second charac-teristic of qualitative inquiry: the enormous quantity of data that must be thoughtfully reviewed, reflected on, and summarized. The researcher must make sense of pages and pages of narratives, observations, and transcripts to carry out the analysis process. Managing the data, tracking the source and type of each piece, triangulating findings, and locating supportive quotations are all complex due to the sheer quantity of material that must be reviewed.

The last challenge centers on the need to reduce or put the data in a manageable format for dissemination of the findings. For the richness of the data to be maintained, the researcher must be thorough and use the words of informants. Yet reporting and publication restrictions necessitate a concise report. Balancing rich description with focus is a challenge for every qualitative researcher.

Qualitative analysis is difficult and complex to do well, mainly because of these challenges. It requires patience, persistence, and a good deal of self-discipline. On the other hand, well-drawn qualitative conclusions enhance the evidence for a holistic view of nursing practice. Ensuring the findings are trustworthy is the job of the qualitative analyst.

Characteristics of Qualitative Analysis

Qualitative analysis may not be standard, but it does have some steps that are common to all approaches. All qualitative researchers must

- Prepare the data for analysis.
- Conduct the analysis by developing an in-depth understanding of the data.
- Represent the data in reduced form.
- Make an interpretation of the larger meaning of the data (Creswell, 2008).

These may look like sequential steps, but the delineation between them is often virtually undetectable because the researcher moves back and forth among data collection, analysis, and drawing conclusions. Unlike quantitative studies, when analysis is postponed until all data have been collected, qualitative analysis begins nearly as soon as data collection has begun. As data are collected, they are reviewed and re-reviewed, and analytic memos are written. New data that are collected are compared to existing data to confirm or refute conclusions and to decide when saturation has been reached. This constant comparison of new findings to existing results is a characteristic of qualitative analysis. This is sometimes called "intensive engagement with the data" to reflect the depth with which the analyst considers the meaning of the information collected (Endacott, 2005). This approach enables the researcher to pursue interesting ideas or to sort through confusing input while informants are still available and data collection is still in progress. The researcher is free to follow where the informants lead instead of taking a predetermined path leading to a single conclusion.

Constant comparison: A method of analysis that involves a review of data as they are gathered and comparison of new data to what has been interpreted to support or reject earlier conclusions.

Using a constant-comparison process allows the analysis to guide subsequent data collection by amending or adding interview questions or changing observational methods. The researcher may even recruit new informants or change selection criteria to illuminate issues raised during analysis. This process, which is essential for the grounded theory approach, is called **theoretical sampling**. Theoretical sampling involves the selection of a second sample of informants with less-restrictive criteria to encourage diverse viewpoints to emerge (Endacott, 2005). These secondary sites or cases are purposely selected to compare with the sample that has already been studied. Although this may sound like a sampling issue, theoretical sampling is, in effect, a source of triangulation, one of the means by which qualitative analysts confirm their results.

> **Theoretical sampling:** Selecting additional members for the sample, often based on loosened inclusion criteria, to ensure divergent opinions are heard; a requirement for grounded theory development.

It is characteristic of qualitative inquiry that data collection and analysis—even sampling and measurement strategies—may be indistinguishable during the research process. Data collection and data analysis are symbiotic in that it is essential to go back and forth between the two to identify the point at which results are trustworthy and data saturation occurs.

Styles of Qualitative Analysis

Qualitative researchers use multiple methods of analysis. Some influential qualitative methodologists provide general direction for the approach to overall analysis. There are generally three major analytic styles that fall on a continuum between structure and lack of structure:

- Template analysis style
- Editing analysis style
- Immersion/crystallization style

At one extreme is a style that provides a highly systematic and standardized approach to analysis, while at the other end is a more intuitive, subjective, and interpretive style. Neither style is right or wrong for a particular study; the selection of an approach and process depends on the research question, the study design, and the sensibilities of the researcher (Grbich, 2007).

The most highly structured style is the **template analysis** style, which includes developing a template that provides an analysis guide for sorting narrative data. This style is appropriate when there is a clear theoretical perspective for a study because it requires using codes that are devised *a priori*. These codes may be developed theoretically or they may be based on established literature. The advantage of template analysis is its simplicity; it is a focused and structured approach to analysis. It is more time efficient than the other analytic styles, and it is a common approach in content analysis. The use of codebooks, interrater reliability assessment, and data definitions are characteristic of this approach, and it is widely used in nursing research.

> **Template analysis:** A style of analysis that includes developing a template to sort narrative data.
> **Editing analysis:** A style of analysis geared toward interpretation of text to find meaningful segments.
> **Immersion/crystallization analysis:** A style of analysis that uses total immersion in and reflection on the text, usually in personal case reports.

The **editing analysis** style is geared toward interpretation of text to find meaningful segments. Researchers using grounded theory, phenomenology, or hermeneutic traditions employ this approach (Boeije, 2009). This approach is common in nursing research and is used to discover the meaning of experiences, relationships, and interactions.

The least structured approach is the **immersion/crystallization analysis** style. This approach is appropriate when a researcher desires total immersion in and reflection on text, usually in case research and ethnography. Stemming from the notion that the researcher is the true analytic tool, this analytic approach requires that the investigator be immersed in the data and rely heavily on intuition to arrive at conclusions (Endacott, 2005). Insights do not necessarily come after the data have been collected, but might occur during data collection as well, and so it also employs constant comparison. As the analysis is being carried out and the conclusions are "crystallizing," the researcher can better decide how to proceed in further data gathering. It is not a style that appears in the nursing research literature as much as the other two styles, but it is still useful in healthcare research. Its primary downside is that it is time-consuming and requires the ability to constantly hold one's biases at bay.

These styles may be employed in a variety of ways. Each has specific characteristics that apply to a particular type of research question and analysis procedure, but there is no single process that all qualitative analysts will use. The primary considerations that follow are generally applicable to qualitative analysis, but a single study may include all of these steps or only a few of them.

The Qualitative Analysis Process

Qualitative data analysis is an active and interactive process. The researcher looks at the data deliberately and in-depth to become thoroughly familiar with them. It is not unusual for the researcher to read and reread the data multiple times in the search for meaning. It is an investigative process that requires integrating multiple ways of knowing to get at the heart of the data. Fitting the data together is similar to putting the pieces of a puzzle together. The researcher becomes embedded in the data, like a detective at a crime scene, looking for clues that might lead to an intuitive conclusion about the data. As the researcher progresses through the process of conjecture and verification, corrections and modifications are made leading to the development of patterns and themes.

Qualitative analysis may be viewed as a cognitive process that evolves through phases:

- *Comprehending* occurs early in the process of analysis. The researcher is attempting to make sense of the data that have been collected and get a sense of the overall tone.
- *Synthesizing* leads the researcher to sift through the data using inductive reasoning to put the pieces of the puzzle together.
  - *Theorizing* brings the researcher to the point of what he or she believes has truly emerged from the data. A continuation of this phase occurs until the best and most parsimonious explanation has evolved. A parsimonious explanation is one that is the most focused while providing the best overview of the final conclusions.
  - Recontextualizing is a process that involves applying the theory that was derived from the analysis to different settings or groups. This further exploration can result in the increased generalizability of the theory that was developed. The premise is that if a theory can be recontextualized, it can be generalized (Streubert & Carpenter, 2010).

Parsimonious: Reduced to the fewest components; a parsimonious model is the simplest one that will demonstrate a concept.

Recontextualizing: A qualitative data analysis and cognitive process undertaken by the researcher to search for meaning that may lead to a theory.

Even though these phases are presented in a linear fashion, they are rarely accomplished in that way. These phases are intertwined with one another and may occur sequentially or simultaneously.

Management and Organization of Data

To make sense of the narrative data, a method of managing and organizing the information must be established early in the research process. The analysis process then can proceed in a logical—if not linear—fashion. Organization and preparation of the data include transcription of audiotapes, optical scanning of artifacts and other documents, the addition of field notes to transcripts, and other preparatory activities.

It is imperative to effectively organize data so they can be thoroughly evaluated and their confidentiality can be preserved. Data that are not well controlled are at risk for misuse and unauthorized access, and so data management is a primary consideration for the qualitative researcher.

Each piece of information that has been collected should be cataloged in some fashion. The source, date of collection, and type of data should be noted with each piece of data. Because qualitative inquiry often generates multiple types of data, the same study may include electronic transcripts, hard copy notes, photography, and audio recordings. Finding a method to track and maintain all the data presents a challenge. The data management process should be determined early in the study so data can be cataloged, reviewed, and analyzed as they are collected.

Review the Data for Initial Impressions

Once the data have been sorted and cataloged, the researcher begins with the first of many reviews of the data. The data will be read and reread entirely many times, but the first read-through is helpful for establishing an overall impression of the data. It is recommended that the first reading be just that—a reading and not a review or note-taking session. This initial review without preconceptions can give the researcher a sense of the data and time to reflect on their meaning. The researcher should finish the initial review with general ideas about the tone of the data, impressions of the depth and clarity with which informants presented their ideas, and thoughts about where the research should go next.

Identify a Classification System

After a general impression has been gained from the read-through of the data, the initial phase of analysis is to develop a classification system. The researcher may establish a schematic to increase the manageability of the data. A schematic is an outline of the categories of meaning that may be expected from the data. In the template approach, this schematic is predetermined. In other approaches, it will likely be a work in progress. Table 17.1 depicts a schematic for a qualitative analysis.

The development of a schematic as a classification system requires either substantial theoretical and literature background or an intense examination of the data. The development of general categories requires that the analyst elicit

Schematic: A system of organizing data into preset categories to allow for examination and further analysis.

Table 17.1	

An Example of a Coding Schematic

Theme	Codes
To care for me: Was that too much to ask?	▪ Feeling abandoned and alone ▪ Stripped of dignity ▪ Lack of interest in a woman as a unique person ▪ Lack of support and reassurance ▪ Labor and delivery staff failed to communicate with the patients
To communicate with me: Why was this rejected?	▪ Labor and delivery staff spoke as if the woman in labor was not present ▪ Clinicians failed to communicate among themselves
To provide safe care: You betrayed my trust and I felt powerless.	▪ Perceived unsafe care ▪ Feared for their own safety and that of their unborn infant ▪ Felt powerless
The end justifies the means: At whose expense? At what price?	▪ Traumatic deliveries were glossed over ▪ Successful outcome of the baby took center stage ▪ The mother was made to feel guilty ▪ No one wanted to listen to the mother

Adapted from Beck, C. (2004). Birth trauma: In the eye of the beholder. *Nursing Research, 53,* 28–35.

gray matter

The following list gives the five steps for developing themes and codes in qualitative research:
- Reducing the raw data
- Identifying themes with sub-samples
- Comparing themes across subsamples
- Creating a coding scheme
- Determining reliability of the coding scheme

Codes: Labels, descriptions, or definitions assigned to data to allow them to be categorized and analyzed in qualitative research.

underlying consistencies, concepts, and clusters of concepts. This intense examination raises many questions: What is this informant saying? What is going on? What does it mean? What is this similar to? What is it different from?

Develop Codes and a Codebook

At the conclusion of an intense examination of the data and the development of an overall schematic, the researcher develops more-specific categories of meaning based on what has been gathered. These categories of meaning are called **codes**. Codes enable a more-detailed analysis process for the data. Codes are "chunks of meaning," or pieces of data that demonstrate patterns or themes in the responses.

Qualitative data have an infinite range of possible codes; however, there are general categories of meaning that the qualitative analyst can reflect on to guide the code-development process:

▪ *Setting and context codes:* Identify elements of the setting or the environment that form patterns.

▪ *Perspective codes:* Relate the unique viewpoint of informants in relation to the topic under study.

- *Subjects' ways of thinking:* Describe how informants frame thoughts and actions about the topic.
- *Process codes:* Outline the ways things get accomplished.
- *Activity codes:* Describe things informants or others do.
- *Strategy codes:* Relate the strategies informants use to accomplish goals.
- *Relationship codes:* Identify the ways individuals interact and relate to one another.
- *Social structure codes:* Describe the ways individuals interact in groups.

This list is not all-encompassing, but it does give the analyst a lens with which to examine potential patterns and themes in the data. **Table 17.2** depicts an example of a **codebook** for a qualitative study of nursing workload related to

Codebook: A guide for the qualitative analysis that outlines individual codes with definitions, criteria for inclusion, and examples.

Table 17.2

A Codebook Excerpt

Staffing Research: Characteristics of Patients/Families that Affect Workload

Transcript Number: _____

Coder: _____

Date Coded: _____

Theme (Record Phrases Here)	Key Words	Definition: Code Phrases into This Category If They Reflect ...
1.0 Presence	<ul><li>Reassuring</li><li>Listening</li><li>Spending time</li><li>Touching</li><li>Comforting</li><li>Offering companionship</li></ul>	A need for a physical presence and actual proximity of the nurse, unrelated to procedures or tasks
2.0 Integrating Information	<ul><li>Teaching</li><li>Acting as liaison</li><li>Translating</li><li>Interpreting</li><li>Explaining</li><li>Knowing what to expect</li><li>Educating</li></ul>	An action related to improving knowledge and understanding about either the disease process or how to achieve health
3.0 Family Dynamics	<ul><li>Dysfunctional</li><li>Poor or limited relationships</li><li>Alcohol or drug abuse</li><li>Mental health issues</li><li>Physical abuse</li></ul>	Family dynamics related to interpersonal interactions and physical or mental problems that affect these interactions
4.0 Physical Condition of the Patient	<ul><li>New or worsening diagnosis</li><li>Comorbidity/complexity</li><li>Pain/anxiety/nausea</li><li>Life-threatening conditions</li><li>Chronic conditions</li></ul>	Interpersonal, emotional, and physical conditions that are a result of a presenting or emerging medical problem

caring behaviors. This codebook was developed for the categorization of phrases from transcripts of focus groups of nurses responding to questions about patient and family characteristics that increase workload on a patient care unit of a hospital.

Code the Data

When a codebook has been developed, the analyst then codes the existing data by classifying each unit of analysis into a coded category. This requires that the researcher determine the unit of analysis within each piece of data. The **unit of analysis** is the most basic segment, or element, of the raw data or information that can be assessed in a meaningful way regarding the phenomenon (Munhall, 2010). A unit of analysis might be a word, a phrase, an artifact, a photograph, or a descriptive paragraph. The researcher then reviews the data again, this time identifying and labeling each unit of analysis. **Table 17.3** depicts an excerpt from a transcript in which the units of analysis—in this case, phrases—have been identified and labeled. This transcript is from the study of nursing workload described earlier.

> **Unit of analysis:** The smallest element of the data that can be analyzed; in qualitative analysis, this is usually a document, phrase, or word.

The units of analysis are then reread and categorized into the appropriate code. An example of the coded excerpt appears in **Table 17.4**. Each phrase number is assigned to a specific code in the codebook. By reviewing the transcript, the reader can see how phrases are coded into categories of meaning in the codebook in Table 17.4. Each identified unit of analysis is assigned to a specific code or placed in a "leftover" category. These leftovers may emerge as individual codes, or they may be isolated responses that are later ignored. Qualitative analysis is rarely about single instances of occurrences, but rather looks for overall patterns and themes in the data. Codes that have a large number of entries are likely the basis for emerging themes; codes with very few entries should be scrutinized to assess whether they represent common meanings or isolated anecdotes. During the coding process, it is not unusual to require modifications to the code labels, definitions, or key words as new data are constantly compared and analyzed in relation to existing data.

Evaluate the Codes to Identify Overall Themes

The coding process is used both to generate descriptions and to begin interpretation of themes and patterns in the data. Using codes for description involves a detailed rendering of information that was common to the people, places, or events in the research setting. Descriptive codes are particularly useful in case studies and ethnography. Identifying themes requires in-depth scrutiny of the codes and the data. As a result of this scrutiny, themes emerge that encompass several codes. A qualitative study may have a substantial number of codes—it is not uncommon for researchers to report anywhere from 10 to 60 codes for an analysis—but only a small number of themes should emerge. Often an analyst will arrive at one central theme, with a small number of subthemes, based on several dozen codes.

> **Themes:** Implicit, recurring, and unifying ideas derived from the raw data in qualitative research.

Themes are, as the word implies, overall patterns that are recognized in the data through categorization and analysis of individual units of meaning. These

Table 17.3

An Excerpt from a Transcript

Houser: What are the things that patients depend on you for that you would call caring, not doing?

Nurse: I think one of the big things I see over and over again, is that patients and their families rely on us as nurses to be some sort of interpreter between physicians and them. [1] I mean a lot of us have stood in the room when the doctor leaves and the patient will look at you and say, "Huh? What did he say?" And you know you kind of bring it down to their level [2] and whatnot. So I think one of the things they truly rely on us for other than starting the IV or giving the shot is to be that intermediary, the communicator [3].

Houser: Nurses have called that translating. Or being an interpreter. Is that what you are meaning?

Nurse: Yeah. Yeah. In a sense.

Nurse: Sometimes just sitting in the room.

Nurse: Uh-huh. If you sit, usually if you sit and listen [4] as opposed to standing and listening that makes a different impression. The time might not be any different. But because you sat the impression is that you listen. Whereas if you stand sometimes the impression doesn't always come across as that.

Houser: What several of you have said is it requires a presence. This is not something that can be done over the intercom or can be delegated. Are there other things?

Nurse: Specifically taking care of their pain [5] in a timely fashion. Even if you are real busy pain is real important to people, hunger [6] is only about the next thing.

Nurse: That is really hard to do when you are busy.

Houser: Can you describe some characteristics of patients that seem to need more in the way of caring?

Nurse: Well I think the patient that grieves in general and it doesn't necessarily have to be about death. It could be about their own death. Maybe they have just gotten the death sentence. Maybe they lost a body part. [7] I myself and most of the ICU nurses will sit down with that patient [8] and try to draw them out. As far as helping their grief. And often you see their vital signs just get better. Just by that talking with them and showing them there is another human being that wants to share that pain and grief [9] with them.

Nurse: The families, a lot of families, they have fear too. And some families bring in baggage. [10] They haven't seen grandma or mom in six months and they got a call from the neighbor, who said, "You know I think you better go see her." And then realize maybe they should have seen mom sooner than six months ago. And so they are dealing with the guilt [11].

themes should be common threads that appear frequently in the analysis, and they should be fairly self-evident by the end of the laborious analysis process. Themes are not single anecdotes, but rather recurring meanings that appear woven throughout all the data that are collected. It is through identification of these overall themes that qualitative analysis makes the greatest contribution to evidence for nursing practice. Table 17.5 demonstrates how a group of codes may be organized into themes. These themes were the result of a

Table 17.4

A Coded Excerpt

Staffing Research: Characteristics of Patients/Families that Affect Workload

Transcript Number: _____

Coder: _____

Date Coded: _____

Theme (Record Phrases Here)	Key Words	Definition: Code Phrases into This Category If They Reflect ...
1.0 Presence: Phrases Coded: 4 8	▪ Reassuring ▪ Listening ▪ Spending time ▪ Touching ▪ Comforting ▪ Offering companionship	A need for a physical presence and actual proximity of the nurse, unrelated to procedures or tasks
2.0 Integrating Information: Phrases Coded: 1 2 3 9	▪ Teaching ▪ Acting as liaison ▪ Translating ▪ Interpreting ▪ Explaining ▪ Knowing what to expect ▪ Educating	An action related to improving knowledge and understanding about either the disease process or how to achieve health
3.0 Family Dynamics: Phrases Coded: 10 11	▪ Dysfunctional ▪ Poor or limited relationships ▪ Alcohol or drug abuse ▪ Mental health issues ▪ Physical abuse	Family dynamics related to interpersonal interactions and physical or mental problems that affect these interactions
4.0 Physical Condition of the Patient: Phrases Coded: 5 6 7	▪ New or worsening diagnosis ▪ Comorbidity/complexity ▪ Pain/anxiety/nausea ▪ Life-threatening conditions ▪ Chronic conditions	Interpersonal, emotional, and physical conditions that are a result of a presenting or emerging medical problem

study investigating environmental elements that affect workload on a patient care unit. Conclusions based on recurrent themes are specific enough to be applicable to practice yet common enough to transfer to other settings and people.

The processes described so far in this chapter belong to one type of general approach to content analysis. The analytic process may be modified, adapted, or otherwise changed when a specific tradition has been employed as a research method. Each of the traditions has some unique characteristics that must be considered in the analysis procedures. Table 17.6 compares the unique characteristics of the three traditions that require substantial adaptation of the analysis procedure: ethnography, phenomenology, and grounded theory.

Table 17.5

The Organization of Codes into Themes

Overall Theme	Individual Codes
Leadership	■ Behaviors support staff work ■ Nurses serve as role models ■ Attitudes that inspire others ■ Skills reduce demand on staff
Expertise of staff	■ Skill and knowledge in clinical specialty ■ Demonstrates good judgment ■ Committed to quality patient care ■ Patient-centered attitude
Staff stability	■ Vacant positions ■ Rate of turnover ■ Acquisition of new employees
Resources	■ Access to financial, material resources for patient care ■ Equipment in working order ■ Enough people, time to get job done

Table 17.6

Comparison of Qualitative Analysis Traditions

Tradition	Common Approaches to Analysis	Research Outcome
Phenomenology	■ Reflection on the data ■ Explication of themes ■ Discernment of patterns that form the essence of the experience	Full, rich description of the essence of a human experience
Grounded theory	■ *Open coding:* Generating categories of meaning ■ *Axial coding:* Positioning each category in a theoretical model that demonstrates the overall relationships ■ *Selective coding:* Creating a story from the interconnectedness of the categories ■ *Theoretical sampling:* Adding informants as the theory unfolds to illuminate/refute specific conclusions	Integrated, parsimonious theory with concepts that have analytic imagery
Ethnography	■ Triangulation of multiple sources of information ■ Use of thick description	Well-described cultural scene

Software for Qualitative Analysis

Overall, the analysis process involves coding segments of data into meaningful categories and developing overarching themes. This coding process is based on units of analysis that may be entire paragraphs of information, and so it can become laborious from a practical standpoint. The process is often done manually, but it may be computerized.

Computer software for qualitative analysis is less common than quantitative analysis software. Often, researchers have no choice but to resort to manual data management, and do so nearly 65 percent of the time according to one study (Shin, Kim, & Chung, 2010). This can be a cumbersome, time-consuming undertaking. Yet many qualitative researchers prefer manual analysis because they believe it enables them to remain immersed in the data (Holloway & Wheeler, 2009).

Use of computerized qualitative analysis continues to raise issues for qualitative researchers. There is sometimes a perception that a process that is viewed as being holistic, interpretive, and humanistic becomes mechanical when it is automated. Others are concerned that the efficiencies of automation will tempt qualitative researchers to use larger samples and sacrifice depth for breadth (McLafferty & Farley, 2006).

Others believe that using a computer for qualitative analysis makes the process quicker and easier without losing touch with the data. Computerized analysis may make coding less burdensome so the researcher is free to find creative ways of looking at the data. The computer offers assistance in processing, storing, retrieving, cataloging, and sorting through data, and so leaves the researcher with more time for review and reflection on meaning. These programs allow the transcribed data to be entered and coded based on a dictionary of codes that has been developed by the researcher in an identical manner to one that is manually based (Banner & Albarran, 2009).

Computerized qualitative analysis provides some very real advantages. Multiple copies of data can be made, so the researcher is not tied to a paper system. Blocks of data can be sorted and moved to other codes, and the ease of assigning data to codes may enable the researcher to try several coding schema before settling on a single one. The capacity to categorize the same data into multiple codes may also help the researcher see patterns that would not emerge when all units of analysis had one exclusive code assigned. During this process, automation allows the researcher to maintain the original data in its intact form so that it can be reread in its context rather than as individual units of analysis. Most computerized systems also have a search capacity to identify specific words or phrases that support the coding process. Using these systems can enhance reliability by applying standard rules that are built into the programs (Banner & Albarran, 2009). Table 17.7 lists some of the most common qualitative software analysis products with related features.

The use of qualitative analysis software is likely to remain the subject of controversy for some time due to the interpretive nature of qualitative inquiry. It is clear, however, that qualitative analysis software can help the researcher be more efficient in data analysis, while leaving the interpretation to the researcher. Software can sort, document, and copy, but it cannot yet perform reflection, analysis, and interpretation. Those elements

| Table 17.7 |

Software for Computerized Qualitative Analysis

	Media Accepted	Capability	Analytic Memos	Marked Codes
Atlas.ti	Text, graphics, audio, web, and video	Strings of words, categories, phrases, and individual words	Can be attached to documents, codes, and other memos; can be written for all object types	Displayed in right margin
HyperResearch	Text, graphics, audio, and video	Text searches for phrases or words	One memo per coded segment	Displayed in left margin
MAXqda	Text	Text searches for phrases, words, or memos	Can be attached to text passages or codes	Displayed in either margin
The Ethnograph	Text	Simple string searches	Can be attached to a project, data file, or line of text	Displayed within the text
QSR NVivo9	Text	String, category, and text searches	Memos can be linked to documents, passages, or codes	Displayed in either margin

require the human component: a skilled researcher who can reduce a large amount of data to a manageable, meaningful form.

Reliability and Validity: The Qualitative Version

Quantitative researchers are concerned with reliability and validity because the generalization of cause-and-effect findings to populations requires a level of evidence based on statistical significance. Applying quantitative standards for reliability and validity to qualitative studies results in frustration for researchers and a lack of studies used as evidence for nurses (Tan, Stokes, & Shaw, 2009). The qualitative researcher should not focus on quantitatively defined indicators of reliability and validity, but that does not mean that rigorous standards are not appropriate for evaluating findings. Guba and Lincoln (1989) established standards for qualitative research that call for an overriding concern based on trustworthiness or the "true value" of the data that have been collected. They recommend four criteria for researchers to use to establish trustworthiness of qualitative conclusions:

- Credibility
- Dependability
- Confirmability
- Transferability

These criteria are familiar to the reader because they also apply to design decisions. This discussion will focus primarily on how trustworthiness is ensured during the analysis process. The qualitative researcher has several means of ensuring each criterion is evident in a final study.

Credibility of Results

Qualitative researchers are concerned with the credibility of the study results. How confident is the researcher that interpretations represent truth? Several techniques can be used to ensure that credibility exists.

First, a prolonged engagement with the participants involved in the study supports in-depth analysis. Time is also needed to test interpretations and conclusions for misinformation or misinterpretation. Documenting the amount of time spent in these activities should be part of the analytic report.

Second, triangulation is useful for the enhancement of the credibility of conclusions. Triangulation occurs when the analyst uses a variety of sources and data to ensure confirmation of interpretations and conclusions (Farmer, Robinson, Elliott, & Eyles, 2006). Four types of triangulation were described in the previous chapter, and any or all of them may be applied during analysis. The researcher should report both the type and source of triangulated results.

Peer debriefing: An external check on credibility of results in which objective peers with expertise in the qualitative method of analysis review and explore various aspects of the data.

Third, performing external checks on the analysis is another method widely used to establish credibility. One check is peer debriefing. Peer debriefing involves reviewing methods, procedures, and conclusions with objective peers who have expertise in the study methods or content. In addition to peer debriefing, study participants may be requested to validate the preliminary findings and interpretations. Member checking is not necessarily used by all qualitative researchers, but it is a solid method for checking the credibility of any themes or categories that the researcher may have identified from data analysis.

Dependability of the Analysis

If the data are not dependable, then credibility suffers. The dependability of the analysis is supported when multiple raters are able to achieve similar results when applying the codebook to identified units of analysis. Interrater reliability or intercoder reliability is used by qualitative researchers to ensure dependability of the data analysis. Measures of interrater reliability quantify the amount of agreement between two coders using the same codebook to categorize units of analysis. Two methods are available to assess quali-

Cohen's kappa: A measure of interrater or intercoder reliability between two raters or coders. The test yields the percentage of agreement and the probability of error.

tative agreements. Simple agreement is the percentage of time that both coders agreed on a categorization; Cohen's kappa takes this analysis one step further and generates a p value for the probability that random error was responsible for the agreement. Agreement of at least 80 percent is considered acceptable for qualitative coding, with an associated p value less than 5 percent that the agreement was due to chance (Fain, 2008).

Considerable controversy surrounds the use of this quantitative method to assess agreement among qualitative raters—or even the need to do so. However, qualitative studies that have subjected an interpretive process to an objective evaluation are often more widely accepted as evidence by the scientific community. In addition, documenting reliability of a codebook can help later if replication of the study is attempted. A codebook that has been substantiated through measures of interrater reliability can confidently be considered a reliable set of codes for future use as a template (Endacott, 2005).

A less quantitative technique that lends itself to assessing dependability is the inquiry audit. This process includes an examination of the data and any relevant documents by an outside reviewer. It involves asking one or more external research peers to view the data separately and conduct two independent inquiries during which interpretations and conclusions can be compared (Creswell, 2008).

> **Inquiry audit:** A review of data and relevant documents, procedures, and results by an external reviewer.

Confirmability of the Analysis

Confirmability is characteristic of findings that reach congruence between two or more independent researchers. An inquiry audit can also support confirmability as well as dependability of analysis. More common is the use of an audit trail. This is a carefully documented record that enables an independent auditor to follow how the researcher arrived at his or her conclusions. To further enhance auditability, the researcher should maintain a decision trail. This trail details the researcher's decision rules for data categorization and the inferences made in the analysis (Fain, 2008).

> **Decision trail:** A detailed description of the researcher's decision rules for data categorization and inferences made in the analysis.

Transferability of the Findings

When findings from the data can be transferred to other settings or groups, transferability has been reached. For this to occur, it is imperative for the researcher to provide enough information to allow judgments about the context of the data. This information is referred to as thick description and refers to the richness and complete description of the research setting, transactions, and processes observed during the inquiry (Holloway & Wheeler, 2009). This level of detail enables the reader to draw conclusions about whether the findings can be transferred to a particular set of patients in a specific setting.

Reporting Qualitative Results

The qualitative report, which is often written in first person, is interesting and engaging to read because of the informal writing style and the liberal use of quotations from informants. The report must still provide information about the topic under study, however, and most qualitative researchers reflect on the "fittingness" of the results as well. Fittingness refers to how well the study findings fit the data and are explicitly grounded in the lived experience that is being studied. It is also a reflection of the typical and atypical elements of that experience. References to theoretical and literature support are often used here. Direct quotes from the informants are used to support this aspect of confirmability (Fain, 2008).

A common way to illustrate and support themes is with what has been described as "low inference descriptors," that is, examples of participants' verbatim accounts. Integrating quotations from informants within the written report of the findings demonstrates that they are grounded in the data. Liberal use of quotations assures the reader that the author has not "cherry picked" quotations that support his or her point of view, and so supports credibility. When reporting supporting quotations, the researcher should find quotes that represent the feelings and thoughts of all the informants best—not dramatic or particularly vivid examples that represent a single person's viewpoint (Creswell, 2008).

Conclusions in qualitative reports are generally reported in a similar fashion:

- The sample and setting are described using codes and thick description.
- The main themes and subthemes are identified.
- Each theme and subtheme is described in detail.
- Quotations from informants are used to illustrate the themes and subthemes.
- The overall implications for nursing practice are described.

This last section is where questions are raised as to how these results can apply to practice, education, and research. What is the impact of the results on nursing theory? What additional aspects of the topic under study need exploration? Did the results generate a hypothesis for subsequent testing with a quantitative design? The qualitative report ends with suggestions for future research and should provide sufficient detail that transferability can be assessed.

Reading the Qualitative Analysis Section of a Report

Qualitative analysis is often more difficult and time-consuming to accomplish than quantitative analysis, but its report is usually engaging and interesting to read, and it provides intuitive insights into human behavior. There are few consistent standards to apply to the qualitative analysis process; there are no rules about which test to use or how to interpret an outcome. The result is that the qualitative evaluation process is also more difficult and time-consuming because it is harder to determine if the author "got it right."

However, it is helpful if the research process is transparent so the reader can trace the decision processes the author used to carry out the study (Boeije, 2009). The reader of qualitative research is dependent on the reporting of the study author to make the link between data and results. There are no numerical tables to review or statistical values to scrutinize, but neither is there an objective way to determine if interpretations of the data were conducted correctly. The qualitative reader, then, is challenged to determine if a study meets his or her standards for credibility, dependability, confirmability, and transferability. Critique is also difficult because the researcher can only provide excerpts of data, and so the reader must take on faith that the researcher used good judgment when coding the narrative data, eliciting themes, and integrating the findings into a meaningful whole.

The author should explicitly identify the approach to data analysis and the specific methods used to accomplish it. The reader should be able to see a clear link among the research question, the tradition used to answer it, the data collection procedures, and the analytic process. These should all be consistent and appropriate for the purposes of the study.

Where to Look

Where to look for qualitative results:

- The report of qualitative data analysis is typically the third or fourth major heading in a qualitative research report. It is usually easily identified and called "Results" or "Findings."
- The authors should describe the process that was used to analyze the data in the methods section, although it is occasionally reported simultaneously with the results. A reasonably informed reader should be able to reconstruct the analysis process given the author's description.
- If the authors used a predetermined schematic, it should be provided in a table or figure. The process for arriving at the schematic should be described in the methods section.
- The report should begin with the major themes that were identified and subsequently describe the more detailed codes that make up each theme. Some authors use a figure or a table to report

all of the themes and associated codes; charts, graphs, and numerical summaries are not typically found in this type of study.

- Each theme should be accompanied with a definition of the theme and a list of associated codes. Direct quotes from informants should be presented to illustrate and support each of the reported themes. Examples of verbatim responses are expected for each code, and liberal use of quotes is one method of ensuring trustworthiness.
- The methods used to establish the credibility, dependability, and confirmability of the results should be described thoroughly, although it is not standard as to where in the report they are described. Approaches to establishing reliability can be described in methods, results, or even in the conclusions. It is common for multiple methods to be used to ensure overall trustworthiness of each element.

When critiquing qualitative analysis, the main objective is to determine if the researcher used the appropriate process to validate inferences and conclusions. Evidence of bracketing serves to minimize the effects of preconceptions and biases. Purposive sampling and inclusion criteria—and perhaps the presence of theoretical sampling—support the credibility of the study. Documentation of triangulation and measures of interrater reliability are helpful in supporting dependability of the conclusions. Peer debriefing, member checking, and an inquiry audit also increase confidence in the results, and an

Checklist for Evaluating Qualitative Results

✔ The report of the sample provides enough details to judge the adequacy and characteristics of the sample.
✔ The procedure used to analyze the data is described in sufficient detail.
✔ The reader can trace the decision processes that the author used to carry out the study (for example, an audit trail or decision trail is present).
✔ The analytic method used is appropriate for the qualitative tradition/design.
✔ The authors report methods for ensuring the following:
  - Credibility of the findings
  - Dependability of the methods
  - Confirmability of the conclusions
✔ Sufficient descriptions and reports of the sample are provided to ensure appropriate transferability.

audit trail supports confirmability. The authors should explicitly describe these procedures and any others used to support confidence in the results.

Using Qualitative Analysis in Nursing Practice

The results of qualitative studies can be applied in nursing practice in a variety of ways. These data provide rich insights into the experiences of patients, their families, and other caregivers. Using the results of qualitative studies in practice requires that the nurse be able to critically appraise the transferability of the data. The nurse must review the descriptions of the setting and the informants to determine if they are similar enough to be confidently applied to another group of individuals.

The nurse reader should focus on the themes that were elicited to determine application to evidence-based practice. These themes often provide guidance in the development of counseling procedures, teaching plans, discharge preparation, and other means of helping patients manage their health. Results of case research can help nurses understand how individuals may experience threats to their health, uncommon conditions, or exacerbations of their disease states. Phenomenology is helpful in understanding the ways that patients experience events and situations so the nurse can design better supports for them. Ethnography can assist the nurse in designing culturally sensitive care. Grounded theory, in particular, helps the user understand and analyze situations, to predict changes in them, and to influence outcomes.

Regardless of the type of study, the results should be scrutinized for trustworthiness to determine which findings can be used in evidence-based practice. In Chapter 16, a systematic process for evaluating the appropriateness of a qualitative study was advanced. The analysis should be subjected to the same critical review. In other words, the study should satisfy general assumptions about the evidence and withstand scrutiny of the methodological quality of the analysis.

Henderson and Rheault (2004) support the use of qualitative results in evidence-based practice, but they also recommend that a stricter standard be applied to qualitative analyses that will be used as evidence for practice. They recommend using the following criteria for determining whether to include qualitative results in a practice guideline:

- The methods of analysis should be described in detail.
- Two or more researchers should independently judge the data.
- Triangulation of data sources, methods, or investigators should be evident.
- A code–recode procedure should be described.
- Peer examination or external audit should be reported.

In addition, they recommend rating qualitative results similarly to those of experiments using levels and grades. Based on the four elements of trustworthiness (credibility, dependability, confirmability, and transferability), levels of qualitative evidence can be linked to recommendations. **Table 17.8** demonstrates the levels of qualitative evidence and associated strength of recommendations that are suggested to integrate qualitative analyses into practice.

Table 17.8

Decision Rules for Incorporating Qualitative Research into Evidence-Based Nursing Practice

Decision	Considerations
The study satisfies general requirements for inclusion in an integrative review.	▪ The journal in which the research appears is peer-reviewed. ▪ The problem addressed in the study meets the inclusion criteria for the review.
The study meets screening criteria as a qualitative study.	▪ The study involves observation of social problems in a naturalistic setting. ▪ The researchers interpret data to arrive at conclusions. ▪ Observations are linked to theory. ▪ Researchers adhere to ethical guidelines for research involving human subjects.
The level of evidence is evaluated based on standards for trustworthiness.	▪ Level 1: Meets the standards for credibility, transferability, dependability, and confirmability. ▪ Level 2: Meets three of the four standards. ▪ Level 3: Meets two of the four standards. ▪ Level 4: Meets one of the four standards. ▪ Level 5: Does not meet any of the standards.
The strength of recommendations is based on the quality of the evidence.	▪ Grade A: Recommended; supported by one or more Level 1 studies. ▪ Grade B: Optional; supported by at least one Level 2 study. ▪ Grade C: Optional; supported by multiple Level 3 or 4 studies.

Source: Adapted from Henderson, R., & Rheault, W. (2004). Appraising and incorporating qualitative research in evidence-based research. *Journal of Physical Therapy Education, 18*(3), 35–41.

Creating Qualitative Analyses

There are few rules for qualitative analyses; however, some general guidelines can help the novice researcher conduct a trustworthy analysis that results in meaningful themes.

- *Establish the goal of the analysis.* The design of the study will provide guidance as to the overall goal of the analysis. The goal of analysis may be to determine content, find meaning, describe a culture, or develop a theory. Beginning the analytic process with a general goal provides the analyst with direction and structure as the analysis proceeds.
- *Organize the data.* There will almost certainly be an enormous amount of data to manage, so developing an organizational system early in the process helps keep the process manageable. Determine a way to identify each piece of data by source, timing, and type as it is collected, and store it in a secure location.
- *Begin analysis early.* Data should be evaluated and analyzed as they are collected. This constant-comparison method enables the researcher to make changes in the data collection plan while informants are still available.

- *Read individual pieces of data in their entirety for tone.* The first read of a data source should be purely to get a sense of the tone of the overall response, not for analysis.
- *Reread each piece of data for meaning.* Subsequent readings begin to reveal meaning. As the data are read, analytic memos should be written in the margins of transcripts, and relevant quotations and examples should be identified. At this stage, the analyst will begin identifying units of analysis such as words, phrases, or entire documents for later analytic coding.
- *Develop codes.* Potential categories for codes were introduced earlier in this chapter. During this phase of analysis, units of meaning are categorized into codes.

There is an infinite number of ways to code data, but Creswell (2008) provides some structural guidance to the process. His approach includes the following steps:

Margin notes: Reflective notes manually inserted into qualitative transcripts that describe ideas about meaning that occur to the analyst during reading.

1. Select a document from the data.
2. Reread the document to get a sense of the whole. Ask questions, such as "What is this about?" The concern at this point is not substance, but underlying meaning. Write thoughts in the margins. These margin notes should describe the ideas about meaning that come to mind during reading.

 CRITICAL APPRAISAL **EXERCISE**

Retrieve the following full text article from the Cumulative Index to Nursing and Allied Health Literature or similar search database:

Waters, A. (2008). An ethnography of a children's renal unit: Experiences of children and young people with long-term renal illness. *Journal of Clinical Nursing, 17,* 3103–3114.

Review the article, focusing on the sections that report the analytic procedures and results. Consider the following appraisal questions in your critical review of this research article:

1. What is the specific tradition used for this research study? What characteristics of the study are specific to this tradition?
2. What was the sample for this study? How were the subjects selected for recruitment?
3. Describe the data collection strategies. Were these appropriate for the study objectives? How were these strategies related to the specific tradition/design that was applied?
4. What type of coding was applied to the analysis? Was the coding scheme emergent or predetermined?
5. Describe how the results were reported. What were unique ways in which these results were depicted?
6. What was appropriate about the reporting format? How could it have been strengthened?
7. Were the conclusions linked to the results, or did they go beyond what the data could support?

3. Make a list of all the ideas that have been written in the margins. Cluster together the ideas that have similarities. Form these topics into columns such as "major topics," "unique topics," or "leftovers."

4. Take the list and revisit the data. Make note of the segments of the data that represent each of these categories. Evaluate this preliminary organizing schematic to see if the codes capture most of the data segments. Review multiple pieces of data to determine if the code categories are sufficient or if additional categories emerge.

5. Find the most descriptive label for each topic and turn it into a category. Write a definition for it and identify representative words in informants' language.

6. Group topics that are redundant, overlapping, that reflect similar concepts. Look for ways to reduce the total list of categories.

7. Label the final categories of meaning and develop a codebook that outlines each code, its definition, and any criteria for placing data into the category. The result of this process leads to the development of a **dictionary** to guide the further analysis of the remaining data.

> **Dictionary:** Specified definitions of codes included in the qualitative analysis codebook.

Once all data have been coded, the analyst scrutinizes the data for overall themes. These are identified and reported, with supporting quotations from informants. Qualitative analysis is complete when no new codes or themes emerge from data analysis.

Summary of Key Concepts

- The sheer volume of data that is characteristic of qualitative inquiry produces challenges for both managing data and drawing sensible conclusions.
- The goal is to reduce the data to meaningful units that can be described, interpreted, and reported in an understandable way.
- Qualitative analysis is challenging because no standard rules exist for interpreting the data that are generated, and concise conclusions must be drawn while retaining the rich description that is a qualitative characteristic.
- Although not standard, some steps apply to most qualitative analysis, including
  - Prepare the data for analysis.
  - Conduct the analysis by developing an in-depth understanding of the data.
  - Represent the data in reduced form.
  - Make an interpretation of the larger meaning of the data.
- As data are collected, they are reviewed and re-reviewed, and analytic memos are written. This process is described as constant comparison. Using a constant-comparison process allows the analysis to guide subsequent data collection by amending or adding interview questions or changing observational methods.
- The three general styles of qualitative analysis are the template analysis style, the editing analysis style, and the immersion/crystallization style.

- To make sense of the narrative data, a method of managing and organizing the information must be established early in the research process.
- After a general impression has been gained from the read through of the data, the initial phase of analysis is to develop a classification system.
- With the conclusion of an intense examination of the data and the development of an overall classification schematic, the researcher develops more specific categories of meaning called codes.
- Units of analysis, such as a phrase, word, or document, are categorized into specific codes that reflect overall meaning.
- The coding process is used both to generate descriptions and to begin interpretation of themes and patterns in the data.
- The most common qualitative analysis procedure is simple content analysis. The method may be adapted to the specific tradition, such as ethnography, phenomenology, or grounded theory.
- The use of automated systems for coding is the subject of controversy, but it is becoming more common. Computerized systems for coding can enhance reliability of the data, although researchers must be careful not to substitute breadth for depth of analysis.
- Standards have been established to determine the trustworthiness of qualitative data analysis. These standards include credibility, dependability, confirmability, and transferability.
- Qualitative results are reported as themes, supported by their descriptive codes and verbatim reports from informants. Quotes should be used that represent patterns, not individual anecdotes.

For a full suite of assignments and additional learning activities, use the access code located in the front of your book to visit this exclusive website: http://go.jblearning .com/houser. If you do not have an access code, you can obtain one at the site.

References

Banner, D., & Albarran, J. (2009). Computer assisted qualitative data analysis software: A review. *Canadian Journal of Cardiovascular Nursing, 19*(3), 24–27.

Boeije, H. (2009). *Analysis in qualitative research.* Thousand Oaks, CA: Sage.

Creswell, J. (2008). *Research design: Qualitative, quantitative, and mixed methods approaches* (3rd ed.). Thousand Oaks, CA: Sage.

Endacott, R. (2005). Clinical research 4: Qualitative data collection and analysis. *Intensive and Critical Care Nursing, 21,* 123–127.

Fain, J. (2009). *Reading, understanding, and applying nursing research* (3rd ed.). Philadelphia: F. A. Davis.

Farmer, T., Robinson, K., Elliott, S., & Eyles, J. (2006). Developing and implementing a triangulation protocol for qualitative health research. *Qualitative Health Research, 16*(3), 377–394.

Grbich, C. (2007). *Qualitative data analysis: An introduction.* Thousand Oaks, CA: Sage.

Guba, E., & Lincoln, Y. (1989). *Fourth generation evaluation.* Newbury Park, CA: Sage.

Henderson, R., & Rheault, W. Q. (2004). Appraising and incorporating qualitative research into evidence-based practice. *Journal of Physical Therapy Education, 17*(3), 35–40.

Holloway, I., & Wheeler, S. (2009). *Qualitative research in nursing and healthcare.* San Francisco: Wiley Blackwell.

McLafferty, E., & Farley, A. (2006). Analysing qualitative research data using computer software. *Nursing Times, 102*(24), 34–36.

Munhall, P. (2010). *Nursing research: A qualitative perspective* (5th ed.). Sudbury, MA: Jones & Bartlett.

Shin, K., Kim, M., & Chung, S. (2010). Methods and strategies utilized in published qualitative research. *Qualitative Health Research, 19*(6), 850–858.

Streubert, H., & Carpenter, D. (2010). *Qualitative research in nursing: Advancing the humanistic imperative.* Philadelphia: Lippincott Williams & Wilkins.

Tan, T., Stokes, T., & Shaw, E. (2009). Use of qualitative research as evidence in the clinical guideline program of the National Institute for Health and Clinical Excellence. *International Journal of Evidence Based Healthcare, 7,* 169–172.

part VII

Research Translation

chapter *18*

Communicating
Research Findings

CHAPTER OBJECTIVES

The study of this chapter will help the learner to

- Discuss the usual sequence of peer review that results in publication.
- Determine the appropriate target audience for a research study.
- Prepare an abstract for submission to a conference or journal editor.
- Develop a compelling poster presentation.
- Prepare and deliver a podium presentation.
- Describe the submission steps for manuscript publication.

KEY TERMS

Abstract	Podium presentation	Poster presentation

Introduction

Imagine there was a treatment that could solve a patient's biggest health problem, and the nurse had no way to find out about it. Or that there was a proven method for improving nursing satisfaction, but it had been kept a secret from all but a few people. There may have been a discovery to help people change their health behaviors for the better, but it is locked away in a file cabinet. The truth is, it is possible that any of these scenarios could be true. Thousands of research studies are conducted each year that are never communicated to an audience larger than a single organization, classroom, or workplace. The body of knowledge available as evidence for nursing practice would immediately expand dramatically if all research study results were communicated to the right audiences.

❝❝ *Voices from the Field* ❞❞

I did a research project for my master's degree that was a mixed method, focusing on the way that conflict between nurses and physicians is related to quality outcomes. I was fortunate that I won the outstanding graduate research award that year, and one of my professors encouraged me to publish my research. She sent me an announcement that was a "Call for Abstracts" for an international research conference, and I decided to submit. I was hopeful I could do a poster presentation, so I was a little stunned when they notified me I would be doing a podium presentation.

I was really excited about presenting, because the attendees were going to be nurses from around the world, and I was interested in meeting them and listening to their research. It was focused on evidence-based practice, so I thought we would have a good deal in common. I talked with nurses from Taiwan, Africa, Europe—the only way you could tell they were from somewhere else was the language, because we are all the same. Nursing is really about heart and caring and how you can help people get healthy. That part is universal.

They send you guidelines to give you an idea how to prepare. I had 15 minutes for my presentation, so I knew I had to revise my graduate research presentation to get it down to that time. I rehearsed it out loud, then I did some revision, then I timed myself several times. I rewrote it and rewrote it, always asking myself—am I getting my point across? I shared it with some friends and my husband and I asked them for suggestions. What was clear? Was anything confusing? What kind of questions did they think of? Then when I got to Montreal, there were rehearsing rooms, so I practiced it again several times. I printed my slides with the talking points. I felt pretty comfortable with the content, but I thought, just in case I get nervous, I will have something I can look at.

It was such an honoring experience to be with so many nurses, from all over the world. Some of the speakers had interpreters. The nurse would speak in English, then the interpreter would interpret questions, and the nurse would answer in English. I thought, that would be so harrowing, to have to present in another language. I thought how committed they must be, to go through learning the English language, just to share your research.

I actually did not find it scary because I had rehearsed so much, and the more I listened to the other presenters, the more I thought—they don't have anything on me. I knew my research topic inside and out; I knew a lot about this topic. I just pretended that I was a professional presenter.

It was really gratifying; there were so many people interested in the topic, and they were excited by the research. There were quite a few questions, not like they were questioning my techniques, more like comments; they were excited about the findings. It was fun to be able to respond to questions, to know you were the expert. I was able to share my research with a lot of different people. It was great.

It was a terrific opportunity. I think when you do a project like mine, the way it becomes more valuable is to share it with other people. That is when it becomes something of real value.

Yvonne Shell, MS, RN

Part of the purpose of research—applied or otherwise—is to make a contribution to the body of empirical knowledge that is the foundation of a profession. There are many ways to communicate research so that it can be incorporated into practice. Local, regional, and national conferences often solicit both poster and podium presentations, and journals are always receptive to solid research studies on relevant clinical topics. Contrary to what many clinicians may think, journals are often anxious to publish works by staff-level practitioners because those closest to clinical processes are often in the best position to determine how to improve them.

Inexperienced researchers may feel their work is not sophisticated or important enough for publication or presentation. In reality, good work is good work, no matter who conducts it. The process of getting a research study reviewed is a systematic one that can be used by any researcher, seasoned or novice. A common approach for a new researcher is to begin by submitting research for peer review as a poster in a regional or national conference. He or she then submits research for podium presentations and, finally, publication in a peer-reviewed journal. Regardless of the venue chosen for peer review, the basic steps are the same.

Finding the Right Audience

The first step in communicating the findings of a research study is to select the right audience for the work. The target audience should be carefully considered before writing the abstract or preparing the manuscript. The best venue is one that has a clearly defined focus that fits with the goal of the research. Some research studies have a clear audience—a study on reducing infections would obviously be appropriate for conferences and journals that focus on infection control—but others are not so clear. Some journals publish lists of priorities or solicitations for articles on their web pages or in the journal itself. Conferences generally identify an overall theme and include a list of conference objectives or goal statements that cover the types of information that are of interest. The more closely the study topic is matched with a topic of interest for the journal or conference, the more likely the submission will be successful.

The best audience is one that can put research results into practice. Many clinical conferences or periodicals will provide access to the clinicians who are in the best position to apply research results.

Preparation of an Abstract

Conferences have very specific requirements for submissions, including spacing, margins, and method of submission. The form for submission generally requires an abstract of the work, which conference organizers use to make decisions about acceptance for a poster or podium presentation. An abstract is a summary of the most important aspects of the research. An abstract also appears in the beginning of a publication and as a summary in searchable databases, so it should be constructed carefully.

Abstract: A summary of the most important aspects of the research that is used to apply for presentation; it also appears in the beginning of a publication and as a summary in searchable databases.

The researcher should pay particular attention to limits on the number of words and to the deadlines. Personnel who screen submissions for reviewers often discard abstracts that violate fundamental instructions, so an abstract may not even reach reviewers if it is too long or in the wrong format. Submissions after the deadline are generally not reviewed at all, so abstracts absolutely must reach the conference organizers prior to the deadline.

The abstract of the research study is the only description that most conference reviewers will see, and it may be the first description that a journal editor sees, so it should be clear, compelling, and concise. The abstract should report the most important elements of the research in a way that generates interest and even excitement about the project. Think of the abstract as an advertisement for the research, focusing on the strongest points and most interesting findings.

The abstract submission guidelines will include a limit for the number of words or even characters. Some limit the abstract to as little as 100 words; others allow up to 500 words. Exceeding the word length generally results in being screened out, so this is a critical consideration. It helps to put each required element as a heading in bold font so that the reviewer can find the various sections easily and determine that all are present without having to read the abstract multiple times. Many times no specific guidelines are provided. In this case, use the generally accepted standards for what is included in an abstract; they appear in **Table 18.1**.

The most successful authors write the abstract, and then edit it multiple times until the word length is achieved. Focus on the results and implications for practice. The abstract should provide the most important information that communicates the study's strengths and usefulness.

The peer review process can take from 2 weeks to several months. When an abstract is accepted, the work of preparing the presentation begins.

The Compelling Poster Presentation

Poster presentation: A research report presented as a visual display, so it can be read and viewed by large groups of professionals in an informal setting.

A **poster presentation** at a conference is a research report presented as a visual display so it can be read and viewed by large groups of professionals in an informal setting. The author stands near the poster at specified times to discuss the details of the research and answer questions. A poster presentation gives the author an opportunity to interact with participants and discuss his or her research. Poster presentations are a good place for a novice researcher to start the communication process because they are less intimidating than a podium presentation and require less preparation than a formal manuscript. Nevertheless, abstracts for poster presentations are peer reviewed and accepted based on merit, and so begin the scholarly review process that is the hallmark of professional research.

Once an abstract has been accepted as a poster presentation, the process of poster development begins. The elements of the poster must be chosen, developed, and translated into physical form. Allow adequate time for this process; it requires the help of specialists in both research and media development, and time is required for others to make their contribution.

Table 18.1

Anatomy of an Abstract

Element	Specific Guidelines
Introduction	■ Begin simply, usually with no more than a sentence or two. ■ Explain why this research is important. ■ Include provocative sentences or an interesting lead-in that will "grab" the readers so they will want to read the whole abstract. ■ Call this section "Introduction," "Summary," or "Background."
Objective	■ Report the primary purpose of the study; this can be one or two sentences that describe the aim of the study in detail. ■ If the research question is a restatement of the purpose statement, do not include both. ■ If the purpose is achieved with an unconventional research question, then include both. ■ Call this section "Objective," "Purpose," or "Aims."
Methods	■ Describe the design of the study, the methods used to achieve the purpose, and the procedures applied to control internal validity. ■ Include the sampling strategy and the analytic plan. ■ Identify the independent and dependent variables, which may also be called "predictors" and "outcomes." ■ Present enough detail so the reader understands the fundamental process for the research, but do not overload with detail. ■ Include only minimal statistics, but these usually include the sample size and the calculated power. ■ Explicitly identify the actual statistical tests that were run.
Results	■ Summarize the most important results (whether they were statistically significant or not). ■ Keep in mind that a lack of effect may be as important as the presence of one. ■ Report some statistical results here, but limit these to test statistics and associated p values. ■ Do not use this section to comment on the meaning of the results, but simply report them.
Conclusions	■ Focus on the most important implications of the findings and the usefulness for practice. ■ Address application issues here.

Each conference will have specific requirements for the size of the poster, the length of time it can be displayed, and the amount of time the author is expected to be present. A researcher should take advantage of all the space available for the poster and plan to be present whenever allowed to maximize exposure and communication of the findings.

The purpose of a poster is to translate ideas and images into graphic form, and so a good poster will show viewers what was done instead of telling them (Hedges, 2010). It is helpful to develop a mock-up of the poster using graph paper and sticky notes to get an idea of the layout that will be effective as well as how much space is needed for each element.

The poster should serve as a stand-alone description of your research. The researcher should determine the information that is critical to understanding the research and its

---

SKILL Builder | Strengthen Your Poster Presentation

- A poster presentation is a visual medium, so try to show what was done instead of using text. Arrows, flowcharts, diagrams, photographs, and schematics may all be used to demonstrate the research instead of describing it.
- Use bullets in the text. These emphasis points make the material easier to follow and read, and add interest to the presentation.
- When in doubt, edit out. Cluttered posters are hard to read and may be disregarded. Make sure every item on the poster is necessary. There should be very little—if any—literature review. The purpose is to stimulate discussion, not formally report every detail of the research and its background.
- Use a neutral-color background for the poster. It is easier on the eyes than bright colors and will not distract from the information on the poster or clash with the colors in charts. Use white space effectively to differentiate parts of the poster and accentuate the elements.
- Self-explanatory graphics should dominate the poster. Although the author may be present to discuss the work in more detail, not every individual who looks at the poster will have an opportunity to discuss it. The work should stand alone as a general report of the research.
- Text and graphics should be readable from a distance of 4 to 6 feet. Sans serif fonts (fonts without embellishments) are easiest to read. Vary the font size according to the importance of the information.
- The flow of the poster should be from left to right and top to bottom. Labeling each element with a number helps the reader follow the sequence of the poster in a logical way.

---

clinical implications; good poster development begins with this content and expands on it as space allows. The usual components of a poster include the following:

- *Introduction:* The introduction attracts attention to the poster, summarizes the identified need for the research, and describes the significance of the study. Statistics reporting the prevalence of the clinical problem and the clinical implications are helpful.
- *Research purpose and question:* The purpose statement and research question help focus the study and identify the exact aim of the work.
- *Methods and design:* This section should include a concise description of the design, procedures, measures, and analytic tests used in the study.
- *Results:* Results should be presented primarily in visual form using tables or graphs, with limited text.
- *Conclusions:* Although brief, the conclusions are the heart of the poster. This section should highlight the most important findings and implications for clinicians.
- *Acknowledgments:* It is appropriate to include recognition of staff who helped with the research or the poster and the sponsors of the project. It should be noted if funding was received that supported the project.
- *References:* A brief reference list, focusing on the most important citations, can be included at the end of the poster.

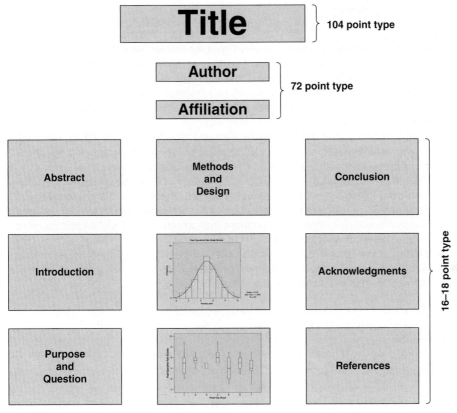

FIGURE 18.1 A Sample Poster

FIGURE 18.1 represents the typical layout of a poster, with associated text font sizes and content. There are, however, infinite ways to lay out a poster so that it is readable and draws the viewer in to find out more.

A poster can be an effective way to interact with those who are interested in the research and to present the study in an informal setting. Podium presentations, on the other hand, provide the opportunity to reach a large audience in a relatively short period of time, while providing more information than is possible in a poster presentation.

> **Podium presentation:** An oral presentation of the key elements of a research study presented at a professional conference.

An Effective Research Presentation

The communication skills that are needed to present research effectively are no different from those needed for any type of group presentation: effective preparation, practice, and focused content development. To prepare for a podium presentation, the researcher needs to know the type of talk that is expected, the composition of the audience, the amount of time allotted, and the objectives for the presentation (Happell, 2007).

SKILL Builder | Strengthen Your Podium Presentation
_____

- Podium presentations often have very tight time frames. When the outline is developed for the presentation, allocate a portion of the time allowed to each section. Develop the detail for each section with these time constraints in mind.
- Practice, practice, practice. It is the novice presenter who goes over the time limit. Keep in mind that 2 to 3 minutes of talking time per slide is the average, so do not overload the presentation with too many slides.
- Have colleagues attend a practice session and provide a critique. Often, someone unfamiliar with a research study can identify gaps or confusing information. Feedback about presentation style as well as content enhances confidence.
- Using a presentation package such as PowerPoint can enhance delivery—or detract from it. Although slides can help hold the attention of the audience, busy backgrounds or slides crowded with text can actually pull attention away from the report. A basic rule of thumb is no more than seven lines to a slide and no more than seven words to a line.
- If detailed statistics or tables are part of the information, put them on a handout instead of a slide. Simple graphs are helpful, but too much detail cannot be read from a distance and distracts the audience.

What Type of Presentation Is Expected?

The types of research presentations can vary from informal roundtable discussions to highly formalized keynote speeches. The kind of presentation will drive the content; different types of presentations have different objectives. Presentations at general clinical conferences will be focused on practice implications, whereas presentations for research conferences may focus on methods and procedures. The goals of the conference can help guide the particular focus of the presentation.

Who Will Be the Audience for the Presentation?

The composition of the audience will drive the development of the presentation. Whether the audience is composed of generalists or specialists will dictate the level of detail provided. The number of participants and where they come from is also important; an international audience needs a different presentation style than a domestic one (Hardicre, Coad, & Devitt, 2007). It is also helpful to know how the audience may apply the information, and whether they will focus on usefulness of the information rather than theoretical considerations. An in-depth knowledge of the audience will help customize the presentation to a particular set of needs, resulting in a better response on the part of the attendees and a greater chance of research utilization.

What Are the Presentation Objectives?

Research results should be presented logically. Most research presentations are brief, so a researcher has to focus on those points that are the most important. The following outline is a suggested format for a podium presentation:

1. An introduction to the problem or clinical issue
2. The purpose or primary aim of the research and the research question
3. Design of the study, including a description of the methods and procedures
4. The findings from the study, including the type of analysis and the major results
5. A discussion of the results, including the major limitations, as well as the most important findings for clinical practice
6. Implications for future research and for clinical practice

The relationship between each stage of the research should be clear to the listener. The conclusion should summarize the overall importance of the study, the main concepts discussed, and the major implications for practice.

Planning for Publication

Poster and podium presentations reach an audience that goes beyond a single hospital or organization. Still, the number who can learn about and use research findings is limited to those who are physically present. Publication in a professional journal reaches the largest target audience and is an attainable goal even for novice researchers.

The first step is to find an appropriate journal. The journal should be selected before the manuscript is written so it can be tailored appropriately to the reader. Reviewing several articles from journals that are being considered can be very helpful (Happell, 2008). Journal web sites provide authors with directions for submitting manuscripts and for monitoring the peer review process. These are generally straightforward and labeled "directions for authors" or "authors' guidelines." They provide valuable information for preparing an acceptable manuscript. **Table 18.2** describes the most common elements of a research manuscript if specifics are not provided by the journal.

The review process takes from 4 to 12 weeks. A request for revision should not be a disappointment; most authors are asked for revisions prior to full acceptance. Some requests for revision may be substantial, but should not be viewed as a rejection. The successful author uses the suggestions for revision as a learning tool and considers them as a step toward publication rather than a rejection (Wollin & Fairweather, 2007). Even the most seasoned authors make revisions to ensure the article meets the expectations of peer reviewers and editors. Feedback can be used to continuously improve both writing and research.

A note is in order about converting an academic paper to a publishable manuscript. Although considerable condensing is required, the author needs to maintain the key substance and meaning of the work. Specifically, the literature review will be substantially shorter for an article, with a focus on the most relevant citations (Heyman & Conin, 2005). To keep the literature review reasonable, do not include any statements that reflect common knowledge in the field or that contribute nothing unique to the study. The writing style should be focused on clarity of expression and using active voice and simple language. Organize the information logically and take care to remain objective.

Table 18.2

Anatomy of a Manuscript

Element	Contents	Considerations
Abstract	Summary of purpose and research question Overview of methods and procedures Major results Implications of the results General conclusions drawn	Generally write after the manuscript is complete. Should be 300 words or less. Report the most important parts of the study. Can stand alone as a description.
Introduction	Detailed statement of the problem Relevance to clinical practice Brief review of the most relevant literature Theoretical framework for the study Specific purpose of the study, research question, and hypotheses (if appropriate)	Provide the context for the research question. State the problem and purpose in the first few paragraphs. Limit the literature review to the most relevant sources.
Methods and Procedures	Specific study design and rationale for selection Sampling strategy, including selection criteria and method Description of sample, including sample size Measurement methods with documentation of reliability, validity, and procedures Procedures for implementation of the treatment and placebo Data collection and analysis procedures	If well-known measurement or treatment is used, give less-detailed description. Use diagrams and photographs to clarify procedures for intervention or measurement. Provide description and references only for unique statistical tests.
Results	Textual description of the statistical tests Tables and figures that summarize the results Decisions for each hypothesis	Do not duplicate tables and figures in the text; information presented in each should be unique. Use this section for reporting only; discussion of the findings comes later.
Discussion	Interpretation of statistical results Discussion of clinical relevance of the findings Contribution of the results to practice Comparison of results with previous works of others Discussion of study limitations and strengths Suggested areas for further study	Do not use commentary to reiterate results, but expand on them and relate findings to practical uses.
References	List of all references cited in the manuscript	

Summary of Key Concepts

- Clinical research in practice requires tremendous effort on the part of the nurse researcher; results should be broadly communicated to generate the most value.
- Research may be communicated through conference posters or podium presentations or through publication in professional or scholarly journals.
- Constructing a thoughtful summary abstract is the first step in submitting research for peer review and consideration for presentation.
- Preparing a poster presentation is often a good first step because it is less complex and enables more face-to-face interaction in an informal setting.

- Podium presentations allow for research to be communicated to a broader audience that can apply the results directly to practice.
- Publication offers the greatest exposure for research and is possible even for novice researchers.

For a full suite of assignments and additional learning activities, use the access code located in the front of your book to visit this exclusive website: http://go.jblearning .com/houser. If you do not have an access code, you can obtain one at the site.

References

Happell, B. (2007). Conference presentations: Developing nursing knowledge by disseminating research findings. *Nurse Researcher, 15,* 70–71.

Happell, B. (2008). Writing for publication: A practical guide. *Nursing Standard, 22,* 35–40.

Hardicre, J., Coad, J., & Devitt, P. (2007). Education and development: Ten steps to successful conference presentations. *British Journal of Nursing, 16,* 402–404.

Hedges, C. (2010). Research corner. Poster presentation: A primer for critical care nurses. *AACN Advanced Critical Care, 21,* 318–321.

Heyman, B., & Conin, P. (2005). Writing for publication: Adapting academic work into articles. *British Journal of Nursing, 14,* 400–404.

Wollin, J., & Fairweather, C. (2007). Finding your voice: Key elements to consider when writing for publication. *British Journal of Nursing, 16,* 1418–1421.

chapter 19

Translating Research into Practice

Introduction

The best research starts with the words "I wonder." Curiosity motivates the process. Designs help researchers answer the following questions: "What is going on now?" "What nursing interventions are effective?" "How do people feel about this?" Statistics answer the logical next question, "Are you sure about that?" After all these questions have been asked and answered, the most important is left for last: "Can we use this knowledge to improve someone's life?" Research without use is a tremendous amount of work for nothing. Even the most theoretical research is used to build models that will, eventually, benefit patients or the nurses who care for them. Our shared profession does not benefit from

❝❝ *Voices from the Field* **❞❞**

I am a nurse educator in a critical care unit. Nearly 2 years ago, my nurse manager asked me to become involved in collecting data on behalf of our hospital for the Surviving Sepsis Campaign. Hospitals around the world are involved in using a database to track how well we adhere to groups of evidence-graded guidelines called "bundles" to reduce mortality and improve outcomes in patients with severe sepsis or septic shock. A bundle is a group of interventions related to a dis-ease process that, when executed together, result in better outcomes than when implemented individually. For example, the Sepsis Resuscitation Bundle has five interventions that include measuring a serum lactate, obtaining blood cultures prior to antibiotic administration, admin-istering broad-spectrum antibiotics within a specific time frame, adequate fluid resuscitation and use of vasopressors as appropriate, and goals for central venous pressure if indicated. There is also a Sepsis Management Bundle, which has four interventions.

I collect data on sepsis patients that come through our ICU. The data let us identify areas that nurses can work on to improve the efficiency and safety of our care. For example, we were able to identify that we were not achieving optimal glycemic control within the desired time frame, and that prompted development of a new and more effective insulin order set. The data have provided us with an excellent tool to examine our processes, not only to see how well we are implementing the guidelines, but also to identify goals to improve treatment, diagnosis, and management of sepsis.

A sepsis order set was created as a tool to help physicians and nurses follow these evidence-based practice standards of care for sepsis patients. We wanted physicians to be able to obtain these orders and use them quickly. It has been a challenge to make everyone aware—doctors and nurses—that the order set is available, and to increase their utilization of it. It can also be a challenge to get practitioners to follow all of the elements of each bundle consistently, not pick and choose individual elements. The evidence shows that if you follow all of the elements in these bundles you can improve outcomes. We are continually striving to increase compliance with the bundles.

Absence of baseline data was an issue. At first, it was difficult to know if we were showing any improvement, simply because we did not know where we started. However, after the first year of data collection, we decided to use that initial data as our baseline to compare future results against. Just getting this baseline has been a huge boon for us; at least now we know what our compliance with the bundles was. I recently completed the second year of data collection, and we are able to see improvement in adherence to each bundle intervention as well as an encouraging decrease in mortality of sepsis patients. Having the time to collect the data can be a huge barrier. With budget constraints, just finding the time is a challenge. I spend quite a bit of time doing data collection.

We use a lot of educational strategies to encourage consistent implementation of the inter-ventions. Two years ago we did a basic overview of the guidelines and why each intervention was important; this last year we reviewed the bundles again and added training on how to correctly calculate an APACHE II score. A lot of the physicians use the APACHE II score to guide decisions, so we needed to teach the nurses what information to look for and use when calculating the score, and how it relates to sepsis. We also have changed our process so that a smaller group of nurses is responsible for calculating the APACHE II, in an effort to reduce operator error. We still need to do more education, and that is also a time barrier.

We have learned a lot from this process. Originally, there were two of us collecting data and it was challenging to attempt to collect data in a uniform manner. Now it is very streamlined; I have a consistent method, so I am gathering data consistently myself and that has increased my confidence in the results.

I know I sound like this has been a slow process—and it has—but some very good things have happened as a result. We do interdisciplinary rounds, and one of the nurse managers is part of those rounds. As part of the process, questions are asked that help to identify if a patient is showing signs of sepsis. So just by including those clinical indicators in the discussion during rounds, we have started to build awareness about screening patients for the early signs of sepsis. It has enabled multiple members of the care team to get involved in a nonthreatening way.

There have been a few obstacles that slow us down, but we have had successes. We need to celebrate the small successes, focus on "here is what we have accomplished"; there has been a lot that is positive. But changing practice is hard and slow; you need a lot of patience and a methodical approach.

The data talk. If you have no data, then you cannot convince people to change, but if you have data, you can present the data and convince people of the positive impact they can make by using the bundles. It really is great because we have so much data available to us now on the use of bundles and their relationship to sepsis outcomes. This has been very helpful to me in my own practice. It has motivated me to look at research, data, and practice guidelines in a different way.

Christy Bullock, RN, BSN

contributions to knowledge that are never put to use. Translating research into practice, then, is the final and most important step in the research process (Bradley et al., 2004).

The previous chapters have described methods of critiquing and conducting research. This chapter will turn to the relationship of research to nursing practice. Even well-designed and executed research studies do not help patients in and of themselves. Research as evidence is only helpful when it is translated into nursing practice. As the accessibility of research and evidence for practice has increased, so has the need to ensure that knowledge translation occurs. Woolf (2008) argues that translational research has come to mean more than translating bench research into treatment potential, but rather "translational research refers to ensuring that new treatment and research knowledge actually reach the patients or populations for whom they are intended and are implemented correctly" (p. 211).

Nurses are being asked to provide the evidence for patient care and to translate existing research knowledge into practice. This paradigm shift is one that is affecting all healthcare professions. The heightened demand for benefit from research has driven such initiatives as the National Institutes of Health (NIH) Roadmap and the Clinical Translational Science Awards, and increased requests for NIH and Agency for Health Research and Quality (AHRQ) grants to support studies of translational efforts (Woods & Magyary, 2010).

Many driving forces conspired to create the current climate. Any time change is instituted, plans for reducing resistance and methods of facilitating strengths and capitalizing on opportunities must be considered. New skill sets—deeply rooted in systematically generated evidence—are needed by nurses at all levels of experience and in virtually all clinical settings.

Why Incorporate Research into Practice?

Several social trends have combined to create an environment that requires knowledge translation, also called research utilization or research uptake, as a basis for nursing practice. These forces have worked together to create a push for nursing practice based on evidence.

Consumerism

Competition for patients has resulted in the phenomenon of consumerism. The consumerism trend in health care is manifesting itself in many ways. As employers seek greater value for their healthcare dollar, they advocate for consumers. As baby boomers age, they increase their exposure to the healthcare system and bring higher expectations with them. The availability of medical information on the Internet has created a situation in which consumers are more informed about and more in control of their care. Consumers are also starting to experience increased healthcare costs as employers ask them to shoulder a greater portion of the cost of increased premiums, and individuals are demanding value for their money. Patients have choices, are more informed about health issues, and frequently demand information about the pros and cons of treatments recommended to them and the evidence that supports the recommendation.

Cost Implications

Poor care has been shown to result in longer hospital stays and higher readmission rates, so research-based interventions that are shown to have better outcomes may reduce healthcare costs by reducing hospital stays and readmissions. By giving the right amount of the right treatment to the right patient at the right time, one can reduce workloads and make better use of resources to result in better health outcomes. Reduced morbidity and mortality result in reduced costs to society as a whole by lessening the numbers of workdays lost and years of potential life lost. Society can apply resources more judiciously and appropriately to improve cost-effectiveness of interventions. Evidence that supports the effectiveness of interventions helps determine its cost implications as well.

Quality

The recent increase in attention paid to quality in health care is strongly related to cost and effectiveness. This reflects limited resources, changes in health insurance coverage, a shift from paternalism to participation in decision making by the patient (patient-centered care), and consumerism (patient demands and expectations). The Institute of Medicine defines quality of care as the degree to which health services increase the likelihood of desired health outcomes and are consistent with current practice knowledge. Knowledge translation fits with both parts of the definition. Application of current evidence should result in improved health outcomes, while at the same time, evidence is being translated into up-to-date practices.

Patient Safety

Patient safety and risk reduction are two of the top concerns of any healthcare system. Prevention of harm is strongly related to high quality. There are many opportunities for knowledge translation to prevent errors, to maintain safety, and thereby to improve health outcomes and contain costs. The Joint Commission, which accredits hospitals, has made developing a culture of safety a top priority.

Regulatory Requirements

The Joint Commission and other regulatory agencies have specific standards requiring the use of evidence as a basis for healthcare delivery. Joint Commission accreditation is a nationally sought measurement of quality among hospitals and other healthcare agencies. The Joint Commission requires adherence to an exhaustive number of protocols and documentation to validate the outcomes of treatment. Therefore, it is important for healthcare agencies to be able to show their evaluation process and to prove they have positive outcomes. By implementing research-based strategies, they improve the likelihood of achieving positive outcomes and discarding outdated strategies that do not prove effective. By citing the research on which their protocols are based, healthcare management organizations verify to the Joint Commission the quality of their healthcare delivery. From the regulatory agency's point of view, research allows the creation of recognizable standards of care and evaluation criteria for a given health problem. This allows for a more objective and valid measurement of successful versus unsuccessful outcomes.

> **Joint Commission accreditation:** A nationally sought measurement of quality among hospitals and other healthcare agencies.

Magnet Status

Hospitals seek Magnet status as a means of documenting their commitment to an environment conducive to professional nursing practice. Obtaining Magnet status requires fostering nursing research. The American Nurses Credentialing Center (ANCC) awards Magnet status to hospitals that meet criteria measuring the strength and quality of nursing service. A Magnet hospital is one where nursing outcomes are excellent, nurses have high job satisfaction, staff nurse turnover is low, and there are appropriate grievance resolution policies. Magnet status indicates nursing involvement in data collection and decision making for patient care delivery. Nursing leaders at Magnet hospitals value staff nurses, involve them in shaping research-based nursing practice, and encourage and reward them for advancing their practice. Magnet hospitals foster open interprofessional communication and a personnel mix appropriate to attain the best patient outcomes and staff work environment.

Health Policy

The final and most significant goal of health care is to improve health at a community, national, and global level. Research-based healthcare measures, evaluated by objective criteria, allow evaluation of the impact of health care on entire populations. The Healthy People initiatives are examples of efforts to improve health at a population level. Every 10 years, the Healthy People goals are reviewed and revised according to how well the previous goals were met.

The Nurse's Role in Knowledge Translation

Nurses are in a unique position to foster the translation of research into practice. Woods and Magyary (2010) identified two critical skills for knowledge translation: team science and transdisciplinary efforts. In the past, traditional models of research dissemination involved researchers working in isolation, focusing on a single problem grounded in a single discipline, and shared only when the research was complete. Contemporary models of research have been transformed into teams of investigators representing diverse disciplines that are better able to investigate multidimensional patient problems. True transdisciplinary work requires understanding the contribution of relevant disciplines, integrating their individual perspectives, and focusing on a shared problem. Nurses are often central to organizing and leading these transdisciplinary research teams, and therefore are capable facilitators of knowledge translation.

Contemporary research translation also requires a variety of methods for data gathering that are relevant for clinicians. Ensuring that interventions will be acceptable to patients requires a focus on more than quantitative analysis. Attention to the acceptability and desirability of evidence-based treatments is also needed. The nursing profession has long relied on mixed methods of inquiry, and so mixing research paradigms is not foreign to the discipline. Indeed, integrative reviews—or the systematic evaluation of both quantitative and qualitative studies in determining practice guidelines—was embraced early by the nursing profession.

A key element of research translation, though, relies on the human component. A growing body of evidence suggests that a therapeutic alliance between caregiver and patient may be the most important predictor of intervention success. Partnership building and effective communication with patients are proving to be some of the most significant predictors of successful treatment outcomes (Woods & Magyary, 2010). Nurses are in a particularly unique position to ensure that emphasis is placed on how relationships contribute to the effects of treatments when translating evidence-based clinical guidelines, protocols, and standard order sets. This may be particularly important in culturally diverse populations.

A significant way in which nurses can contribute to knowledge translation is to ensure that the context of application is considered in the design of interventions. Including contextual factors—such as compliance issues, level of care, or burden of treatment—in planning and evaluating intervention studies may have the greatest impact on subsequent utilization (Wallin, 2009).

Identifying Problems for Knowledge Translation

Problems that are suitable for knowledge translation are identified in a multitude of ways. Direct patient care, patient and colleague questions, conferences, journals, hospital and other healthcare delivery agency data, professional organizations, government agency research priorities, and quality reports can all generate inquiry. In daily nursing practice, nurses face problems that are easily translated into questions that can be answered with research evidence.

One way to capture these day-to-day musings is to create a method for doing so, such as placing a notebook or file cards in various places where nurses spend their time (e.g., the documentation station, the nurses' station, next to telephones, and in break rooms). These can be collected and discussed at staff meetings to prioritize problems suitable for research.

Patient questions and outcomes can also prompt the identification of research problems. Focus groups of patients, often undertaken for marketing purposes, can be a source for identifying research issues. Follow-up calls with patients after discharge can elicit areas of research to prevent readmission. Conferences and journals can be wonderful sources of information as well as research questions. Studies can be replicated and presented at conferences, which provide an opportunity to interact with researchers in an informal way. Professional organizations and government agencies, such as Healthy People, often have research priorities that are also good sources of research problems. An excellent source for research questions is the unit report. Length of stay for various diagnoses, nosocomial problems, and patient safety issues are only a few issues that become apparent in the unit report.

Finding and Aggregating Evidence

The help of experts in electronic retrieval of documents should be sought to make best use of nurses' time and abilities. Time and training must be provided for nurses to learn how to critique an article and how to evaluate whether findings are useful. There may be a case for nurse managers to support a differentiated practice model, where baccalaureate-prepared nurses use their educational preparation to critique and evaluate research, and master's and doctorally prepared nurses can help initiate projects and translate knowledge into practice (McCloskey, 2008). The Doctor of Nursing Practice degree holders are the

Potential Research Questions Generated During Nursing Care Delivery

A diabetic patient is admitted to the unit for a partial amputation of the right leg due to impaired circulation. Each part of the nursing process can potentially generate questions for evidence-based practice:

Assessment

When the nurse first admits a patient, a complete assessment is performed. Research questions related to intake assessment might include the following:

- Is there a difference in outcome for patients who are homeless compared with those who are not?
- Which co-morbid conditions are associated with increased length of stay for diabetic patients?

The nurse uses ongoing assessment to monitor patient progress during the hospital stay. One of the most important areas to assess is the skin. Surgical wound healing and potential skin breakdown are areas filled with opportunity for researchable questions:

- Which patients are more likely to have skin breakdown?
- What are the earliest and most effective interventions to prevent breakdown?
- What is the effect of skin breakdown on length of stay?

Diagnosis

Circulation is one issue of primary concern, as is protection from neurovascular compromise and infection. Diagnosing early signs of impaired circulation can help the nurse prevent further tissue damage. Enhancing wound healing and creating an environment for effective rehabilitation and ambulation are also important for this patient, leading to the following questions:

- What is the relationship between nutrition education and wound healing?
- What is the impact of early ambulation provided by nurses on wound healing in diabetic postsurgical patients?

Planning

The care plan includes goals for the patient, nursing orders, and a time frame. When planning care for the patient, the nurse often relies on tradition, although many of these basic procedures have been tested with scientific rigor. The following questions are examples of research questions about care practices that have been "assumed to be effective":

- What is the relationship of frequency of repositioning to skin integrity for postsurgical, diabetic patients?
- Is there a difference in length of stay between postsurgical diabetic patients who have pressure-sensitive bedding compared with those who do not?

Implementation

When implementing care, the nurse has numerous tasks to perform with each patient. How do we know the best way to position a certain patient? How do we know the best way to perform skin care? Here are some questions that can be investigated through the research process:

- What is the relationship between the frequency of skin care and skin integrity for a postsurgical diabetic?
- Is there a difference between postsurgical diabetic patients who receive skin care in the morning compared with those who receive it in the evening?

Evaluation

The evaluation phase lends itself well to research-based testing because it is essentially checking for the effectiveness of interventions. Again, the questions can be as varied as those for the previous phases:

- What is the relationship between specific nursing interventions and length of stay?
- Is there a difference in understanding and health outcomes between patients who are offered patient education throughout their stay compared with those who receive education at discharge?

ideal liaison between practice and research, and can be placed in charge of creating knowledge translation projects.

Experts at creating synthesized reviews should be made available to assist and mentor nurses. Organizations interested in encouraging nurses to perform literature searches should have access to databases and a mechanism for obtaining requested literature. A collaborating librarian is most helpful in these circumstances and can assist with finding the more obscure materials.

The strongest evidence for nursing practice is provided when multiple studies report the same results. However, multiple studies must still be evaluated for quality and the results aggregated in a way that reveals recommendations for practice. Several processes are available for evaluating, aggregating, and summarizing multiple studies as evidence.

> **gray matter**
>
> Five primary methods are available for aggregating the results of research studies for translation into practice:
> - Systematic review
> - Integrative review
> - Meta-analysis
> - Meta-synthesis
> - Practice guidelines

The Systematic Review

One of the cornerstones of evidence-based practice is the systematic collection and analysis of all available research on a topic: the systematic review. These reviews are critical for evidence-based practice because they summarize the numerous and sometimes contradictory findings in the literature in an unbiased, methodical way (Mistiaen, Poot, Hickox, & Wagner, 2004). A systematic review is a highly structured and controlled search of the available literature that minimizes the potential for bias and produces a practice recommendation as an outcome (Bettany-Saltikov, 2010). Systematic reviews can focus on patient concerns, the prevalence of problems, or the effectiveness of diagnostic procedures. However, in recent years, much attention has been paid to the effectiveness of healthcare interventions.

> **Systematic review:** A highly structured and controlled search of the available literature that minimizes the potential for bias and produces a practice recommendation as an outcome.

With regard to systematic reviews of healthcare interventions, the Cochrane Library (www.cochrane.org) is widely recognized as one of the most useful sources of high-quality reviews. The reviews conducted within the framework of the Cochrane Collaboration are highly valued because of their thorough searches and their methodological rigor. These reviews are focused heavily on quantitative analysis and experimental designs and so provide solid evidence for the effectiveness of interventions.

Because the Cochrane Library had its start in medicine, it is sometimes criticized for providing little evidence for nursing care. However, these concerns appear to be unfounded based on the work of Mistiaen et al. (2004). These methods researchers found ample evidence of systematic reviews for nursing practice, including studies of psychological interventions, technical procedures, nutritional counseling, educational interventions, organizational studies, and studies of the effectiveness of exercise and positioning. All these were either focused on or had direct relevance to nursing practice.

Although Cochrane is the most familiar source of systematic reviews, other databases contribute systematic reviews of interventions. Table 19.1 lists some common databases of systematic reviews.

The strength of the systematic review as a basis for practice recommendations is its unbiased, exhaustive review of the literature, followed by a rigorous methodological

Table 19.1

Databases of Systematic Reviews

Database	Focus
CCTR (Cochrane Controlled Trials Register)	Systematic reviews, randomized controlled trials, and protocols for systematic reviews
CRD Database of Abstracts of Reviews of Effects (DARE)	Systematic reviews
CRD Health Technology Assessment (HTA)	Systematic reviews of the application of technology in database health care
GEARS (Getting Easier Access to Reviews)	Consumer access to systematic reviews
NHS EED (NHS Economic Evaluation Database)	Systematic reviews
Best Evidence 3	Systematic economic evaluations of healthcare interventions
TRIP Database	Clinical search tool designed to allow health professionals to rapidly identify the highest quality clinical evidence for clinical practice

evaluation and the use of objective rules to link findings to recommendations (Hemmingway & Berenton, 2009). Each step of a systematic review has guiding rules that inhibit the potential for bias in article selection, evaluation, or elimination from consideration. This avoids the potential that a practitioner will solicit and summarize only those articles that support his or her current beliefs about practice, rather than testing them. This neutral, objective, and unbiased review of the literature is the hallmark of a systematic review (Pettrigrew & Roberts, 2006).

As the name implies, planning the search strategy for a systematic review involves a sequence of carefully considered questions:

1. *Determine the background for the review:* Why is it important to have a systematic review for this intervention? How was the need identified?
2. *State the main review question:* What is the goal of the review? Is the review to test a specific existing intervention or to come up with "best practices"?
3. *Develop inclusion and exclusion criteria:* Who are the patients of interest? What age groups, diagnoses, or other conditions are of interest? Which specific patient groups will not be included? Which interventions and outcomes are of interest?
4. *Devise a search strategy:* What are the sources of studies that will be searched (including published, unpublished, and "gray literature" such as conference proceedings)? What are key journals that must be hand-searched?
5. *Develop study selection criteria:* What search terms will be used? What types of studies are acceptable (for example, experimental, descriptive, qualitative)? What time frame will be considered?

6. *Determine study quality criteria:* What quality indicators will be used to appraise articles for inclusion? What quality level is acceptable overall? What quality problems warrant exclusion from the study?

Once the search strategy is devised, it is carried out faithfully as planned. Studies that are excluded at any stage of the review must have an objective rationale for elimination. The systematic reviewer maintains a record of each abstract and article reviewed, along with documentation of the reason for elimination if a study was dropped from consideration. This ensures that the reviewer is using objective and defensible reasons for selecting studies for final recommendations and minimizes the potential effects of researcher bias on the outcome. FIGURE 19.1 depicts the process for making decisions about the inclusion of specific studies in the final recommendations from a systematic review.

Case in Point: A Systematic Review

Although we often focus on systematic reviews as a basis for clinical care, in reality, this type of aggregate evidence can be used to guide leadership and educational decisions as well. Harder (2010) conducted a systematic review of the evidence on the effectiveness of the use of simulation in teaching and learning in the health sciences. Many institutions have adopted simulations to help educate their students and to reduce the burden of clinical placements in healthcare facilities. Yet evaluation of the effectiveness of this method of education needs to be systematically conducted.

This review focused on the use of high-fidelity simulations using computerized human patient simulator manikins for instruction in clinical skills. The author set criteria for studies that included quantitative comparative studies but excluded purely descriptive or qualitative studies. The outcomes of interest were clinical skills performance and perceived confidence and competence. Five sets of preset terms were used to search three comprehensive databases, yielding 61 studies that were evaluated using preset quality criteria. Twenty-nine studies were eliminated because they did not meet the detailed inclusion criteria, and an additional 9 did not evaluate the intervention appropriately. The final set of 23 articles was evaluated and used in the final review.

The use of simulation increased the students' clinical skills in the majority of the studies. These students were also better able to manage scenarios that were not previously encountered. Three of the studies did not identify a statistically significant improvement over nonsimulation methods, but the authors concluded this may have been due to the way that competence was measured. Even when the differences were not statistically significant, students who experienced simulation reported higher confidence levels prior to entering the "live" clinical experience. Identifying the relationship between self-confidence and subsequent clinical performance was identified as an area of potential future research.

This systematic review is typical of the approach taken by most quantitative reviews. The *a priori* search terms and identified databases were typical of the methods used to reduce the potential for bias in the search. The fact that a large number of potential citations was reduced by more than half is not unusual. The inflexible inclusion criteria and rigorous methodological quality that is required of studies often result in a small number of studies that are actually appropriate for inclusion in the final review.

Source: Harder, N. (2010). Use of simulation in teaching and learning in health sciences: A systematic review. *Journal of Nursing Education, 49*, 23–28.

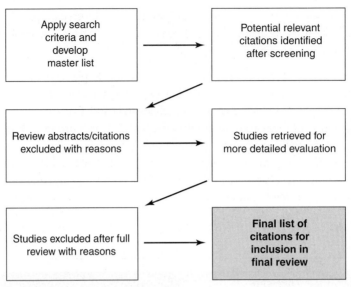

FIGURE 19.1 The Study Selection Process

The outcome of a systematic review is a recommendation for practice. These reviews are considered the strongest evidence in practice because findings are presented only when multiple studies of strong methodological rigor have supported practices (Bettany-Saltikov, 2010). Many recent changes in practice—from the way neonatal skin is cared for, to the way pain is controlled in adults, to the way diabetics' blood glucose is managed—have come from systematic reviews. Nurses are in key positions to both use and generate systematic reviews. However, many systematic reviews, particularly those in Cochrane, have been criticized for relying exclusively on randomized trials and quantitative studies. Nursing is a humanistic profession, and so attention to the whole person demands that systematic reviews for many nursing practices must accommodate more than experiments and incorporate qualitative findings into reviews.

The Integrative Review

Reviews of evidence in the healthcare literature are some of the most established methods of aggregating research into coherent, concise recommendations. Integrative reviews, on the other hand, are broader reviews that allow for the simultaneous inclusion of experimental and nonexperimental research to more fully understand a phenomenon of concern (Whittemore & Knafl, 2005). Integrative reviews achieve a wide range of review goals: They allow nurses to define concepts comprehensively, review evidence holistically, and analyze methodology from multiple perspectives. The integrative review has the potential to play an extraordinarily important role in the development of evidence-based nursing knowledge.

The integrative review is a methodology that synthesizes empirical, theoretical, and experiential research to provide a comprehensive understanding of the human response

Integrative review: A methodology that synthesizes quantitative, theoretical, and qualitative research to provide a comprehensive understanding of the human condition.

to health, illness, and interventions (Weaver & Olson, 2006). Integrative reviews have the potential to contribute to nursing knowledge, inform research, guide practice, and form policy initiatives with a solid foundation on what is known about both science and human behavior. However, combining diverse data sources is complex and challenging. A well-done integrative review adheres to the guidelines for systematic reviews that ensure control of bias in study selection and evaluation. However, integrative reviews require an expansion of two key areas of a systematic review: the criteria used for selecting specific research designs and the standards used to judge the quality of the evidence. Qualitative designs must be considered for applicability to the problem under study and specified

Case in Point: An Integrative Review

The diagnosis of cancer and the treatment decisions associated with it may cause stress and anxiety for any patient. These reactions are particularly disturbing when the diagnosis is delivered to parents regarding their child. The emotional tensions created by such a devastating experience may affect the parents' relationship during the course of their child's illness. The researchers daSilva et al. (2010) used an integrative review to examine the evidence related to the effects of childhood cancer on the parents' relationship.

These authors chose an integrative review because of the emotional nature of the question and the need for a holistic view of the research question. Key search terms were used to retrieve articles from six research databases that included both nursing and psychological literature. Although both quantitative and qualitative research designs were included in the search, all studies were evaluated based on accepted methodological quality standards, informational value, and the focus of study.

More than 800 studies were retrieved with the initial search, but after excluding articles that did not meet the focus criteria or the quality standards, only 14 studies were included in the final review. All studies were descriptive and included 4 quantitative and 10 qualitative studies.

Four themes emerged from the aggregation of the evidence. The parents' relationship did indeed change during the child's illness, with the greatest change between 4 months and 1 year of diagnosis.

When the child had been ill for more than 2 years, the parents noted little change in their relationship. Communication between parents emerged as a critical determinant of the impact of the illness on their relationship. As one would expect, good communication helped nurture a positive relationship, whereas lack of communication influenced negative effects. Gender differences were reflected in the different role expectations of mothers and fathers and in the family's coping. A final theme described the role changes that parents went through as their child's illness required them to reorganize their lives.

This integrative review demonstrates the primary distinction of this aggregation approach—the inclusion of both quantitative and qualitative studies in the review. Conclusions reflected numerical data (the ratings of marital communication, for example) and verbal data (perceptions about changing marital roles). This is an excellent example of the way an integrative review can support optimal nursing practice because it makes clear that the child is not the only one affected when a diagnosis of pediatric cancer is present. The nurse is in a pivotal role to ensure that the parents are supported so their relationship is healthy enough to support their child through the challenges of cancer treatment.

Source: daSilva, F., Jacob, E., & Nascimento, L. (2010). Impact of childhood cancer on parents' relationship: An integrative review. *Journal of Nursing Scholarship, 42,* 250–261.

as acceptable. Appraisal of study quality must be based on standards for qualitative trustworthiness, not those used for quantitative evaluation. Using quantitative standards to evaluate qualitative study will result in frustration for the reviewer and a dearth of qualitative studies that make the final cut.

The translation of final study findings to recommendations must also be modified in integrative reviews. The link between studies and recommendations must be amended to include grading for both types of studies. If carefully and objectively completed, an integrative review can play a critical role in evidence-based practice initiatives, portraying the complexity that is inherent in the human condition.

Meta-analysis

Meta-analysis: A statistical method of aggregating the results of quantitative studies so an overall effect size can be evaluated.

Meta-analysis is a statistical method of aggregating the results of quantitative studies. When experiments are replicated on similar populations using standard measures, it is possible to sum up the aggregate impact of the intervention on an outcome. The strength of a comprehensive meta-analysis is its ability to reveal structural flaws and sources of bias across primary research studies (Noble, 2006). When the results of multiple studies are compared, methodological weaknesses become apparent and true effects are revealed. Much as a sampling distribution of the means is a curve made up of many, many group means, a meta-analysis is a result that is the compilation of many, many effect sizes. It is extremely useful in health care for judging the clinical and practical significance of any effects the intervention may have had.

Meta-analyses are complicated to run, and they yield complex output. The challenge of meta-analysis is to find a sufficient number of studies that used similar populations, measures, and statistics. Meta-analysis is particularly challenged to quantify the size of a common treatment effect because of the clinical diversity of the trials and the potential differences among patients in the trials (Noble, 2006). Available software programs can analyze disparate types of data for commonalities. The numbers that are yielded by a meta-analysis describe typical responses and provide a numerical basis for judging the magnitude of effect across all studies (Berenstein, Hedges, Higgins, & Rothstein, 2009). Interventions that have demonstrated *statistical* significance across several studies may have, in aggregate, a relatively small effect. In these cases, meta-analysis reveals that the nurse can conclude with a great deal of certainty that the intervention improves things, but not much.

On the other hand, when an intervention is very effective, it will demonstrate a strong effect over and over again. In these cases, meta-analysis will reveal the amount of improvement that can be expected, and the nurse can use these findings with confidence.

Qualitative Meta-synthesis

Qualitative meta-synthesis: The development of overarching themes about the meaning of human events based on a synthesis of multiple qualitative studies.

Qualitative meta-synthesis is the development of overarching themes about the meaning of human events based on a synthesis of multiple qualitative studies (Walsh & Downe, 2005). It is an appealing approach for qualitative researchers because it has characteristics of methods that elevate the level of evidence provided by the outcome. Multiple sites, multiple samples, and replication of qualitative studies

Case in Point: A Meta-analysis

Transitions and new experiences characterize the college years. Frequently, these translate into stress, social strain, financial concerns, or feelings of being overwhelmed. Although counseling services are common on college campuses, less than one third of distressed students obtain such services. Nam et al. (2010) set out to understand gender differences in attitudes toward seeking professional counseling in the college setting.

The authors set criteria for including and excluding studies based on the subject characteristics, type of study, and statistics reported. Only quantitative studies comparing gender responses were included. After a systematic search of five databases using specified search terms, 1847 studies were identified for possible consideration. By limiting studies to those that used one of two help-seeking scales as a dependent variable, the final sample included 14 empirical articles.

Although the studies provided different statistics, the authors chose to convert all of the effect size statistics to a correlation coefficient, which produced a common effect size. These authors included all of their statistical transformations in the article, making it easier for the reader to determine their method for producing comparable measures of effect size.

The result demonstrated a medium effect size of gender on help-seeking behaviors. Female students had more positive attitudes toward seeking help than did their male counterparts. These gender differences were mediated by ethnicity. The largest effect of gender was in Caucasians, with men have a much larger avoidance of psychological counseling than women. Asian or Asian American men had the smallest difference in attitudes toward help-seeking. However, it was of note that neither women nor men of Asian or Asian American descent sought help at a significant rate, because these students often view seeking psychological help as a sign of shame.

The meta-analysis conducted by these authors is typical in that only quantitative studies that reported effect size statistics were included. These are almost exclusively comparative designs, because these are generally the only studies that can report effect sizes. This means, necessarily, that a much smaller sample of articles will remain after screening. In this case, more than 1800 originally identified studies were narrowed down to 14 for the ultimate analysis. This study is also typical in that nonstandard measurements, sampling procedures, and diverse statistics made the analysis complex and difficult to accomplish. The result, however, is particularly strong evidence in that both aggregate statistical significance and the size of the effect can be quantified.

Source: Nam, S., Chu, J., Lee, M., Lee, J., Kim, N., & Lee, S. (2010). A meta-analysis of gender differences in attitudes toward seeking professional psychological help. *Journal of American College Health, 59,* 110–116.

enhance trustworthiness and, therefore, the confidence with which one can generalize the results (McCormick, Rodney, & Varcoe, 2003). Meta-synthesis is conducted much as meta-analysis is, but the focus is on recurrent themes rather than aggregate effect sizes. Meta-synthesis represents a family of methodological approaches to developing new knowledge based on rigorous analysis of existing qualitative research findings (Thorne, 2004).

Practice Guidelines

All aggregate studies provide strong evidence for nursing practice. They are at the top of the pyramid of evidence because replication and consistency enable confidence. The practicing nurse, however, will find that practice guidelines are

Practice guidelines: Research-based recommendations for practices that are graded as mandatory, optional, or supplemental and that may be stated as standards of practice, procedures, or decision algorithms.

Case in Point: A Qualitative Meta-synthesis

Linnarsson, Bubini, and Perseius (2010) focused on a range of studies describing the needs and experience of the significant others (SOs) of critically ill or injured patients. The authors noted that a great deal of qualitative nursing research has been done on this subject, going back to the early 1970s. The aim of this analysis was to aggregate the common themes of these studies to understand the experience of SOs and how it affects them. A second aim was to identify the needs expressed by SOs and how they should be prioritized.

The authors identified a range of search terms and databases *a priori*. Specific inclusion and exclusion criteria were established. For example, the authors excluded families of children and dying patients because those populations generate such unique findings that common themes would be difficult to determine. The quality of the studies was appraised using a standard approach for qualitative critique. The initial exploratory search identified 198 studies, of which 15 were included in the final analysis. The authors interpreted and synthesized the key findings of these 15 articles into five common themes.

Families reported a sense of chaos and uncertainty that was described as an emotional "roller coaster." This experience was characterized by a general feeling of anxiety, distress, and fear. A second theme was the need for honest and consistent communication. Most desired was information that prepared them for what might happen. These significant others referred to an alertness to implicit as well as explicit information, listening and observing for messages through tone of voice and body language as well as words. The way that information was given was crucial for the SOs to be able to keep up hope. A third theme was the need to protect and guard the loved one. This was generally demonstrated by staying near and keeping vigil. The SOs took pride in being able to help the patient, and being part of the care—especially touching—was important to them. A fourth theme was the desire to form an alliance with caregivers. Establishing a personal relationship with the nurse fostered communication and confidence. When this communication and connection failed, it often led to SOs acting out or withdrawing from the situation. A final change was the disruption in social normality experienced during this time. Although the SOs often found support networks with other families of critically ill patients, there was a need for support from others such as family, friends, and colleagues. A failing social network created distress, but a successful one often created a powerful intensified family bond. Significant others particularly found strength in listening to others' experiences, helping them find their own strategy for coping.

This study has clear implications for clinical practice, especially regarding the nurses' ability to influence the SOs' experience. Facilitating interaction between the patient and their loved ones, communicating clearly while balancing hope and reality, and fostering social networks are all nursing strategies that can help these families cope.

This was a typical meta-synthesis in that only qualitative studies were selected for inclusion. The themes and codes from all the studies were synthesized into a single model that was supported by all fifteen articles. This was a particularly strong study because a great deal of research had been done in this area, and clear themes emerged across all of the studies. It is not unusual for authors to exclude populations that may introduce themes that are too unique for aggregation. This meta-synthesis was typical in that a relatively large number of studies was reduced considerably after sampling criteria and quality standards were applied. This aggregation and rigorous evaluation process gives the nurse greater confidence in using these findings in practice.

Source: Linnarsson, J., Bubine, J., & Perseius, K. (2010). Review: A meta-synthesis of qualitative research into needs and experiences of significant others to critically ill or injured patients. *Journal of Clinical Nursing, 29*, 3102–3111.

among the most practical and understandable ways to read aggregate evidence. Practice guidelines are often developed by a group of clinical experts who are convened by a professional or academic body. The team conducts a rigorous and systematic review of existing research and judges how to best apply the research. Guidelines provide recommendations for practices that are graded as mandatory, optional, or supplemental and may be stated as standards of practice, procedures, or decision algorithms. There are many sources for practice guidelines at the government clearinghouse at www .guidelines.gov, which has the most comprehensive source of publicly available evidence-based guidelines.

The results of aggregate studies offer the most direct link between research and practice. Still, evidence-based practices require change, and that requires a systematic approach to ensuring efficient, timely research uptake.

Models for Translating Research into Practice

Translating research into evidence requires the ability to find, appraise, and synthesize research results into recommendations. However, a myriad of other support systems must also be available to ensure knowledge translation. Systems for communicating findings in a comprehensive and accurate way must be available. Ongoing support from nursing leadership is a requirement, and systems for monitoring the effects of the change must be in place. Using a tested model for a systematic organizational approach to knowledge translation enhances the potential for ongoing success. However, no single model will fit every patient care environment. Six models of research use will be presented here: the Iowa Model of Evidence-Based Practice, a guide for practicing nurses; the Johns Hopkins Nursing Evidence-Based Model, based on clinical–academic collaboration; a model for integrating evidence into a Magnet hospital environment; a framework for outcomes-focused knowledge translation; the Collaborative Model for Knowledge Translation, which focuses on interaction between researchers and practitioners; and the Ottawa Model of research use.

The Iowa Model of Evidence-Based Practice

The Iowa Model is based on a five-step process.

1. *Identify a nursing problem and conduct a search of the literature.* Topics can include clinical care issues, cost-effectiveness, or operational issues, among others (Titler, 2001).

2. *Determine whether the issue is a priority for the organization.* Considering the resources required to conduct research, this is an important determination. Higher priority issues will be those that fit organizational, departmental, and unit goals; those that are high volume or high cost; or those that are driven by market forces. Administration will be able to guide nurses to determine which topics are most appropriate.

3. *Form a team to develop, implement, and evaluate the project.* There may already be a research committee in place that can provide oversight. The authors of the model suggest that representatives of all stakeholders and disciplines be involved in the team. For example, a pain management project should include pharmacists, physicians, nurses, and psychologists, whereas the team for a project concerning effective bathing should include nursing staff and experts in skin care.

4. *Assemble the relevant literature.* Existing systematic reviews are important to secure. In addition to published literature, the authors suggest looking at bibliographies, abstracts published as part of conference proceedings, master's theses, and doctoral dissertations.

5. *Begin the process of critiquing the literature.* Guidance from advanced practice nurses should be sought in this stage as the literature is synthesized. A group approach helps distribute the workload and helps staff nurses understand the scientific basis for implementing changes. At this point, the group decides if there is enough research to guide practice. The following are some of the questions to consider when reviewing the literature:

- How consistent are the findings across studies?
- What are the types and the quality of studies?
- How relevant are the findings to clinical practice?
- Are there enough studies using a population similar to that of the organization in which the findings will be applied?
- How feasible are the findings in practice?
- What is the risk–benefit ratio?

The Iowa Model is widely recognizable, easy to understand, and straightforward to implement in a clinical setting. It does require time, support from management, and training in research critique as elements for success. Often, training and mentorship can be provided by individuals who have a research record and the capacity to provide practical advice. Seeking out a collaborative relationship with an academic organization often provides this support.

The Johns Hopkins Nursing Evidence-Based Practice (EBP) Model

Clinical–academic collaborations can form the basis for effective evidence-based practice uptake because the relationship is mutually beneficial. Clinicians can get the education and mentorship needed for bedside science projects, and researchers often gain access to the living laboratories that make for the best applied studies.

The Johns Hopkins Nursing Evidence-Based Practice (EBP) Model was developed by a collaboration between hospital nursing staff and nursing faculty (Newhouse et al., 2005). This model incorporates the impact of internal and external environmental factors on nursing problems. The core of this model (represented in **FIGURE 19.2**) is the use of best available evidence. All sources of evidence are used to consider a nursing issue in the domains of practice, research, and education. A multidisciplinary approach is used to identify problems, search out evidence, and implement a plan. There are three phases to the model: practice question, evidence, and translation.

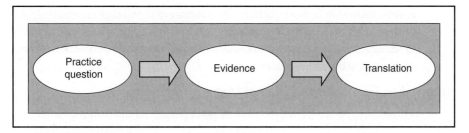

Practice question
    Step 1: Identify an EBP question
    Step 2: Define scope of practice question
    Step 3: Assign responsibility for leadership
    Step 4: Recruit multidisciplinary team
    Step 5: Schedule team conference
Evidence
    Step 6: Conduct internal and external search for evidence
    Step 7: Critique all types of evidence
    Step 8: Summarize evidence
    Step 9: Rate strength of evidence
    Step 10: Develop recommendations for change in processes of care or
             systems on the basis of strength of evidence
Translation
    Step 11: Determine appropriateness and feasibility of translating
             recommendations into the specific practice setting
    Step 12: Create action plan
    Step 13: Implement change
    Step 14: Evaluate outcomes
    Step 15: Report results of preliminary evaluation to decision makers
    Step 16: Secure support from decision makers to implement recommended
             change internally
    Step 17: Identify next steps
    Step 18: Communicate findings

FIGURE 19.2 The Johns Hopkins Model of EBP Implementation
Source: Used with permission, Lippincott Williams & Wilkins. From Newhouse, R., Dearholt, S., Poe, S. et al. (2005). Evidence-based practice: A practical approach to implementation. *Journal of Nursing Administration, 35*(1), 37.

1. In the practice question phase, a clinically relevant practice question is generated that is endorsed by administration. The scope of the research question is defined, and a nurse is assigned to lead the project. A multidisciplinary team is recruited, and a team conference is held.

2. In the evidence phase, an internal and external search for evidence is conducted. The evidence is critiqued, summarized, and rated for strength (credibility based on the types of studies and their outcomes). The last step in this phase is to develop recommendations for modifying processes of care or systems based on the strength of the evidence.

3. The final phase, translation, may be the most important. An evaluation is conducted to determine the appropriateness and feasibility of translating the recommendations into the clinical setting. An action plan is created, and the change

is implemented as a pilot program. The outcome of the change is evaluated, and the results reported to decision makers. A decision is made by administration as to whether to support institution-wide changes in the process, and this is communicated to the stakeholders.

Knowledge Translation as Part of Magnet Recognition

Magnet hospitals, in particular, are required to have operational and clinically influential evidence-based practices in place. Turkel et al. (2005) created a model for integrating EBP as part of the Magnet Recognition Process (see FIGURE 19.3). The model consists of five steps:

1. *Establish a foundation.* Critical to step one is the support of leadership. The chief nurse executive (CNE) must create a supportive environment to change the nursing and healthcare culture in favor of EBP. Commitment of leadership is the first criterion required when establishing the foundation for research utilization in practice. The CNE's focus will be to obtain resources to establish and maintain the program. Resources include electronic databases, a consulting librarian, computers devoted to the project, release time for nursing staff, and/or funding for a doctorally prepared nurse consultant. RNs and APNs should work together to come up with areas of concern, create EBP protocols, educate peers, facilitate journal clubs, and conduct research projects. The CNE may form a nursing research committee to guide projects. Using participation in EBP projects as part of the annual performance review or as part of clinical leader advancement will motivate staff nurses to become involved in the work.

2. *Identify areas of concern.* Ideally, the research committee will provide a forum for interested nurses to discuss areas of interest, coordinate journal clubs, and begin to learn about EBP. Topics need to be staff-nurse driven to ensure excitement, buy-in, and acceptance of the outcome. Nursing staff meetings can be a good starting point.

3. *Create internal expertise.* This is the time to begin reading and discussing the literature. The traditional journal club requires a 1-hour group meeting to critique an article that all have previously read. Turkel et al. (2005) propose two alternative formats:
   - The "journal club on the run," where a facilitator is available for an hour, but the nurses rotate in and out at 15-minute intervals. The discussion focuses on the relevance of the article to practice.
   - An electronic, online approach, which allows maximum flexibility for participants who can post their contributions at a convenient time. This approach allows for reflective thinkers to be heard, compared with real-time discussions where only two or three voices are heard. This approach requires collaboration with the information technology department, which will have to create a web page and a listserv.

4. *Implement EBP.* The nursing research committee will need education to help its members come up with a process for reviewing articles, synthesizing reviews, and

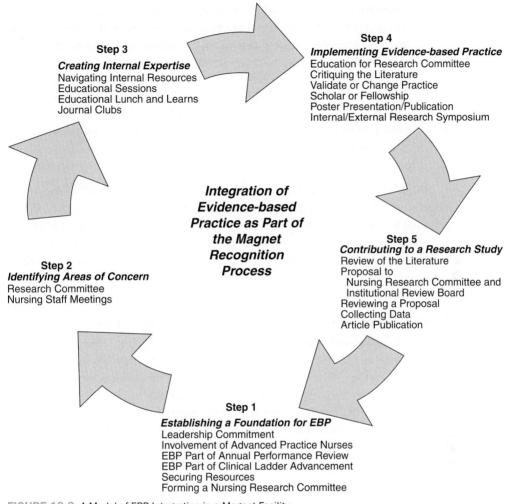

Step 3

Creating Internal Expertise
Navigating Internal Resources
Educational Sessions
Educational Lunch and Learns
Journal Clubs

Step 4

Implementing Evidence-based Practice
Education for Research Committee
Critiquing the Literature
Validate or Change Practice
Scholar or Fellowship
Poster Presentation/Publication
Internal/External Research Symposium

Integration of Evidence-based Practice as Part of the Magnet Recognition Process

Step 2
Identifying Areas of Concern
Research Committee
Nursing Staff Meetings

Step 5
Contributing to a Research Study
Review of the Literature
Proposal to
    Nursing Research Committee and
    Institutional Review Board
Reviewing a Proposal
Collecting Data
Article Publication

Step 1

Establishing a Foundation for EBP
Leadership Commitment
Involvement of Advanced Practice Nurses
EBP Part of Annual Performance Review
EBP Part of Clinical Ladder Advancement
Securing Resources
Forming a Nursing Research Committee

FIGURE 19.3 A Model of EBP Integration in a Magnet Facility
Source: Used with permission from Lippincott Williams & Wilkins. From Turkel, M., Reidinger, G., Ferket, K. & Reno, K. (2005). An essential component of the Magnet journey: Fostering an environment for evidence-based practice and nursing research. *Nursing Administration Quarterly, 29*(3), 254–262.

determining whether the results validate current practice or demand a change in practice. If it is decided to make a change in practice based on the review findings, a proposal should be drafted and sent via established lines of authority for consideration. The committee should disseminate its findings with a poster presentation and/or a publication.

Dissemination is important to increase awareness of the developing EBP nursing knowledge base. Consideration should be given to establishing an annual internal research symposium where units can display their work. Likewise, nurses can attend external research symposia to present their findings.

5. *Contribute to a research study.* With an evolving foundation of EBP knowledge, it is not a difficult task to advance to this final step. Previously critiqued articles from journal clubs can serve as the basis for the literature review. The internal or external nurse expert can review the staff nurses' work and assist with development of a research proposal to be submitted to the research committee and institutional review board. Nurses on the committee can review the proposal with the expert, furthering the members' development of expertise. Nurses can assist with research in the organization by collecting data. This assistance can include distributing surveys, helping with clinical interventions, and identifying potential subjects.

Some models go further into the implementation of knowledge translation and actually collect outcomes to inform the process. By monitoring and acting on outcomes achieved with evidence-based care, nurses are able to continuously adapt their care to the changing needs of patients. Three models add to the basic knowledge translation process by incorporating this outcomes feedback loop into the formal knowledge translation model.

Outcomes-Focused Knowledge Translation at the Bedside

This outcomes-focused knowledge translation model is aimed at influencing nursing-sensitive outcomes such as patient functional status, patient symptoms, therapeutic self-care, pressure ulcers, and fall outcomes. The simplified model includes four elements: sources of evidence, patient preferences, context of care, and facilitation. These four elements contribute to the uptake of evidence at the point of care by the nurse. This results in the nursing intervention and then patient outcomes. Outcomes link back to the initial four elements as feedback to inform the system. This model, depicted in FIGURE 19.4, is easy to interpret and understand and is a good model for use by staff nurses.

Collaborative Model for Knowledge Translation

This model was created to reflect a shift in communication from unidirectional research utilization toward an interactive model of knowledge transfer (Baumbush et al., 2008). Research champions (staff nurses) establish and maintain connections between researchers and nurses, help researchers navigate the complexities of the healthcare system, negotiate entry into various clinical areas, and provide ongoing feedback on how research is perceived and applied in a practice setting. This model has two dimensions: process and content.

The *process* dimension is the dynamic part of the model and is made up of the collaborative relationship between researchers and nurses. This relationship is characterized by accountability, reciprocity, and respect. The process reflects an ongoing dialogue focused on emerging findings and their effect on patient care. This dynamic interchange allows practitioners to use findings in a rapidly evolving healthcare system and helps researchers to refine research questions in the context of real-world care.

Outcomes-focused Knowledge Translation

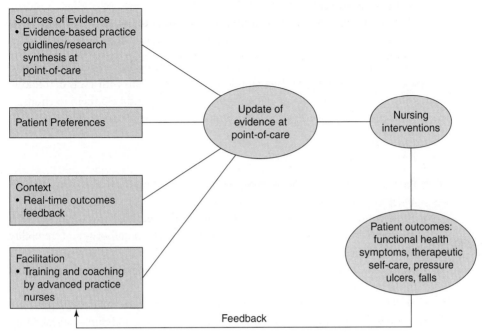

FIGURE 19.4 An Outcomes-Focused Knowledge Translation Intervention Framework. *Source:* Used with permission from Wiley InterScience. From Doran, D., & Sidani, S. (2007). Outcomes-focused knowledge translation: A framework for knowledge translation and patient outcomes improvement. *Worldviews on Evidence-Based Nursing, 4*(1), 3–13.

The second dimension—*content*—translates knowledge from a program of research into practice. This feedback element allows outcomes information to be shared with nurses in a way that can be immediately synthesized into practice.

Ottawa Model of Research Use

A final model of research translation, the Ottawa Model, is an action-oriented model of knowledge translation. It involves three phases: assessment, monitoring, and evaluation (Graham & Logan, 2004).

1. *Assessment* includes examining both barriers to and facilitators for the research uptake project. Some of the aspects considered in the assessment process are patient demographics, clinical and practice characteristics, perceptions of the decision by those impacted, and resources required.
2. *Monitoring* of those impacted by the decision is continuous during implementation and a process for follow-up is put in place. Communication, feedback, and observation are common mechanisms for monitoring progress. The goal of this phase is to reduce decisional conflict among those involved. Thus, implementers may discover that more information, education, and training are required

to realize a positive outcome. Expected outcomes may have to be changed as a result of this process.

3. *Evaluation* allows implementers to review the process and outcomes, and determine the quality of the decision-making process as well as its outcomes.

Translation of research into practice can sound daunting, but without being put to use, research has achieved little. These models provide clinicians with a way of thinking about knowledge translation and evidence-based practice and help them to choose a process that effectively ensures that research ultimately benefits patient care.

Summary of Key Concepts

- It is important to promote nursing research to improve the health of individuals and groups in society.
- The accountability for transferring research to the bedside lies with nurses.
- The translation of nursing research into practice provides authority and credibility to the practice of nursing.
- Nurses must be empowered by the organizations that employ them to examine the basis for their own practice.
- The reward for organizations will be quality patient care, cost efficiency, cost effectiveness, better patient outcomes, and increased patient and nurse satisfaction.
- Organizational outcomes, including those sensitive to nursing, will be scrutinized by potential patients and third-party payers.
- Many methods exist for the identification and aggregation of research for translation into practice, including systematic reviews, integrative reviews, meta-analyses, and meta-syntheses.
- Systematic models for knowledge transfer—including the Iowa model, the Johns Hopkins model, the Magnet model, outcomes-focused knowledge translation at the bedside, the collaborative model for knowledge translation, and the Ottawa model of research use—can guide the implementation of evidence-based practices.

For a full suite of assignments and additional learning activities, use the access code located in the front of your book to visit this exclusive website: http://go.jblearning .com/houser. If you do not have an access code, you can obtain one at the site.

References

Baumbusch, J., Reimer Kirkham, S., Basu Khan, K., McDonald, H., Semeniuk, P., Tan, E., et al. (2008). Pursuing common agendas: A collaborative model for knowledge translation between research and practice in clinical settings. *Research in Nursing and Health, 31,*130–140.

Berenstein, M., Hedges, L., Higgins, J., & Rothstein, H. (2009). *Introduction to meta-analysis: Statistics in practice*. West Sussex: Wiley InterScience.

Bettany-Saltikov, J. (2010). Learning how to undertake a systematic review: Part 1. *Nursing Standard, 24*, 47–55.

Bradley, E., Webster, T., Baker, D., Schlesinger, M., Inouye, S., & Barth, M. (2004). *Translating research into practice: Speeding the adoption of innovative health care programs*. New York: The Commonwealth Fund.

Doran, D., & Sidanai, S. (2006). Outcomes-focused knowledge translation: A framework for knowledge translation and patient outcomes improvement. *Worldviews on Evidence Based Nursing, 4*(1), 3–13.

Graham, I. D., & Logan, J. (2004). Innovations in knowledge transfer and continuity of care. *Canadian Journal of Nursing Research, 36*, 89–103.

Hemmingway, P., & Berenton, N. (2009). *What is a systematic review?* London: Hayward Medical Communications.

McCloskey, D. (2008). Nurses' perceptions of research utilization in a corporate health care system. *Journal of Nursing Scholarship, 40*, 39–45.

McCormick, J., Rodney, P., & Varcoe, C. (2003). Reinterpretations across studies: An approach to meta-analysis. *Qualitative Health Research, 13*, 933–944.

Mistiaen, P., Poot, E., Hickox, S., & Wagner, C. (2004). The evidence for nursing interventions in the Cochrane Database of Systematic Reviews. *Nurse Researcher, 12*(2), 71–82.

Newhouse, R., Dearholt, S., Poe, S., Pugh, L., & White, K. (2005). Evidence-based practice: A practical approach to implementation. *Journal of Nursing Administration, 35*(1), 35–40.

Noble, J. (2006). Meta-analysis: Methods, strengths, weaknesses, and political uses. *Journal of Laboratory and Clinical Medicine, 147*, 7–20.

Petticrew, M., & Roberts, H. (2006). *Systematic reviews in the social sciences: A practical guide*. Oxford: Blackwell Publishing.

Thorne, S., Jensen, L., Kearney, M., Noblit, G., & Sandelowski, M. (2004). Qualitative metasynthesis: Reflections on methodological orientation and ideological agenda. *Qualitative Health Researcher, 14*(19), 1342–1365.

Titler, M. (2001). The Iowa model of evidence-based practice to promote quality care. *Critical Care Nursing Clinics of North America, 13*(4), 497–509.

Turkel, M., Reidinger, G., Ferket, K., & Reno, K. (2005). An essential component of the Magnet journey: Fostering an environment for evidence-based practice and nursing research. *Nursing Administration Quarterly, 29*(3), 254–262.

Wallin, L. (2009). Knowledge translation and implementation research in nursing. *International Journal of Nursing Studies, 46*, 576–587.

Walsh, D., & Downe, S. (2005). Meta-synthesis method for qualitative research: A literature review. *Journal of Advanced Nursing, 50*, 204–211.

Weaver, K., & Olson, J. (2006). Understanding paradigms used for nursing research. *Journal of Advanced Nursing, 53*, 459–469.

Whittemore, R., & Knafl, K. (2005). The integrative review: Updated methodology. *Journal of Advanced Nursing, 52*(5), 546–553.

Woods, N., & Magyary, D. (2010). Translational research: Why nursing's interdisciplinary collaboration is essential. *Research and Theory for Nursing Practice: An International Journal, 24,* 9–24.

Woolf, S. (2008). The meaning of translational research and why it matters. *Journal of the American Medical Association, 299,* 211–213.

index

Page numbers followed by *t* or *f* indicate tables or figures, respectively.